Creating a Comprehensive Trauma Center

Choices and Challenges

The Plenum Series on Stress and Coping

Series Editor:
Donald Meichenbaum, *University of Waterloo, Waterloo, Ontario, Canada*

A Continuation Order Plan is available for this series. A continuation order will bring delivery of each new volume immediately upon publication. Volumes are billed only upon actual shipment. For further information please contact the publisher.

Creating a Comprehensive Trauma Center
Choices and Challenges

Mary Beth Williams

Trauma Recovery Education and Counseling Center
Warrenton, Virginia

and

Lasse A. Nurmi

Police College of Finland
Espoo, Finland

With the assistance of Michelle Ledbetter

Kluwer Academic / Plenum Publishers
New York   Boston   Dordrecht   London   Moscow

Library of Congress Cataloging-in-Publication Data

Creating a comprehensive trauma center: choices and challenges/Mary Beth
Williams and Lasse A. Nurmi.
    p.   ; cm — (The Plenum series on stress and coping)
    Includes bibliographical references and index.
    ISBN 0-306-46327-X
    1. Trauma centers—Cross-cultural studies. I. Williams, Mary Beth. II. Nurmi, Lasse A.
III. Series.

RA975.5.T83 C74 2000
362.18—dc21   00-026808

ISBN: 0-306-46327-X

©2001 Kluwer Academic / Plenum Publishers, New York
233 Spring Street, New York, N.Y. 10013

http://www.wkap.nl/

10 9 8 7 6 5 4 3 2 1

A C.I.P. record for this book is available from the Library of Congress

To my "next generation," in the hope that their lives will be less impacted due to a more prepared, prevention-focused world. This next generation includes:

> Natalia Vallette
> Bishop Alexander Vallette
> Nikolai Stefan Vallette
> Mikaela Alexia Correia
> Joshua Charles Correia

MBW

To my son, Joonas, and to my father, Tauno Nurmi, who survived the horrors of World War II.

LAN

While interviewing center directors for this volume, I was inspired by and dedicate my work to those who have the courage to survive and continue on, in spite of their turmoil, traumas, and victimization. My own path to professionalism is dedicated to my parents, Cheryl S. Ledbetter and Jerry R. Ledbetter. Thank you.

ML

Preface

Early Thoughts on Creating Comprehensive Trauma Centers

This volume has been many years in writing. When Dr. Donald Meichenbaum first suggested it and I approached my coauthor Lasse Nurmi, it did not seem to be as formidable a task as it has become. Interviewing the centers in this book has taken years—to get responses, to summarize those responses, and to return the summaries for further comment. Many centers have been created in that time; others have suspended operation. This volume does not claim to present even a majority of those centers. However, the ones contained herein are representative of "what is out there."

The idea to create a comprehensive trauma center is not new. The initial section of this forward examines thoughts I proposed as part of my comprehensive examination for my doctorate. Many of the ideas proposed then (1989) seem to fit now. It is my dream to put them into practice someday in the future.

THE COMPREHENSIVE EXAMINATION QUESTION

In 1989, one question on the written comprehensive examination questions for my doctorate was, "If you were to create a comprehensive trauma center in your suburban area, making use of what you have learned in your [doctoral] experience, describe the organization of that center, the mission, structure, personnel, funding, objectives, and services it would offer." Some of the conclusions reached then now seem applicable to the task at hand: designing comprehensive trauma centers (CTCs) for the 21st century.

The CTC envisioned in 1989 was a new type of human service organization: a purpose-driven organization that was results-riented. It began with an individual or group of individuals who had a vision and saw the need. This

CTC made available a greater range of services for victims of traumatic stressors and served as a hub for networking and coordinating other trauma-related agencies, organizations, practitioners, groups, and networks.

Then, as today, the goal/aim of a CTC is to provide a variety of services to victims/survivors without duplicating or undermining existing community programs or practices by complementing the existing community/regional service delivery system and coordinating services with other programs (rape crisis networks; shelters, victims' rights organizations; criminal justice, social service, and community mental health agencies; business organizations; and private practitioners).

At that time again, as now, I realized that much groundwork had to be done prior to the implementation of a CTC. First, it is necessary to assess the need for services within the chosen geographical area. Questions presented to other agencies include "Who else provides comprehensive trauma treatment services at present? What services are necessary? What services are missing? Are there waiting lists for services in various agencies? Are there persons who specialize in the treatment of trauma in the area? Who does critical incident debriefing or critical incident stress management? Who is familiar with trauma and its treatment? I also recognized that any comprehensive trauma center, to be effective, needs legitimization and/or sponsorship—whether from a board of directors, a community group, an association or respected professionals, or an institution of higher learning.

Given the "state" of trauma in the world in the closing years of the 20th century, trauma and its impacts are sources of major problems in many large metropolitan areas. In 1989 the awareness of traumatic events and their impacts seemed to be increasing and the numbers of persons impacted by those events was also increasing as technology began to link people together through computers and the media. The social fabric of many geographical areas even then was conducive to the development of trauma centers, but in many of those areas, services to trauma survivors were generally fragmented, particularly if they were less developed or more rural. As today, providing education about trauma and the need for specific trauma centers, or at least trauma-based programs within larger centers, is one way to help professionals understand the specialized nature of trauma treatment. While I did not know the term "salutogenesis" in 1989, Antonovsky (1979) had already conceptualized treatment of trauma based on a salutogenic framework of health and wellness.

MISSION STATEMENT

The mission statement is the social justification for any organization's existence and identifies the reasons for that existence. The mission of a CTC, as envisioned in 1989, was to provide clinical services to persons, groups, families, communities, organizations, and others who had been traumatized as well as conduct preventive interventions, research studies, and educational activities. This CTC, as a proactive organization, was dedicated to providing quality care using innovative, trauma-centered, research-based treatment techniques and strategies. The mission also was to help victims/survivors of trauma to reempower themselves, to restore wholeness and meaning, and to integrate the trauma(s) they have experienced into their lives so that they were no longer at the mercy of those external events. As this book illustrates, mission statements of the organizations now in existence are similar in scope and objectives.

OBJECTIVES AND GOALS OF A CTC

In 1989, I envisioned that the major objectives and goals of a comprehensive trauma center were:

1. To provide appropriate, complete treatment that was technically competent and of high quality.
2. To combat norms and values that legitimize and glorify violence, blame victims, and recognize sexism.
3. To provide professional training and community education about trauma and traumatic stress.
4. To consult with other groups, individuals, and agencies about the assessment, diagnosis, and treatment of all levels of traumatic stress disorders.
5. To lobby for change, when appropriate, at a variety of legal, political, and social levels.
6. To conduct scientific research that examines the efficacy of various treatment methodologies, gathers statistics about the occurrence and etiology of stress reactions, investigates longitudinal patterns of adaptation, and contributes to the theory of traumatic stress.
7. To develop a computerized database for research use.
8. To develop and conduct primary and secondary prevention activities in combination with follow-up research as to their efficacy.
9. To increase public understanding of the impact of trauma within a framework of wellness and salutogenesis.
10. To help persons who have been traumatized restore meaning, wholeness, and a sense of purpose and control to their lives.

If the center at that time was to develop and achieve these objectives—as well as others—and conform to its mission statement, all members of the organization (including a board of directors should one exist) had to acknowledge, understand, and accept them. In addition, the center's multiple constituencies needed to be informed of the mission statement and objectives.

ESTABLISHING A SERVICE DELIVERY SYSTEM

According to Sugarman (1989, p. 19), the well-managed human service delivery organization had to have appropriate "organizational mechanisms and programs for accomplishing its goals" including "a formal organization, policies, procedures, resource budgets, staffing, and fiscal and management information systems" giving consideration to the efficient use of people and machines, scheduling of staff time, and workflow. In 1989, I had formulated or envisioned no diagrammatic model for this CTC; I envisioned numerous configurations of staffing arrangements and I recognized that a CTC consisted of an executive director or directors and several staff therapists. One possible pattern was a group practice of professionals with expertise in various aspects of treatment, cognitive consistency and complementarity, and a basic agreement as to their rights, duties, and expectations. Support staff (ideally a secretary/bookkeeper/insurance technician) also were needed. In this group practice, each professional was responsible for setting his or her personal schedule within the parameters of available space. Two weekly staff meetings for all staff were mandatory. The first of these discussed policies, schedules, working arrangements, delegation of duties, and specific cases. The second was educational with rotating leadership, allowing each staff member to present an article, conference summary, or some topic relevant to growth of the entire staff.

A carefully written agreement established the extent and limits of responsibility of each staff member. It specified percentages of fees paid for center overhead and amounts that each clinician received for services provided (as based on standard acceptable fee schedules). Initially, each staff member carried personal malpractice insurance unless a group policy was more cost effective. The organization would also investigate rates for group health insurance for employees or arrange to obtain occupational health services for staff. Each staff member was responsible for filing income taxes and withholding appropriate money to pay those taxes.

Initially, the ideal staffing pattern included:

1. A chief executive officer who was licensed, offered direct services, functioned as a proactive leader, and was the driving force of the organization.
2. A PhD psychologist who was certified, licensed, and had testing and clinical expertise.
3. A PhD researcher/statistician with grant writing expertise.
4. A psychiatrist/MD on call for consultation, referrals, and medication management.
5. An American Association of Marriage and Family Therapists licensed marriage and family therapist (LPC) to focus on family issues.
6. A licensed, certified therapist with experience in the area of substance abuse and groupwork.

7. A licensed, certified therapist, preferably male, with experience in survivors' issues, men's issues, and veterans' issues.
8. A licensed, certified therapist, or clinician with expertise in crisis intervention and critical incident stress management.
9. A licensed, certified clinical social worker with case management expertise, knowledge of comprehensive service, and wraparound service planning.
10. A licensed, certified therapist (LCSW or PhD psychologist) with expertise in the treatment of traumatized children.

One or more of these individuals had training in curriculum development; others had experience in program development, consultation, and training.

I envisioned the CTC in 1989 as a high-growth organization with an opportunistic focus. Staff would take risks and be flexible in orientation of use of time and self. Staff rotated "on-call" responsibilities and expectations of successful intervention were high. Staff met together as peers but functioned with high levels of autonomy; the staff as a whole developed and implemented trauma protocols for the various types of trauma victims/survivors. These mutually agreed upon protocols functioned as a generic framework for treatment, allowing for individual variation and phenomenology. Staff therefore was aware of appropriate referral facilities and refers when appropriate.

Availability of Services

The center had 24-hour availability to respond to crises or disasters. Should a major disaster occur, the center had an on-call team ready for immediate critical incident stress management interventions. If more personnel were needed than the center had available, then other agencies could be contacted to help provide this service. During crisis situations, all staff members would carry beepers and the center answering service.

The center offered direct services:

1. Crisis intervention services to individuals, families, groups of survivors, and communities; critical incident stress debriefings and critical incident stress management.
2. Individual therapy and support for child, adolescent, and adult trauma survivors, their families, and significant others.
3. Couples and family therapy.
4. Diagnostic assessments of posttraumatic stress disorder (PTSD) for treatment determination, forensic practice, and use of the assessments for claims for compensation, for example.
5. Specialized fee-based therapy groups that were both short and long-term for specific trauma populations.
6. Phone counseling (not a hot line) for individuals in crisis either by the client's personal therapist or an on-call staff member to provide

information, help alleviate distress and function as a type of crisis intervention.
7. Substance abuse evaluation and referrals.
8. Educational workshops for victim/survivors about the trauma process, the phenomenology of trauma, the traumatic reaction process, and community referral services, systems, and supports.

The center offered consultation, education, and training:

1. Inservice training programs to various community and professional groups including police, schools, and others
2. Experiential, skills-building workshops for specific professional groups; training materials for the programs
3. Case consultation
4. Licensure supervision
5. Critical incident stress management for traumatized professionals
6. Curricula development for specific organizations or groups of professionals
7. Speaker's bureau
8. Teleconferencing

And the center offered adjunct services:

1. Advocacy at various hearings and legislative forums
2. Maintenance of a referral and resource file
3. Provision of an in-house center library for client and professional use at the center (the library could serve as a clearinghouse for information on traumatic stress)
4. Administration of research grants and research projects through affiliation with local universities, students who are doing doctoral work or postdoctoral work, and agencies; utilizing information gathered to contribute to the scientific literature
5. Inclusion of an outdoor challenge, outward-bound, wilderness component that might include a Ropes course on-site or available for use, annual retreats for various survivor groups, and/or center or a retreat center program
6. Provision of an annual conference or workshops on trauma-related topics for professionals using well-known speakers (nominal fee basis)
7. Sponsorship of self-help groups and/or provision of consultation for those groups
8. Development of a volunteer component using recruited, trained volunteers who work under specific contractual agreements; volunteers were job matched and trained in crisis intervention, peer support, stress management, community resources, and advocacy; they could provide direct services that do not require a high level of expertise or licensure yet provide invaluable assistance to traumatized persons

Thoughts from the Primary Author

These thoughts about a trauma center, though over a decade old, seem appropriate today to a large degree. The impact of trauma on survivors and the role of trauma in mental health treatment are better known today. While each individual practitioner within a trauma center had his own style, philosophical orientation, or specific theory base (e.g., psychodynamic, contextualistic, cognitive–behavioral), he also acknowledges the importance of appropriate treatment within a trauma framework. Each staff member belongs to at least the International Society for Traumatic Stress Studies and has certification through the Association of Traumatic Stress Specialists.

A CTC as superficially described in this preface, continues to be my dream but, after interviewing the centers in this book, I recognize it is only one model of service delivery. As the reader will soon see, many other models of service delivery exist. I now know that the most appropriate model for a given area is culturally specific and must adhere to the needs of its environments. As this volume is completed, the dream may become a reality through collaboration with the Masters Group and the eventual creation of a trauma center for preteens and teens in rural northern Virginia. Transformation of the theories presented in this book into practice will then become the scope of a future volume.

MARY BETH WILLIAMS

THOUGHTS FROM THE PERSPECTIVE
OF A POLICE PSYCHOLOGIST

As a police psychologist and senior instructor at the Police College of Finland, I believe that every possible professional helper should recognize the symptoms of traumatic stress and be aware of how to behave when he or she sees people who are victims of crime, accidents, and other traumatic events. These first responders need to think of the phenomenon of traumatic stress when they decide how to behave and what to say as they meet individuals in the shock phase of an acute stress reaction. For example, the Ministry of Social and Health Affairs now has developed new instructions for persons who are working as dispatchers as to how to behave and what to say in a crisis situation.

All employees of police organizations also need to know all possibilities for ways for society to provide to people who are victims because they, too, can serve as referral agents as well as responders. Police officers and officials who are on site need to be familiar with the health care system, health care centers, crisis response teams, and, if available, CTCs. Having knowledge of both official (public, governmental) and private resources should be part of the everyday life of a helper. Becoming aware of the existence of a trauma center, as well as how that center works, can become a preventive intervention.

A CTC is an institution that lies between a first responder intervention and professional mental health organizational response. To be sure, a CTC generally cannot do everything for all survivors; still, a trauma center led by qualified professionals can provide trauma-based therapy, can use the services of peer supporters, and also can have available a variety of professionals in a multidisciplinary team. Among those on staff may be social workers and clergy.

In Finland people are now aware of crisis teams that are sponsored by and part of public mental health care. When a crisis occurs, people know to go to those teams to ask for help. However, they also need to know where to go for trauma-related help beyond crisis intervention. The trauma center in Oulu run by Paivi Saarinen and Soili Poijula is the only pure trauma center in Finland that offers such help. However, there are so many traumatic events that happen every day in my country (unexpected deaths, car accidents, close calls, traumas happening to those nearby) that there is a need for a greater number of places to go with specialists trained in trauma intervention on staff—specialists who can understand and deal with acute stress as well as longer term reactions.

This book is important because it is the first of its kind to give a picture of what is happening in the organizational world of trauma at the present time. It describes 66 centers that exist throughout the world and how they work. It gives persons who want to create their own trauma centers suggestions on how to lead those organizations. Leaders of new organizations generally are enthusiastic and have many ideas. They also need to take into consideration how to manage trauma-related organizations, how to structure those organizations, and also how to organize responses to bigger traumatic events (disasters) as well as the more everyday traumas. Identification of who organizes such responses, who leads, and who serves as contact person(s) is part of this response. When a larger disaster occurs, many organizations and individuals have "good will" and want to respond in the best way possible. In spite of this good will, if there is not a planned organizational response, these individuals may work against each other and not know how to work together. It therefore is the job of the trauma center and its leadership to get the work of disaster response done in an efficient manner.

Over the years, as I have dealt with ever greater numbers of traumatic events, my own view of trauma has changed. Before I could "sort of" believe that I could determine whether an individual would not need support, even if that individual as a responder had "only" been watching what had occurred. Now I realize that it is impossible to determine or say which person or group may or may not need help or support. My view now takes into account more than first-line victims; tertiary victims also can have reactions very close to those of first-line victims. The more we know about the field of trauma, the more we have to learn, including more abut the factors that might put individuals at risk for traumatic stress responses or PTSD.

I believe that one important function of a CTC is to do research on risk factors, to collect information on different types or responses to differing traumatic events over time, and to study what makes people feel alike and connected to each other during an after a traumatic event. Surviving an accident (e.g., the sinking of the ferry *Estonia*) can make a bond among individuals that did not know each other ahead of time. Learning how that bond occurs and what bonds them through their common experience of tragedy is an important task.

The majority of people come through a tragedy "OK." They may need a minimal amount of support to help them go forward and get on with their lives, they may need crisis intervention, they may need some form of critical incident stress management (defusing, debriefing), they may need a few counseling sessions. The CTC is the best location to study the differential responses of individuals to traumatic events, to make differential diagnoses, and then provide differentiated responses. No trauma center is able to provide long-term individual treatment for everyone. As the readers will note repeatedly in this volume, particularly in war-related traumatic situations, provision of psychosocial support may be the best (and only feasible) intervention for the greatest number of persons. In this and other situations, provision of peer support and provision of social interventions that support daily life and help individuals go forward, are purposeful ways to help lessen traumatic impacts. Through provision of information (brochures, papers, handouts), presentations, computer websites, media presentations, debriefings, and support (among others), trauma center staff can triage and provide services to those impacted.

LASSE A NURMI

Contents

1

The Comprehensive Trauma Center as an Organization

Basic Concepts from Organizational Theory

WHAT IS AN ORGANIZATION?

A comprehensive trauma center, first and foremost, is a goal-directed, social entity composed of persons working to provide essential organizational and interpersonal client-oriented work-related functions to survivors of trauma. An organization, as a social collective with some level of coordination and communication, has goals that direct its activities and the activities of its members, as well as an overarching mission recognized by all (Miller, 1995). An organization creates processes to achieve those goals through a structure of patterned relationships and coordinated interactions. All aspects of the organization are influenced by the environment(s) surrounding it and of which it is a part.

The comprehensive trauma centers described in this volume, as organizations, are of many types and forms. Many are still in the process of formation, have less formalized structures, and may have few staff members. Some are new ventures, designed to provide services for generic or specific groups of trauma survivors. Their visionary leaders creatively organize tasks to be performed and administer the organization. These centers tend to be more flexible and informal and often have less division between leaders and followers.

Other trauma centers are growth organizations that have been in existence for some time and now are expanding and developing new operating systems. An example of this is the Traumatic Stress Institute (TSI) in South Windsor, Connecticut, which added Trauma Research, Education, and Training Institute (TREATI), an educational, nonprofit component, to its organization. Growth organizations frequently become more complex in structure as they expand. Only a few organizations are larger and have more elaborate

structures, more specialized tasks, and more developed administrative components such as TSI (Mintzberg, 1979).

A third type of organization is the professionalized organization. This
prosperous organization is more formal. It has more defined roles and planning is more administrative (Sperry, 1996). None of the centers described in
this volume can be classified as professionalized as of yet.

A comprehensive trauma center (CTC) exists for a purpose and an end;
that end varies with the goals of the organization and of its employees. The goal
may be to provide services to disaster victims, to children who have experienced or witnessed trauma, to victims of a specific type of traumatic event (e.g.,
sexual abuse), or to all victims, regardless of the traumatic event (Young, 1993).
How the work is organized and performed in a CTC, both in formal and
informal ways, may be identified by answering questions including:

- What tasks are to be performed?
- What social networks (informal structure) help or hinder accomplish-
  ing those tasks?
- What tasks are standardized?
- What processes are standardized?
- What alliances exist with other organizations to accomplish those tasks
  or with the stakeholders (clients) themselves? (Hunty, 1993)

Any comprehensive trauma center has structural and contextual dimensions. Structural dimensions of a CTC include written documentation of procedures, policies, manuals, curricula, brochures, rules, and other materials;
specialization of tasks; standardization of work activities; hierarchy of authority
and power; professionalism or level of formal training and education; and
personnel configuration of administration, support staff, and line therapists/
physicians/and so forth (Daft, 1986). Contextual dimensions include the size
(number of employees), technologies (therapy, counseling, forensics), environments outside the actual boundary of the CTC, and the goals of the
organization.

ENVIRONMENTS AND CTCs

The comprehensive trauma center, by necessity, interacts with the environments around it and the events that happen in those environments. It is an
open system that takes in inputs from the environment (traumatic events,
trauma survivors), transforms them (through the work of the organization),
and then sends them back to their environments in a changed (hopefully, at
least somewhat healed) format as outputs. In other words, as an open system, a
CTC imports energy from the environment and depends on the environment
for new sources of energy (Pfeiffer, 1994a). It then transforms that energy into
usable outputs through reorganization or throughput. This is the work that

gets accomplished. The organization's output is the outcome of the work that gets used by other systems. Inputs also include theory, information, research results, financial resources, and physical resources. (Inputs provide the CTC with the energy it needs to maintain itself and perform the functions for which it was created.)

There are various types of environments in which a CTC functions. The enabling environment includes government agencies, regulatory agencies, licensing organizations, and host agencies (e.g., a university or hospital) with which (or within which) a CTC functions. The functional environment of a CTC includes suppliers (of materials, funds), employees, and customers (clients/patients). The normative environment of the organization includes professional organizations* of which employees are members (American Psychiatric Association, American Psychological Association, National Association of Social Workers, International Society for Traumatic Stress Studies, Association of Traumatic Stress Specialists, and others) and competitors who offer similar services. Organizations also are impacted by diffused environments of the local communities in which they exist (including the culture of that community), the general public, and the media (Miller, 1995). If a comprehensive trauma center is to function effectively within its many environments, it has to deal with demands made on it by those environments; however, these demands may be in conflict with its goals, values, and way of doing business.

MODELS OF ORGANIZATIONS

A model is a simplified representation of reality as to how work gets done (Sink & Tuttle, 1989), how the organization is impacted by the environments around it (Likert, 1967), or how tasks, clientele, and interventions interface. Some models are descriptive; few deal with cause (organizational conditions) and effect (resultant performance). The various models of organizations presented here describe organizational structures which include relationship systems, methods of communication, procedures to make decisions, rules for practice (norms), accountability systems, and reward systems. The model created by the authors is described in the concluding chapter of the volume.

The Burke and Litwin (1989) model (see Fig. 1.1), according to Pfeiffer (1994b), attempts to specify the interrelationships of organizational variables and looks at the dynamics of organizational behavior and change. Change can be transactional (fine-tuning and improving the organization) or transformational (significant and even fundamental). The "most influential organizational dimensions for change are external environment ... and then mission-strategy, leadership and culture" (Pfeiffer, 1994b, p. 37).

The Burke–Litwin model describes both the climate of a center and the culture of the organization. The everyday interactions within the center and between center and clientele constitute that climate and are the transactional

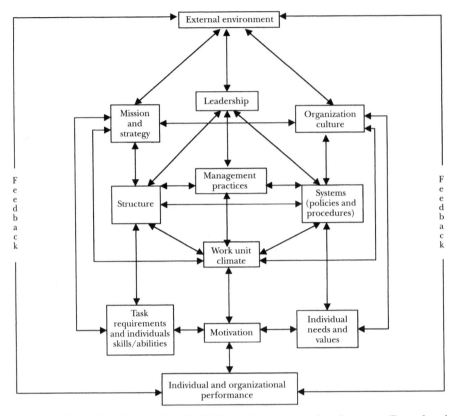

Figure 1.1. The Burke–Litwin model of individual and organizational performance. (Reproduced with permission from Pfeiffer, 1994b.)

aspects of the organization. They include structure, task requirements, and individual skills/abilities, management practices, work unit climate, motivation, systems policies and procedures, and individual needs and values. This model also looks at transformational components of the organization that are necessary if genuine change occurs. Transformational factors include the external environment, leadership, mission and strategy, and organizational culture. This model is complex and fits within general systems theory inputs, throughputs, and outputs. It also recognizes that organizational change occurs more from environmental impact and that strategy, leadership, and culture are more significant in leading to change than are structure, management practices, and systems. The model depicts primary variables that need to be considered in attempts to predict and explain the behavioral output of the organization, the most important interactions between variables, and how the variables affect change. Transactional variables are presented in the lower half of the model.

The second model is Weisbord's (1976) six-box model (Fig. 1.2). The degree of interaction between a CTC and its environment is complex and is determined by the boundaries of that center. Within those boundaries are the six boxes, or interrelated processes of all organizations, each of which has a formal system determined by mission statement, flow charts, job descriptions, and an informal system designed to meet the needs of the staff of the CTC. The first box is the purpose of a CTC and includes formal goals and informal goal commitment. The second box is the structure and includes the formal organizational structure and informal ways the work of the center gets done. The third box is that of relationships and includes formal chains of command and working units/teams as well as informal aspects of the quality of work

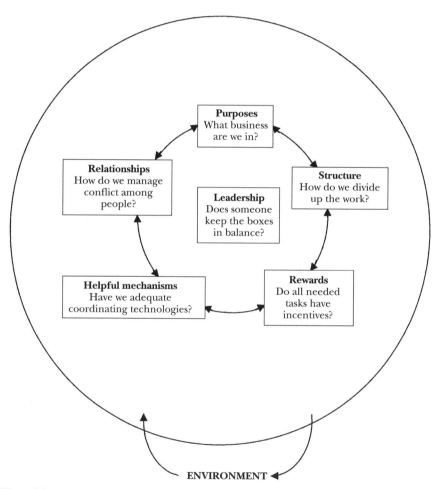

Figure 1.2. Weisbord's six-box model. (Reproduced with permission from Weisbord, 1971, by permission of Marvin R. Weisbord, Block Petrella Weisbord, Inc., Plainfield, NJ.)

relationships. The fourth box includes the rewards and incentives (salaries, benefits, travel, etc.) as formal components and the informal reward system for work that is done well. The fifth box is leadership. The primary tasks of leadership are "defining purposes, embodying purposes in programs, defending institutional integrity and managing internal conflict" (Pfeiffer, 1994b, p. 172). Leadership also has both formal and informal components. The final box includes helpful mechanisms such as procedures, policies, staffings, memos, and so forth, that help the work of the other boxes. The framework of this model, when used, can help the leadership of a CTC examine how well the center fits its environment, how well the center is structured to carry out its goals and mission, and how well in tune are formal and informal systems.

The third model is the cube: a global model for a comprehensive trauma center (Pace, Stamler, Yarris, & June, 1996) (Fig. 1.3). This model describes clear distinctions among services, targets of client groups (individual, group,

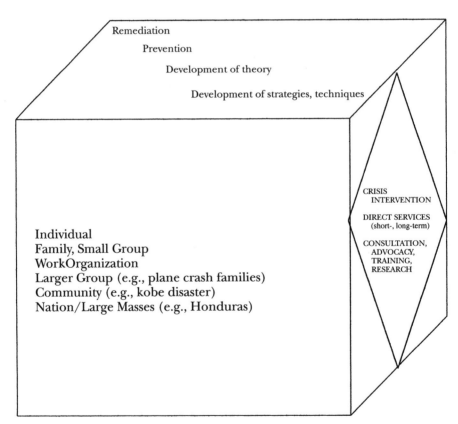

Figure 1.3. The global trauma response model. (Adapted from Pace, Stamler, Yarris, & June, 1996.)

community), purposes (preventive, remedial, development of theory, research, consultation), and methods (direct intervention, consultation, training). It provides a framework for service delivery within a global model. In this model, the individual is only one target for intervention. Resource allocation is made on the basis of expressed need for service within a flexible framework; some individuals need more or less intervention and accommodation than others. In other instances, the group (family, work setting, neighborhood) is the focus. In other situations, the focus is the entire community. This model also recognizes the role of consultation and training.

THE VISION AND MISSION OF A CTC

The organizational vision of a CTC includes its long range objectives. A shared organizational vision is a powerful energy force that gives form to ideas as to what a CTC is trying to accomplish. Also at the core of any organization are its values and philosophy. The philosophy contains the organization's purpose and reasons for existence. For a CTC to be successful, these core elements must be held in consensus by staff; if they are not, working together may be difficult if not impossible. For example, is the reason for existence of a particular trauma center to provide fee-based services to clients or is it to obtain funding for research? A lack of consensus about the primary purpose of a center can lead to tension and ineffective performance.

A mission statement is a brief statement of the objectives of the organization. The mission statement crystallizes the organization's vision and serves as a guidepost for making decisions about structure, power, and use of resources. As Schwartz (1998) noted, "A good mission statement can help ... define ... business, articulate vision, and guide ... operations" (p. 26). One of the most important tasks of an organization is to develop a mission statement that is clear. The mission statement, however, is not a business plan or operational strategy. Ideally, it is developed by the entire staff of an organization and therefore is articulated, supported, and followed by that staff (Sperry, 1996). In addition, it guides the comprehensive trauma center's code of conduct and standards of acceptable behavior (Schwartz, 1998). On one hand, the mission statement is broad enough to lead to flexible implementation; on the other, it is specific enough to act as a template to make decisions (Sink & Tuttle, 1989). Guidelines for developing a mission statement for a comprehensive trauma center include the following:

1. Keep the statement simple.
2. State the business of the comprehensive trauma center first.
3. Follow that statement with the values, principles, and philosophy of the CTC; these components of the mission statement indicate how the mission is accomplished.
4. Test the mission statement throughout the entire CTC and then make

corrections, additions, and deletions until everyone in the organization can "buy into" it.

5. Share the mission statement with all possible environments and clientele groups; put it in a policy manual, in brochures, and on the walls of the center; make sure all potential employees receive a copy of it and agree with it before they are hired.
6. Use the mission statement for guidance in decision making.
7. Encourage staff to develop personal mission statements in light of the organizational statement. Ask each staff member to examine:
    a. What is most important to him or her in the work at the center.
    b. What gives life/work meaning.
    c. What does he or she want to do and accomplish as part of the CTC.
8. Challenge the mission statement when it needs challenging.
9. Use the mission statement as a measure of success or failure for center activities and staff performance (Schwartz, 1998).

The mission statement often includes information about the explicit values and beliefs of the organization and its guiding principles that are shared, permeate the organization, and are consistently lived by employees in the context of their work (Ivanevich & Matteson, 1995). The organizational values of a CTC may include cooperation among staff, openness of staff and clients, respect and dignity for those being treated, solicitation of feedback from clientele, authenticity, commitment to healing, autonomy of staff to the greatest extent possible, and proactive responses to crisis situations (Jones, 1981). It is important to keep values explicit, to share them with constituents, to model and support commitment to them, to include value considerations at staff meetings, to question values when staffing cases, to update value statements and mission statements when needed, and to set organizational goals consistent with values. Thus, values lie at the core of a comprehensive trauma center (Jones, 1981) and define the reason for its existence and its purpose. They impact the philosophy of the center as well.

The leader/manager of a CTC has the responsibility to monitor the degree to which staff members agree on and base practice on a common set of assumptions, philosophies, purposes, and values. These values, as explicit as possible, need to fit with the common standard of practice within the CTC and also need to be consistent with organizational goals and are modeled by that leadership (Jones, 1981).

THE CTC AS AN ETHICAL ORGANIZATION

The work of a CTC must be done within an ethical framework. Lax and Sebenius (1986) proposed a set of questions that help identify what is ethical within an organization.

1. What are the mutually accepted, understood rules of the CTC? Are they being followed? (This is the principle of mutuality.)
2. Can those who make decisions defend and discuss their actions openly?
3. Are the actions applicable to all comparable situations? (This is the principle of generality.)
4. Does the action show care for the legitimate interests of others. (This is the principle of caring.)

ORGANIZATIONAL GOALS

The goals of a CTC give the reasons for its existence. According to Senge (1990), these goals include:

- Commitment to learning
- Commitment to the development of knowledge about trauma based on accurate information
- Belief in ethical treatment provision
- Respect for individual differences in staff and clientele
- Priority for health of employees
- Appreciation for growth of employees
- Flexibility
- Resilience
- Commitment to the production of good service
- Commitment to lowering stress in the organization

Though goals may change over time, they also serve as a measure of the legitimacy of the organization to those outside its boundaries. They give direction to the staff of the organization and guide their work for decision making. They also provide standards for assessment of performance (how many clients have been seen? how many problems resolved? how many debriefings conducted?). Types of goals within a CTC include:

- *Official goals*: formally defined outcomes which describe the organization's mission, its reasons for existence, and the values underlying that existence
- *Operative goals*: the actual operating procedures of the CTC that tell exactly what it is trying to achieve and include the primary tasks
- *Overall performance goals*: profitability, number of clients seen in a specific time
- *Resource goals*: numbers of grants, donations, contracts
- *Market goals*: advertising, television spots, brochures
- *Employee development goals*: training, supervision, vicarious traumatization workshops
- *Productivity goals*: output and the primary tasks of the organization

A comprehensive trauma center is effective to the degree that it attains these and other goals.

CULTURE AND THE CTC

Every organization has an identity. The identity of a comprehensive trauma center is influenced by the world of trauma around it (i.e., the events); the "customer base" of traumatized individuals, groups, or communities; and the products (counseling, research, training) the CTC provides. Identity also includes location, size, and motivation for existing (Ackerman, 1984). If staff, customers, governmental agencies, funding sources, and others understand the identity of a CTC, they then have explanations for the behavior of that organization and have some idea of what makes a particular CTC distinctive. Identity also leads to a clearer decision-making process and can mobilize staff toward more effective implementation of plans of action.

An organization's culture includes the ways of thinking, acting, and believing that members of that organization have in common; it is the basic assumptions, shared values (what is important), and causal and normative beliefs (how things work) that guide the organization's behavior (Cooke & Rousseau, 1989). The CTC exists within a specific cultural context and therefore has cultural factors that must be considered in the development, management, and performance of its mission. Some of these factors are the norms and expectations that govern social interaction within the culture, including the role of social distance, openness, the use of space and territory, the view of time, and eye contact/touch; these norms structure information sharing, socializing, and self-expression. If cultural factors are not taken into consideration, the effectiveness of how an organization "does business" may be compromised or even made impossible. Any culture consists of what its members stand for, believe in, and share, as well as commonly accepted meanings and views about beliefs, attitudes, and motives (Mallack, 1993). Wanger and Spencer (1996) write, "strong cultures provide stability and predictability for their members, as they supply people with clear direction, ground rules for behavior, and ideas about how to respond or make the most appropriate decisions" (p. 70). Schein (1985) adds that culture includes norms (rules of behavior), dominant values, philosophy guiding policy and practice, and observed behavioral regularities. Cultural norms structure information sharing, socializing, and self-expression.

A CTC's organizational culture is the "relatively enduring set of values and norms that underlie (its) social system" as well as a "meaning system" that allows members (clients, patients) to attribute "meaning and value to the external and internal events that they experience" (Pfeiffer, 1994a, p. 30). An organization has at least four core cultures that when taken together combine to represent the character or personality of that organization. The four cultures are control or power (decision making), collaboration/structure/ role (dynamically within a team in a people-driven manner), competence/ achievement (success, commitment), and cultivation of possibilities and creative options or support (mutual caring, belonging) (Schneider, 1994). The culture of an organization is more effective when it supports its mission.

Bolman and Deal (1997) note that some authorities believe that "organizations *have* cultures; others insist that organizations *are* cultures" (p. 231). There also is discussion whether leaders shape culture or whether culture shapes leaders. They continue that "over time, every organization develops distinctive beliefs and patterns. Many of these are unconscious or taken for granted, reflected in myths, fairy tales, stories, rituals, ceremonies, and other symbolic forms" (p. 231) In order to diagnose a center's culture, outsiders and insiders observe how people act, dress, speak, spend time, and relate to/with one another.

Myths of an organization, according to Campbell (1988) and Cohen (1964) have many roles. They "provide the story behind the story. They explain. They express. They maintain solidarity and cohesion. They legitimize. They communicate unconscious wishes and conflicts. They mediate contradictions. They provide narrative to anchor the present in the past" (Bolman & Deal, 1997, p. 220). The CTC may have many or a few myths: leaders are in control of all that happens; traumatic events are preventable; experts in traumatic stress are truly objective; there is only one "best" way of treatment. These myths develop over time; some are shared and become part of the "remember when" folklore and history.

The CTC also has stories that are told and retold. Stories communicate the myths of the center and become part of the traditions. As Bolman and Deal (1997) noted, stories "convey the value and identity of the organization to insiders and outsiders" (p. 222). Another aspect of culture is ritual. The CTC develops group ritual to carry meaning and give structure to the work of the organization. There may be initiation rituals for new staff members to make them "one of us" in the center. There may be rituals to use with varying groups of clients, based on the culture of those clients. There may be rituals surrounding loss and death, whether the death of a program, the death of a staff member, or the death of a client. Rituals tend to become more public through ceremony. Ceremonies tend to be official; they "socialize, stabilize, reassure, and convey messages to external constituencies ... (they) offer meaning and spiritual connection ate important transitions" (Bolman & Deal, 1997, p. 227). The events around which ritual and ceremony are built often give "order and meaning and bind an organization together" (p. 229). Trice and Beyer (1992) identify nine rites or cultural practices for organizations, six of which also are in occurrence in tribal societies. These six are rites of passage, degradation, enhancement, renewal, conflict resolution, and integration; the other three are rites of creation, transition, and parting.

Symbols are the most basic and most frequently encountered tangible forms of culture; the building blocks of culture management. The language of an organization (in a symbolic sense) includes its jargon, specific slang, songs, gestures, signals, signs, humor, jokes, rumors, metaphors, proverbs, and slogans (Trice & Beyer, 1992). Not all beliefs of a culture can be communicated through symbols. Some are too complex or too vague. Instead, they need mission statements, statements of principles, and vision statements (as narratives), as well as legends (with a figment of truth) and stories.

CLIMATE OF AN ORGANIZATION

While culture defines how a member should behave in an organization, climate includes what actually occurs in a CTC and how it feels to be a member of that organization (Cooke & Rousseau, 1989). Climate is the psychological atmosphere or state that both results from and determines the behavior of individuals (staff and clientele) within a comprehensive trauma center. Descriptions of climate are highly subjective. Climate is strongly affected by organizational conditions and includes degree of employee morale, level of stress, extent of vicarious traumatization or compassion fatigue, as well as extent of trust between staff and between staff and clientele, community, and other organizations. Pfeiffer (1994a) identifies the following 12 dimensions of climate: orientation—members' principal concern; interpersonal relations; supervision and impact on motivation; problem management: how the organization views and solves problems; management of mistakes: attitudes toward errors; conflict management: processes used to resolve conflict; communication: styles and characteristics; decision making; trust; management of rewards; risk taking and the way the center handles risky situations; and innovation and change: who is responsible to instigate change, by what methods, and to what ends (pp. 110–111).

ORGANIZATIONAL FUNCTIONING

Power is the ability to have an effect on someone or something in contrast to authority, which is the right to exercise power (Hunty, 1993). When power and authority are shared, morale is higher and an organization tends to be more cohesive. This power includes informational power (their knowledge about treatment of trauma and their knowledge about access to networks, resources, and services) as well as personal power and positional power.

Morgan (1986) noted that there are many sources of power within an organization. Among them are the following:

1. Formal authority
2. Control of scarce resources
3. Use or organizational structure, rules, regulations
4. Control of decision making

5. Control of knowledge and information
6. Control of boundaries
7. Control of technology
8. Management of meaning and symbols
9. Personal power

Staff members of a CTC have varying degrees of power and influence with clients, community members, and fellow staff. French and Raven (1959) were among the first to state that power resides more in the minds of those who perceive and respond to that power than inherently in a person. They identified five bases of power. The first basis of power is *reward power:* the ability to grant or distribute rewards such as money, recognition, promotion, access to services. Staff of a CTC are more powerful if they can expedite access to resources when a client has been traumatized. If a staff member knows how to obtain emergency housing, respite care, or other services, his or her reward power is perceived to be higher. *Coercive power* is typically based on promises or threats through withholding desired resources or rewards or delivering punishment or sanctions; it often leads to resistance. *Legitimate power* is based on the position or right of leadership and staff to exercise power, make demands, or give orders. It also is known as *position power (authority)*, which relies on formal authority. For example, if staff members do debriefings after crisis events, legitimate power allows them to establish rules of confidentiality, procedure, and process. *Referent power* is based on the desire to be associated or identified with a powerful staff member or members. If a staff member has referent power, she or he frequently is charismatic and attractive to others.

A primary source of power for staff members of a CTC is *expert power*. Expert power is based on the special knowledge, skill, or expertise that staff members have in the assessment, diagnosis, and treatment of trauma. A staff with that level of expertise, particularly in times of crisis, is respected, seen as credible, and can help or teach others. Expert power also may be "informational" when staff members have or can get access to information that is needed in the wake of traumatic events (French & Raven, 1959). In other words, there is power inherent in having the know-how to solve problems and find solutions. There also is power that comes with being able to identify and define the beliefs and values of the organization and with getting everyone to accept the myths, metaphors, and symbols of the comprehensive trauma center as his or her own. One additional source of power in the CTC is *personal power*. Some individuals have personal characteristics that bring them power (Bolman & Deal, 1997).

Teams in the CTC

Much of the work done in a CTC may be accomplished by teams rather than by individuals in isolation. These teams tend to have mutual goals or reasons to work together, are interdependent in their work relationships, are committed to the group effort, and are accountable as teams to those in authority (Reilly & Jones, 1974). Team members need to collaborate and need to be "present" physically and emotionally at team meetings. Through collaboration, teams work toward problem-oriented solutions in a flexible manner or work with other organizations.

Many factors either contribute to or get in the way of this collaboration including theoretical orientation of the organization, mission, methods, values, guiding policies and procedures, turf issues, existence and quality of interagency service agreements or affiliation agreements, history of tension and conflict between the agencies, and individual characteristics of employees (personality, work style, etc.). As team members work together, it is important that they are sensitive and aware of each other's feelings, beliefs, and positions. Work teams are most effective if their members operate in an interdependent manner toward solving the tasks at hand (Pfeiffer, 1994b).

Interprofessional collaboration is higher when team members or agencies have common values regarding intervention strategies, respect for each others values, roles, and expertise; professional expertise; administrative support; established procedures that support collaboration (confidentiality, information sharing); and service plans or affiliation agreements that support collaboration (Behar, Zipper, & Weil, 1994).

Conditions supporting collaboration between CTCs and other agencies include formal interagency agreements, administrative support, a culture that supports collaboration, funding mechanisms that support collaboration, and clarity and compatibility of agency functions and roles. If agencies are to work together with trauma survivors as a team, they will be more successful if they follow the 10 Cs of teamwork (Behar, Zipper, & Weil, 1994, p. 59): cooperation, communication, coordination, collaboration, consistency, confrontation of problems, compromise, consensus decision making, caring, and commitment.

In the ideal center, teams work well together because they follow what Katzenbach and Smith (1993) consider to be distinguishing characteristics of high performance teams:

1. The teams work out specific goals and plans of operation that mesh with the mission, goals, and objectives of the comprehensive trauma center. Team members have clear authority to develop creative interventions.
2. Team members translate mission and purpose into measurable performance goals that explicate the specific "work products," keep the team focused on the work of the center (whatever that work may be), and serve as a yardstick for successful completion of those goals.
3. The teams are of optimal size—between 2 and 25 people.
4. The teams recognize and utilize the expertise and specializations of members in theory and practice-oriented interventions, as well as in decision making, problem solving, and communicating. Teams explore

who is best suited to perform specific tasks and how team members come together to create a "whole" Gestalt.
5. Team members have a commitment to working together effectively.
6. Team members hold themselves collectively responsible for achieving center goals.

In order to become this type of team, Keidel (1995) proposes the following questions:

1. What is the nature and degree of task-related interaction among team members?
2. What is the geographic distribution of the team members? Are there satellite centers, a network of independent practitioners, a centralized location?
3. How autonomous are team members and in what capacities?
4. How is coordination achieved among team members and between team members and leadership?

ORGANIZATIONAL STRUCTURE AND STRATEGY

Each and every CTC has a structure that can be both formally stated and informally implemented and a strategy to get the work done. There are six major aspects of that structure:

1. Reporting relationships and locus of power and influence within the CTC in both formal and informal spheres of influence
2. Methods of communication including formal staffings, meetings, reports, case files, memos, publications, research data, and informal communication methods of rumors, networks, group sharing, and gossip
3. Decision-making procedures include the formal and informal ways that problems are solved within the CTC including regulations (who are clients, how is intake done, how many sessions can be given, when does a referral occur, what tests can be given) as well as informal ways to influence decisions
4. Norms include the formal rules of conduct (hours of work, flextime, punctuality; dress codes if any) and informal norms (working overtime, staff relationships) (Colon, 1995)
5. The accountability system includes formal performance reviews, methods to measure "successful" treatment and financial accounting; an informal accountability system may include collusion between staff to cover up incompetence
6. The reward system also includes formal rewards of compensation, benefit packages, programs for recognition and informal rewards of getting positive feedback or recognition otherwise for a good job

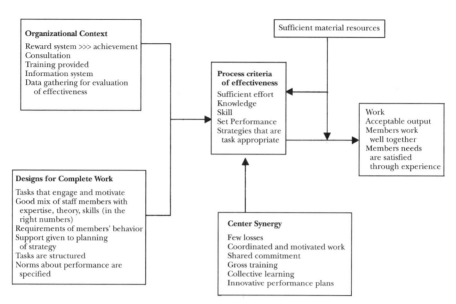

Figure 1.4. Fostering work in a CTC. (Adapted from Ivanevich & Matteson, 1995.)

The structure determines how jobs are designed for a higher degree of performance and greater organizational effectiveness (Ivanevich & Matteson, 1995) (see Fig. 1.4). The content of structure delineates the functions, methods, techniques, data, subject matter, and services of the CTC. The context of structure includes the physical demands and working conditions as well as conditions of accountability. Job requirements (including minimal qualifications) and job designs (the range and number of tasks) also are part of structure. Organizational structure must be established within a framework of various environments: the enabling environment (government, regulatory agencies, licensing organizations); the functional environment (suppliers, employees, customers/clients); the normative environment (professional organizations, competitors); and the diffused environment (the local community, the general public, and the media) (Miller, 1995).

The CTC's strategy defines how the work gets done. It includes functional aspects of personnel selection and marketing as well as the strategic plan for goal achievement (Sperry, 1996). When examining the structure and strategy of an organization, it may be helpful to determine roles of members by answering the following questions:

1. Who makes decisions and by what process?
2. Who communicates with whom and using what network?
3. Who conforms to organizational norms?
4. Who initiates ideas and issues or confuses ideas?

5. Who manages or does not manage conflicts?
6. Who has influence to persuade, force, appease others?
7. Who supports others?
8. Who has empathy?

As Bolman and Deal (1997) have written, the structure of the comprehensive trauma center as an organization must align with the core processes of that center. The core processes of a trauma center range from clinical practice to training to research to gathering of historical archival testimony data (for research and future prevention) to prevention to crisis intervention. The most viable structure for a comprehensive trauma center possible must consider:

1. What the center is trying to accomplish
2. The work that needs to be done
3. Who is in charge
4. Who is to do what
5. How what is done is coordinated
6. What individual staff members care about most—type of work, quality of work, amount of excitement, time on task, for example
7. The special abilities, talents, training, and interests of each staff member
8. The relationships between staff members and staff members and various client groups
9. The criteria that indicates success

THE CTC AS A POLITICAL ORGANIZATION

When the task facing a comprehensive trauma center involves intervening in some manner with politically sensitive client groups, for example, refugees, torture survivors, torture perpetrators, and others, the center must become politically aware. There are many interest groups that want or do not want the issues of these politically sensitive groups brought into public awareness. The political environments in which a CTC must function, seek funding, or utilize scarce resources, as well as political interests, impact how resources are allocated, as well as how goals are set and decisions are made (Bolman & Deal, 1997).

At least some of the staff as well as the leadership of a CTC need to be politically astute. This astuteness means they must have or develop political skills. The first skill is agenda setting. In the political realm, an agenda, according to Bolman and Deal (1997), is a statement of interests and direction that balances the vision of the center and ways to achieve that vision with the political, social, economic, and cultural climate. Knowing how governmental and other cultural influential entities think "and what they care about" can help the CTC "... fashion an agenda that responds to their concerns" (p. 172).

Setting the strategy to achieve the vision recognizes that there are forces that work for or against that agenda.

There also is a need to "map the political terrain." The steps for this mapping, according to Pichault (1993) include:

1. Determining channels of informal communication
2. Identifying the principal agents of political influence (the players, including the opposition)
3. Analyzing possibilities for internal and external mobilization
4. Anticipating strategies others will employ to undermine the work of the CTC

Because the CTC generally must function in a political environment, nothing that the center tries to accomplish will work if there is no political, cultural, or community power base. In other words, if a center is to be effective, it must be supported by others and those in power outside the organization must lend their cooperation and influence. The leadership of the CTC must look to those in authority for help. This help is gleaned from building networks and coalitions and developing relationships with those in authority so that, as Bolman and Deal (1997) point out, "they will be there when you need them ... building a resource base that helps (the CTC) to "secure blessings"—getting necessary approvals and mandates" from outside the organization when needed (pp. 184–185). In order to get things done, it is important to have constituencies that are allies in "high places."

It also is important, from a political point of view, to be able to bargain with those in power when necessary. Creative negotiation, according to Fisher and Ury (1981), focuses on interests not on positions. The interests of the clientele of a CTC are paramount. When those in political power and the leadership/ staff of a CTC have different interests and preferences for action that needs to be taken (which often involves funding issues), it may be necessary to bargain and look at what those in power and those individuals leading the CTC actually want. Any bargaining needs to be done within an ethical frame, although those with political power may not agree to that principle.

INITIAL CONSIDERATIONS ABOUT LEADERSHIP

For a CTC to be effective, it needs to have an effective leader or center director. Arnold and Feldman (1986) summarized the characteristics that make a leader effective:

1. The personal traits of the director make a difference in the way an organization is run, although they are not the only determinant of effectiveness.
2. The most effective leadership style is an employee-oriented style that is considerate and oriented toward employee needs.

3. Effective leadership is contingent on the nature of the situation. It takes into account the training and qualifications of staff, the nature of the job to be done, the nature of the work group (cohesive vs. fragmented), the nature of the organization (rigid and inflexible vs. adaptive and flexible), the nature of the leader (skill, experience), and how these things match with the demands of the situation.

4. Leadership is a process of mutual influence between director and staff.

5. The impact of leadership is limited and is only one of many factors that influence the performance of trauma center staff. Other factors include the characteristics of staff members, the nature of the job to be done, the nature of the clientele, and the nature of the organization.

6. The impact of leadership is able to expand through coaching, job redesign, change in the organization's policies as well as other areas of leverage (Vroom & Yetton, 1973).

7. An effective leader is open, tolerant of others, and "goes with the flow" as she or he tries to increase trust levels in the organization. She or he is available, direct, and focuses on staff members' strengths (Pfeiffer, 1994b, pp. 181–185).

Leaders

- Establish clarity of purpose
- Develop a climate of attention and consideration
- Reframe and integrate ideas
- Assess processes for consensus building and decision making
- Are democratic in style
- Model positive communication and supportive feedback
- Guide interaction
- Balance process and task (Behar et al., 1994)

They are committed to

- Searching for opportunities to change, grow, improve, innovate
- Experimenting, taking risks and growing from mistakes
- Envisioning a positive future
- Appealing to the values, hopes, dreams of others to get them to share the vision
- Fostering collaboration through cooperation and trust building
- Sharing information and power while increasing discretion and visibility
- Setting an example for consistent, congruent behavior
- Building commitment
- Recognizing individual contributions to every success
- Celebrating accomplishments of subordinates

What type of leader is most effective in a CTC? The qualities, characteristics, and skills required in/from a leader are determined to a large extent by the demands of the situation in which she or he is functioning as leader (Fiedler, 1967; Hersey & Blanchard, 1982). Leadership is not what the individual possesses; it is what the individual does with others that makes her or him effective. This perspective leads to the concept of situational leadership. The successful leader is one who attempts to match her or his style of supervision with the subordinate's competence and commitment. The supervision must analyze and understand the members of her or his working team and the demands and objectives of the job (Walsh & Donovan, 1990).

Blake and Mouton (1985), the developers of the "managerial grid," claim that there is one best way to lead a group: The supervisor who is able to combine a high concern for employees and relationships with a high concern for task preference makes the best leader. Blanchard and Johnson (1983) claim that the tough autocrat and the nice democrat are only partially effective. Effective managers manage themselves and the people with whom they work so that both organization and clients benefit and profit from their presence. This is the goal of the manager/leader of a CTC.

The supervisor who is able to balance both concerns is more effective than the supervisor who deals with only one. This balance can be achieved only if the supervisor understands both himself or herself as well as the situational and human dimensions of circumstances and the environment he or she is operating. The ideal leader of a CTC has concern for both productivity and concern for human factors and tries to balance them so that the greatest number of individuals can be helped in the most effective way.

THE WORK OF A CTC IN TIMES OF CRISIS

Although the CTC has day-to-day activities, programs, protocols, and interventions, by the nature of its focus it must be available to meet crisis situations. These crises or traumatic event occurrences vary in nature (from natural disaster to transportation accident to mass murder), intensity, number of victims, predictability (warning signs that a natural disaster is "in the making," e.g., an impending hurricane), priority for intervention, and potential impact on the environments of the CTC. The CTC has crisis teams identified and trained among the staff members of the center. These teams are trained to intervene utilizing various aspects of critical incident stress management (Everly & Mitchell, 1996). Recommendations concerning the operationalization of this aspect of the work of a CTC are found in the concluding chapters.

THE CTC AS A TRAINING FACILITY

Ideally, staffs of CTCs provide training to groups or individuals within their environmental communities or even to persons from other environments and cultures. This training is competency based, that is, based on those aspects of knowledge, attitudes, skills, activities, abilities, and behaviors that are related to effective performance. Performance encompasses general knowledge, specific knowledge that is trauma related, cognitive and affective understanding of the field, skills, values, attitudes, and interests, as well as information about research findings. Training (of staff) as well as others begins with a strong theoretical orientation that takes into account the massive proliferation of information and knowledge presently occurring in the trauma field. Training also provides firsthand experience and information and is designed to respond to the profile of the audience being trained (Rafe, 1991). Some of the questions that trainers can ask include:

- Who is the audience to be trained?
- Why do they want training in trauma and/or its treatment?
- What prior knowledge do they have and how familiar are they with concepts, strategies and interventions?
- What is the level(s) of interest?
- What are the expectations of the training?
- How urgent is their need for training?
- What is most important to them to learn?

Training is a process of mutual inquiry allowing for individual differences (Lindeman, 1926). It must be culturally, ethnically relevant, taking into account differences in communication styles, uses of language, topics to be included, forms of interaction utilized, proxemics, kinesics, paralanguage, and nonverbal communication.

MEASURING THE EFFECTIVENESS OF A CTC

A comprehensive trauma center is effective only if it meets its goals, designs interventions and programs that fit its value system, disseminates appropriate information to clients, public, and funding sources, and times its interventions appropriately. In addition, an effective organization is obligated primarily to its clients and their needs. A successful trauma center must have clear direction, competent task design, participative management and goal setting, maximization of human capital, constancy of purpose, congruence of mission, and shared values (Sink & Tuttle, 1989). Through planning, a CTC will have integrated strategies, goals, objectives, action plans, and performance. The roles played by staff will vary according to those needs and include roles as:

- Facilitator to keep communication open between staff and clients, clients and their environments, and staff themselves
- Healer to give supportive help while listening to the stories of trauma

- Mediator between demands of all interest groups
- Expert-consultant to educate clients, groups and organizations about traumatic stress
- Advocate to help those with less power become more equal
- Arbitrator to take a mutually acceptable role as authority; administrator
- Buffer or separator (Chetkov-Yanoov, 1997)

Because it is a human services agency that generally is budget driven, demonstration of its effectiveness becomes a major driving force. If a CTC cannot be viewed as productive, it will not survive. Productivity within a CTC is measured quantitatively through statistics and qualitatively through self-report of those served (Gummer & Edwards, 1995) and may be used to validate the necessity of its existence.

SUMMARY

This chapter has identified some of the major concepts of organizational theory as it applies to CTCs. As the authors of this volume draw conclusions

---

Vision (Long-Range Objectives)

Guiding Principles (Values and Beliefs)

Mission (Purpose)

Analysis of Input and Output

1. Who must we serve; Whom do we want to serve? (Downstream)
2. Whom are suppliers, vendors, clients? (Upstream)
3. What do we want to be/need to be/should be/are?
4. What services do we provide (outputs)?

Desired Outcomes

Transformative Processes

Structure/Staffing

Facilities/Environments

Technology

Performance Levels

Implementation Plans: Strategies, Techniques, Tactics

Problems/Roadblocks

External Strategic Analysis: Do We Do It?

Figure 1.5. The components of a CTC.

from summaries of various trauma centers and make their own conclusions about what is needed in an ideal CTC, they will refer back to these and other principles and concepts of organization development. The center they envision as ideal, whose components are present here in Figure 1.5, will be described in detail in the concluding chapters of this volume (Sink & Tuttle, 1989). Before a CTC becomes a functioning organization, however, those individuals who are creating it must envision its existence and identify its guiding principles, values, and beliefs. Once this task is completed, they can then create the organization's mission statement and identify what work it is to do (Sink & Tuttle, 1989).

Ideally, a CTC is an evolving, changing, adapting (and hence, cybernetic) organization. A CTC is dependent on some type of financial and material support for its legitimacy and resources, whether government, university, or client fee/insurance fee. It also must function within a matrix of governmental, agency, and organizational agreements, policies, ethical codes, attitudes, and regulations. To succeed, the CTC must be sensitive to needs and demands of all its environments (client/corporate/governmental) and be flexible in its service delivery in a humanistic manner. Only then will it survive into the future (Colon, 1995).

2

The Need for Comprehensive Trauma Centers

The State of Trauma in the World Today

This chapter has been months in its writing. During one revision, the tragic events of the death of Diana, Princess of Wales, were being replayed throughout the world. Her battered body was laid to rest on an island in the middle of a lake on her ancestral homeland and the grief of the entire world mourned her tragic, untimely death. Thousands of bouquets were thrown on her hearse as it carried her on that final ride. Her sons, not as stoic or controlled as others in the royal family, but alive and grief stricken as normal boys, accompanied her to the small spot of earth that was her final destination. One year later, on the anniversary of her death, the world mourned again, replaying the events in great detail as television shows questioned the conspiracy theories surrounding her death, played biographical programs, and repeated their telecasts of the funeral and mourning period.

In the United States, in the Eastern time zone, getting up at 4 AM to watch the cortege was an act of reverence and honor done by millions. In Finland, the time difference put the beginning of the ceremony at 11:00 AM. Both of us, the authors, were among the watchers and mourners. The trauma of Princess Diana's death became our own personal trauma and we, too, took time to mourn. Her death and funeral procession allowed us to express personal grief for her, as well as for those significant persons who had died in our lives and to be part of the worldwide outpouring of sorrow. Her death also illustrates the interconnection of the world of the late 1990s. Out of the sadness of her life, Diana found purpose and mission. Out of her personal trauma came the dedication to help others and eliminate land mines. She taught us that healing and growth come only with perseverance and dedication to something beyond ourselves. This is what traumatology is about and what we, as traumatologists, are about as well.

THE TRAUMA PARADIGM

A paradigm is an accepted, common, standard, traditional way to look at things, collect and process information, and then make decisions and solve problems (Kuhn, 1962). As a conceptual framework, the trauma paradigm presents a way to look at the world that is useful and applicable to a variety of situations and events ranging from the impact of the destruction of TWA Flight 800 on family members of the victims to reactions of individuals who have survived serious car crashes to the posttraumatic stress reactions of soldiers who have participated in or witnessed atrocities. As Joseph, Williams, and Yule (1997) pointed out, a traumatic event presents individuals with stimulus information that can lead to extreme emotional arousal, if that information is perceived as threatening, dangerous, or otherwise intense. Because that emotional arousal interferes with processing of the event, the event and its representations get held in memory as cognitions that are not easily assimilated. Some information about a traumatic event may not be available to conscious recovery and retrieval. Other information is easily retrieved and edited. The cognitions are idiosyncratic to each person who has experienced the trauma and are impacted by the individual's experiences, personality, schemata, subjective appraisal of the event, and the aspects of the event themselves. From these cognitions arise the flashbacks, intrusions, and other criterion A components of posttraumatic stress disorder (PTSD) as well as thoughts about the information and meanings of the trauma (appraisal cognitions). At times these latter thoughts seem to be automatic (American Psychiatric Association, 1994).

According to MacDonald (1996), PTSD is the "primary diagnostic category for psychiatric casualties of trauma" (p. 41) and is one of the most common psychiatric disorders. Marsella, Friedman, Gerrity, and Scurfield (1996) wrote that "PTSD is a clinically meaningful diagnosis because of universals in human experience in response to trauma" (p. 531).

Van der Kolk and McFarlane (1996) noted, "experiencing trauma is an essential part of being human" (p. 3). Tunnecliffe (1997) hypothesized that direct or secondary exposure to trauma, in actually, may be the "norm" of human experience. If that is so, he hypothesizes that the implications of this awareness include the following:

1. All of human history needs to be understood as saturated with traumatic dynamics, with all the limitations we now know trauma imposes on individuals.
2. We need to think of ourselves as currently living in a world saturated with the effects of trauma, even if our lives have been relatively unaffected directly.
3. If trauma causes dissociation, then a very large fraction of our entire species has lived or is living in significantly dissociated states.

4. Alcoholism and addiction may well be largely self-medication for traumatic stress.
5. "Low standards" of popular culture and entertainment, composed chiefly of sex and violence, can be understood as commercial exploitation of traumatic fixations.
6. Every healthy individual or family is a marvelous achievement against the odds; health is not (necessarily) the norm. Perhaps we ought to view each (healthy) one as an optimistic example of what our true, untraumatized potential is.
7. With any planning, scientific, therapeutic, political, educational, or community work, we may be dealing with many in the population who are traumatized.

WHAT IS A TRAUMA?

What is meant by the term "trauma?" Is a trauma "a wound," "an injury," "the thousand mile stare," or a terrifying experience that defies an individual's sense of invulnerability and safety? A major consideration is whether to view trauma and a subsequent posttraumatic stress reaction as an inclusive entity or as separate items of event and effect. Is an event traumatic if no one is traumatized? The PTSD response consists of a number of characteristic symptoms of intrusion and reexperiencing, avoidances, and increased arousal that occur in response to primary or secondary exposure to a traumatic event and leads to functional impairment in a variety of domains. Many of the pamphlets developed by various trauma centers that accompany the descriptions of those centers detail the various aspects of PTSD.

An immediate reaction to a traumatic event is now conceptualized as an acute stress reaction If a traumatic reaction occurs, yet the event does not meet the *Diagnostic and Statistical Manual of Mental Disorders*, 4th edition (DSM-IV) [American Psychiatric Association (APA), 1994] criterion B definition of a stressor, is the person able to be diagnosed as traumatized or afforded the PTSD diagnosis? Or is the individual's reaction something "other than" acute stress or posttraumatic stress? Furthermore, is the person's response reasonable, given the nature of a particular event? Dennert (1998), in a query to the readership of the Traumatic-Stress Internet Forum, asked if the view that the experience of a traumatic event leads to a recognizable syndrome called PTSD is warranted. He suggests caution in attributing the causal force to the antecedent event and suggests that other variables may determine the development of the syndrome, although he does not specify them. Reactions to trauma vary. To be sure, most individuals exposed to trauma do *not* develop PTSD; however, they may respond with some degree of upset and emotion.

Complex PTSD, otherwise known as disorders of extreme stress not otherwise specified (DESNOS), as proposed by Herman (1992) and the PTSD Task

Force, seemed initially to be a severe form of PTSD. Ford (1998) has noted that his research has demonstrated that veterans with DESNOS and PTSD have severe intrusive reexperiencing of their traumas. DESNOS appears to have a great deal in common with traumatic grief, as well.

We, the authors, recognize that the word "trauma" is used to refer to both the event and the response of the individual, group, community, nation, or organization to that event. We also realize that PTSD does occur in and of itself, alone, without accompaniment of other disorders. We also recognize that many factors contribute to its formulation.

A SHORT NOTE ABOUT THE BIOLOGY OF PTSD

Ford (1998) noted that the presence of "either characterological, social resources or neurobiological vulnerabilities or resiliences (from a salutogenic perspective) appear critical to the development and persistence of posttraumatic impairment." Characterological deficits may include attachment problems, and peritraumatic dissociation may be etiologically neurobiologically associated with PTSD. Ignumdson (1998) replied that investigations have suggested a relationship between reduced hippocampal volume and PTSD. Increased levels of stress hormones (e.g., the glucocorticoids) lead to selective neuronal loss in the hippocampus, a region of the brain now seen to be related to acquiring new memories. This region has many glucocorticoid receptors. Some of these reductions in volume appear to be reversible, and a smaller hippocampus might predispose a victim to PTSD symptoms.

More and more studies are now examining the biological basis of the PTSD reaction. A unique feature of trauma, and hence, traumatic stress, is the involvement of the central nervous system, which mobilizes to meet a threat through fight, flight, and/or freeze reaction(s). Prolonged stress can lead to elevated cortisol levels and hippocampal neurons then become more susceptible to future insults since they are not being replaced. If it is true that trauma impacts and causes structural changes in the central nervous system, then those changes in the hippocampus and other brain structures or processes mean that there is less of a possibility that culture can negate the occurrence of a traumatic stress reaction. Researchers at the present time are stating that PTSD is a biologically induced reaction, not a normal reaction. Yehuda and McFarlane (1995) reviewed then current studies to conclude that the chronic PTSD diagnosis is not the usual reaction to an extreme posttraumatic event. However, Davidson, Hughes, Blazer, and George (1991) disagreed and found a 46% rate of chronicity in the PTSD cases that were 1–3% lifetime prevalence of 2985 Americans.

Experiencing a traumatic incident forms a very strong memory network around that incident. When activated, that network leads to the fight–flight response that can cause an individual to overreact to future traumas. Associated secondary conditioning of stimuli accompanies the network and leads to reexperiencing when triggers occur. The network forms during or immediately after the event, when the victim is in a state of high arousal, extreme fear, distress, confusion, disorganization, or/and other similar alterations. This network may remain out of conscious awareness or lie dormant; when triggered by future exposure of direct or indirect linkages, similar responses then occur (Creamer, 1996).

We also recognize that trauma can be approached from a more strengths-based, health-oriented perspective. Calhoun and Tedeschi (1998) noted that a variety of personality characteristics are more likely to lead to posttraumatic growth. Among them are hope and optimism; flexibility, activity, and openness; creativity, inquisitiveness, imagination, and an ability to suspend judgment; viewing crisis as opportunity; ability to give the trauma a meaning; and wisdom.

WHAT MAKES AN EVENT TRAUMATIC? WHO GETS PTSD?

Central to the conceptualization and identification of an event as traumatic are subjective aspects of helplessness, powerlessness, and threat to life and/or physical integrity, as well as conceptualizations about the impact of the event itself. Bowman (1997) concluded that postevent distress reflected a person's beliefs about "the world, sources of danger in the world, beliefs about the self and the amount of power the self has (and) the suitability of emotional displays" (p. 75). Williams (1990), in her doctoral study of 531 survivors of child sexual abuse, found that perception of the impact of the abuse as traumatic was the greatest predictor of a PTSD reaction. Bowman (1997) also noted that causal factors of traumatic reactions are broader than aspects of the event itself; they include a combination of "long-standing individual and group characteristics triggered into life by visible and proximal adverse life events that get invested with attributes with the help of belief systems" (p. 139).

In studies of the impact of pretrauma vulnerability and personality traits, factors found to lead possibly to a greater likelihood of developing a traumatic reaction are a positive family history for psychiatric disorders (Foy, Resnick, Sipprelle, & Carroll, 1987), introversion, early traumatization, early separation from parents, and lower education (Shalev, 1992, 1996). Conversely, being married and having a higher level of education, according to Schaefer and Moos (1998), are related to more positive outcomes. Optimism also is related to personal growth and stronger expectations of positive outcome from a traumatic event. Young (1998), in a presentation to the membership of the Association of Traumatic Stress Specialists (ATSS) in Oklahoma City, Oklahoma, noted that certain elements of traumatic experiences lead to a greater risk of developing a posttraumatic stress reaction. Persons aware of the destruction and loss involved in a traumatic event from a distance or as observers are less likely to be impacted than are persons who have been directly involved in the disaster and, by chance, came out unscathed. These latter individuals may develop survivors' guilt at some point.

The duration of exposure to an event also is a factor in the type of reaction formed. Persons who have some type of control during the event often experience it as rapidly occurring; persons with no control tend to experience it as elongated and taking "forever." If there is a risk of injury, if panic occurs, or if there is a threat to life, the risk of developing a posttraumatic reaction increases. If the victim witnesses injury or is injured, that risk becomes even greater. Individuals who survive only by some freak circumstance (when, by all rights, they should have died) and individuals who are exposed to death and/ or mutilation have the highest likelihood of developing some form of post-traumatic reaction or disorder. Furthermore, the closer one is to the center of the event (the core), the more likely the individual will be traumatized (Green, 1990; Young, 1998).

The existence of a history of prior trauma may or may not be a factor in developing a nonsalutogenic reaction to a traumatic event (Pynoos & Eth, 1986; Resnick, Kilpatrick, Dansky, Saunders, & Best, 1993). For example, while Newman (1976), in a follow-up study of child survivors of the Buffalo Creek disaster, found the children to be more vulnerable to further stress, Warner and Weist (1996) recognized that witnessing urban crime could renew symptoms of early trauma. They also found that many of the exposed youth became desensitized to violence.

Posttraumatic stress disorder does exist in greater numbers in persons who have experienced prior traumatic events than in the general population. While Davidson et al. (1991) found a prevalence of 1.3% PTSD in a community study, Resnick et al. (1993) found a lifetime prevalence in crime victims varying from 19 to 75%. Kluznick, Speed, Van Valkenburg, and Magraw (1986) and Yehuda and McFarlane (1995) found the prevalence rate in prisoners of war was 47–50%.

One important factor recognized by DSM-IV (APA, 1994) and numerous studies is that subjective appraisal of the significant of an event, as well as appraisal of the life threat and injury associated with the event, leads to a greater incidence of PTSD (Foa, Steketee, & Rothbaum, 1989; Kilpatrick et al., 1989). Cognitive appraisal, attribution style, or meaning of the event are similar (Milgram, Toubinana, Klingman, Raviv, & Goldstein, 1988; Warner & Weist, 1996).

When the tragedy or traumatic event impacts an entire community, the extent of negative impact can be immense. If there has been extensive death and mayhem (e.g., in a major earthquake such as the Kobe disaster), if there is massive dislocation and relocation of the population (as in the Armenian earthquake), if there are severe financial losses incurred, if there is extensive property destruction, if there is extensive death (as in the sinking of the *Estonia*), and if local helpers themselves are so traumatized they cannot respond effectively, then the impact becomes even greater (Young, 1998; Zinner & Williams, 1999).

Adequate preparation can protect an individual from the effects of stress, and studies of the role of dissociation during an event and coping during an event are being conducted (Shalev & Mintz, 1989). Other areas of study include the impact of debriefing (Nurmi, 1997) and the amount of subjective distress occurring immediately posttrauma. In spite of these studies and others, at the present time there is no definitive way to predict who will develop a traumatic reaction (whether acute or chronic) and who will not.

Cultural norms and components can impact how a reaction is expressed, defined, or subjectively viewed, however. Additionally, differences in rates of a traumatic stress reaction across cultures may reflect the presence or absence of cultural sensitivity in the way traumatic stress is measured. PTSD is evident in Southeast Asian refugees, Salvadorean war refugees, Navajo and Sioux Vietnam veterans, Finnish police officers, and Slovenian children, among others.

Fullerton and Ursano (1997) have noted that most persons exposed to trauma do well over time. Joseph et al. (1997) have concluded that "for most events, symptoms of PTSD appear to diminish by around 18 months ... events involving massive death and destruction as well as human agency seem particularly likely to have chronic effects" (p. 67).

For some persons, the experiences of trauma can become central to a reorganization or reorientation (Ursano, 1981, 1987) or as a psychic organizer (Holloway & Ursano, 1984). Yet, if only 10% of those exposed eventually become impaired, that percentage can constitute large numbers of individuals. Elliot and Briere (1995) discovered that of the 76% of American adults who had been exposed to a traumatic stressor, approximately 10% developed PTSD. As Shalev (1996) noted, survivors of trauma often demonstrate symptoms of PTSD immediately after a traumatic event. These symptoms over time can become recurrent, obsessive, repetitive, and perhaps even permanent. If a comprehensive trauma center (CTC) exists and can intervene before symptoms can become fixed, permanent damage may be averted or at least moderated.

A number of other factors also have been considered as potentially impactful. These include objective measures of exposure to death, injury, and atrocity; injury of the self; longer duration of exposure; and subjective components of blame, guilt, and perception of negative impact (Green, 1993; McFarlane & deGrolamo, 1996; Williams, 1990). Suddenness, unexpectedness, life-threatening conditions that overwhelm, intrusiveness of the event into everyday life, and purposefulness and deliberateness of human-involved causation also are considered to be potentially more damaging. Ballard, Stanley, and Brockington (1995) noted that as objective intensity of the event increases, so does the likelihood of later psychological problems. Events that have massive death, destruction, life threat, personal injury, and/or human intention are more likely to lead to a posttraumatic stress reaction. For most events, the symptoms of PTSD seem to lessen or diminish at 18 months postevent. However, in these events with massive death and injury, symptoms and effects are more long lasting.

Some people appear to be more susceptible to traumatic impacts and become more reactive and more highly aroused by a traumatic event than others. Joseph et al. (1997) conclude that it is impossible to untangle the effects of objective and subjective factors in a stressor event that led to development of PTSD. Therefore, evidence presently suggests that the intensity of exposure is both objectively and subjectively assessed. The higher that intensity, the more the association with poor outcome, at least right after the event (Goenjian, 1993).

Another important factor that, in some studies, appears to mediate the occurrence of PTSD is social support (Butler, Foy, Snodgrass, Hurwicz, & Goldfarb, 1988; Davidson et al., 1991; Gallers, Foy, Donahue, & Goldfarb, 1988; Kendall Tacket, Williams, & Finkelhor, 1993; Madakasira & O'Brien, 1987, in studies of victims of sexual abuse and children and tornadoes). In light of these findings, a good case is made for the creation of trauma centers to offer varying levels of support and intervention.

THE HISTORICAL DEVELOPMENT OF PTSD AS A DIAGNOSIS

Humans, as open systems, exchange materials, energy, or information with the environments around them. Humans are adaptive systems, generally able to react to events in a manner that allows them to operate and function. Posttraumatic stress disorder, as one model of what happens when traumatic events impact human environments, presents an abstraction of reality as well as a representation of reality. PTSD is a means to simplify and organize reality, as well as a reduction of reality. PTSD, as a model, is conceptually translated into a computer-consumable language through statistical methods.

The initial model of PTSD was a medical model and was phrased in stimulus–response language. In the 1860s, PTSD-like symptoms of stress (nightmares, sweating, hypervigilance) were diagnosed as *neurasthenia* in accounts of the American Civil War; Page (1885) was first to suggest that a person's belief systems might moderate and influence responses to traumatic events. In 1893, Freud proposed that neurosis was based on the occurrence of childhood traumatic events. However, criticism from colleagues led him to shift from a psychoenergetic stimulus–response model to a pathogenic fantasy arousal model to explain the development of sexually related trauma (Crewdson, 1988). Freud maintained his medical model only in his sparse war-related trauma writings.

By World War I, traumatic stress reactions were conceptualized primarily as relating to organic events, and shell shock was viewed as a neurocortical consequence of exposure to heavy artillery. These reactions also were supposedly rare in occurrence. By the end of World War II, even larger numbers of soldiers were demonstrating combat exhaustion, however, and their numbers could not be as easily "explained away" as pure medical reactions (Marmar & Horowitz, 1988). Three hundred percent more psychiatric casualties were treated after World War II than after World War I, primarily with Pentothal, hypnosis, and (sometimes) electroshock and frontal lobe surgery. DSM-I (1952) used the stimulus–response framework, as it described traumatic neurosis as a generally reversible, transient illness that might become permanent. No diagnostic counterpart to traumatic neurosis appeared in DSM-II (APA, 1968).

Cybernetics, named by Norbert Wiener, began in 1942 (Becvar & Becvar, 1988). This communication paradigm of PTSD, applied as information theory, led to a new conceptualization of a traumatic reaction. In the cybernetic paradigm, traumatic reactions were still viewed linearly. The stressor event, as input, no longer led directly to a physiological or psychological output–reaction, because a transformative, internal process occurred between stimulus and response. Furthermore, the traumatic reaction, as output, provided feedback to the victim–survivor and impacts his or her further reactions and symptomatology. In this paradigm, the traumatic event upset the steady state and caused outputs that either maintained stability or led to seeking change. In other words, the extent of a traumatic reaction depended in part on the perception, interpretation, and attribution of meaning of the event. This model of traumatic stress viewed humans as active, transformative systems (Lillenfeld, 1978). The first major researcher–practitioner to apply cybernetically based systems models to posttraumatic stress reaction was Krystal (1968).

Information-processing systems theory expanded and modified cybernetics theory. During the years that cybernetics and information-processing theories developed, public and professional knowledge of PTSD and its phenomenology were restricted. However, DSM-III (APA, 1980) appeared and utilized a PTSD definition primary based on the informational processing model of PTSD as formulated by Horowitz (1976). The core concept of this model was an approach–avoidance reaction as a means to come to terms with the stressor event and to treat further recurrence.

When DSM-III-R appeared in 1987, it included an interactive field model of PTSD. According to McWhinney (1987), "field theory encompasses the sciences of the whole ... (and the) position of maximum interdependence among elements" of biopsychosocial forces. This model is more complex and more inclusive as it examines "patterns and relations and processes as opposed to objects affecting each other" (p. 44). This model took PTSD theory beyond strictly causal information processing and fully considered the belief systems and subjective reality of trauma victims as moderators of reactions, as well as pretrauma factors of familial background, individual temperament, history, culture, and others (Williams, 1992). Biological factors (Yehuda & McFarlane, 1995), ethnicity (Kinzie et al., 1990), cultural experience (Kinzie et al., 1984), and personality variables (Herman, Perry, & van der Kolk, 1989) are only a few of the factors that have been studied. Some researchers show that these factors, as well as exposure to prior trauma, can lead to more serious reactions; others have found that exposure to prior trauma can actually lead to the development of personal strengths (Jensen & Shaw, 1993).

The key issue of the transactional–field model of stress is the appraisal, perception, and subjective evaluation of the impact of trauma as well as the coping and information processing of the stressor inputs (Bloom, 1985; Green, Wilson, & Lindy, 1985). The situational context also is important because the coping process is situation specific. The equation for this model becomes

$$e b \text{ (PTSD)} = f\{p(\text{past})\}, E \text{ (traumatogenic aspects of the event)},$$
$$e \text{ (environment, society, support, cultural factors)},$$
$$+ \; t \text{ (transformative cognitive processes)}$$
$$\text{or } b = f(p,E,e) + t$$

The exact amount of variance in symptomatology due to each of these variables (and their subvariables) is still unknown. Multiple variables operate at the same time in this interactive field model.

The most recent model of trauma looks at salutogenic as well as pathogenic aspects of a traumatic stress reaction and is an evolutionary systems model. In this model, interactions are nonlinear and self-reflexive and an individual uses both environment and internal self-generated schemata to sustain the self. Accepting this paradigm means accepting the assumption that, by changing prescriptions, expectations, beliefs, and frames, the trauma victim–survivor may be able to change the general meaning of the trauma. These paradigms are still being conceptualized, particularly as constructivist approaches interact with biological formulations of the etiology of a traumatic reaction. Closest to this model is the cognitive constructivist contextualistic self-development model of McCann and Pearlman, (1990), operationalized as a forthcoming workbook (Rosenbloom & Williams, 1999).

Thus, the development of trauma theory parallels the development of contemporary systems theories. The evolution of new theory is continual, based on ongoing research in clinical, biological, cultural, and topic-specific arenas. Many questions concerning the impact of differing levels of stressor severity, social support, coping abilities, premorbid conditions, cultural factors, and personality variables continue to be the focus of studies and investigations. Only time will tell if a newer paradigm will be able to explain, perhaps through sophisticated path models or other statistical models, the mechanisms of posttraumatic stress reactions and disorder (Williams, 1992).

THE STATE OF TRAUMA TODAY: STATISTICS AND INCIDENCE

In a shrinking world of global communication and global connection, information about traumatic events is passed from one nation to another instantaneously as countries, groups, and individuals react to those events. The suicide death of 39 members of Heaven's Gate cult became a topic of discussion in countries other than the United States within seconds of its discovery. As a consequence, the layman who may not have experienced a direct traumatic event is immediately made aware of trauma occurring thousands of miles away as well as in his or her immediate environment, even when she or he lives in, watches television in, or uses a computer in some remote location. To illustrate this observation, how many persons around the globe are able to recall scenes of the Waco incineration of the building under siege, scenes of the Oklahoma City bombing site after the blast, images of the funeral of Princess Diana, or images of countless plane crashes or aftermaths of school shootings? These easily reconstructed imaginal pictures reiterate that life is not predictable and may not be safe or meaningful (Janoff-Bulman, 1992). Through this constant exposure, an individual's definition of what constitutes a traumatic event may expand and become more personalized as he or she is exposed to increased chaos and disorder.

Horrific events occur regularly in the lives of many millions of persons throughout the world. The Third National Incidence Study of Child Abuse and Neglect (U.S. Department of Justice, September, 1996), based on a sample of over 5600 professionals in 842 agencies, found that an estimated 1,553,800 children in the United States were abused or neglected under the harm standard during 1993. This was a 67% increase from the 1986 finding of 931,000 children and a 149% increase from the 625,100 children identified in 1980. The estimated number of sexually abused children rose from 119,200 in 1986 to 217,700 in 1993 (an 83% increase). The harm standard includes children only if they had already experienced harm from abuse or neglect.

The endangerment standard includes children who have experienced abuse or neglect that puts them at risk of harm. Using this latter standard, the estimated number of sexually abused children increased from 113,600 in 1986 to 300,200 children in 1993 (a 125% increase). These figures validate the fact that there appears to be a real increase in the incidence of child abuse and neglect and a rise in numbers of seriously injured children. Many of these survivors of abuse and of other types of harm escape somewhat unscathed, while others develop significant levels of traumatic reactions.

What is the extent of the existence of trauma in the world today? Estimates made by the Armenian government suggest that 300,000 children in Armenia have PTSD as a consequence of exposure to war, the 1988 earthquake, and the resulting continuing social disruption. Goenjian (1993) found higher rates of PTSD for children and adults who lived closer to the earthquake's epicenter. Seeing mutilated bodies, hearing screams of persons trapped in the buildings' rubble, and seeing family members search for buried loved ones made after-disaster experiences even worse (Goenjian et al., 1994). Various researchers have determined that a minimum of 8–9% of the population of the United States have symptoms of PTSD (Wolfe, Gentile, & Wolfe, 1989; Green, 1994;

Figley, 1995). Green (1994) also noted that approximately 25% of individuals exposed to a traumatic event overall experience PTSD at some time. Of persons exposed to specific potentially traumatic events, 2% of accident victims, 25–33% of those involved in a community disaster, 25% of individuals with traumatic bereavement, 29% of female assault victims, 75% of persons experiencing nonsexual assault, 84% of women in shelters, and between 35% and 92% of rape victims have been shown to demonstrate PTSD in various studies (Figley, 1995; Green, 1994; Matsakis, 1996; Wolfe, 1989). Resnick et al. (1993) found that one third of over 4000 women queried had experienced some type of crime; one likely outcome of those experiences is PTSD. Rape had a lifetime PTSD prevalence rate of 57.1% in a study by Breslau, Davis, Andreski, & Peterson (1991). In a study by Resnick, Veronen, Saunders, Kilpatrick, & Cornelison (1989), 76% of rape victims met PTSD criteria at some point within 1 year after the event. If the rape involved life threat and physical injury, the rate increased to 80% (Kilpatrick et al., 1989). Williams (1990), in her study of 531 child sexual abuse survivors, found that 37.7% met diagnostic criteria for a DSM-IIIR diagnosis of PTSD an average of 22 years postabuse. Norris (1992), in a sample of 1000 adults, found that 69% had been exposed to a traumatic event. Current prevalence of PTSD for them was 5% for victims of disasters, 8%, tragic death, 12% motor vehicle accident, and 14% sexual assault.

Kulka et al. (1990), at the time of the study, discovered that 15% of all male Vietnam veterans had current PTSD (479,000 of the 3.14 million men who served), almost half a million veterans of this war alone. An additional 22.5% of men had had partial PTSD over their lifetimes with a current prevalence rate of 11.1%. Of the 7,200 women who served in Vietnam, at the time of the study, 8.5% had current PTSD and 21.2% had a lifetime prevalence rate. Combining full and partial rates for PTSD reveals that 53.4% of males and 48.1% of females who served in Vietnam had had clinically significant symptoms of a traumatic reaction. Rates of PTSD were even greater proportionally for veterans who had been wounded or exposed to heavy combat (Card, 1987) or who had witnessed death and/or had been exposed to the grotesque (Chemtob et al., 1990; Solkoff, Gray, & Keill, 1986).

In the United States in a given year, the American Red Cross declares 350–400 national disasters, events requiring assistance from outside the immediate geographical area. Thirty of these disasters generally are declared by the President as national disasters in need of federal assistance (Jacobs, 1995). Joseph et al. (1997) noted that the International Federation of Red Cross and Red Crescent Societies reported 7766 disasters between 1967 and 1991. These disasters killed more than 7 million people and impacted over 3 trillion individual lives. Disasters are not unique to the United States; they can occur at anytime, in any community, in any country in the world (International Federation of Red Cross, 1993). The cost of these major disasters is great (Zinner & Williams, 1998). The Kobe, Japan, earthquake, for example, had damage of more than $150 billion dollars (Emerson & Mineta, 1996). De la Fuente (1990) determined that over 30% of survivors of the 1985 earthquakes in Mexico displayed PTSD in his study.

In spite of the numbers of disasters, disaster mental health intervention is a young field. Cohen (1995) noted that the three aims of postdisaster relief are to restore the capacity of the individual to function, to assist the trauma survivor to reorder and reorganize his or her personal world, and to assist the survivor to deal with any bureaucratic or political programs.

TREATMENT OF PTSD

Studies of what is effective treatment for survivors of traumatic events, whether these survivors are experiencing acute traumatic stress reactions, long-term, subclinical PTS reactions, or full-blown PTSD, have not arrived at clear conclusions as to what works. Therefore, the possibilities for conducting studies of treatment efficacy within a CTC are great. Several of the centers described are doing longitudinal research to add to treatment efficacy literature.

At the present time, though, treatment relies on certain basic principles and stage theories that are more intuitively than factually based. The first and foremost of these principles is the necessity to establish safety within and without the therapeutic environment if a person is going to manage traumatic symptoms and return to functioning within the everyday world (Herman, 1992; Williams & Sommer, 1994). Siegel (1997) wrote that "the overall goal in the treatment of an individual who has experienced trauma is to allow (him) to function as fully as possible and to have a subjective experience in life which is characterized by a sense of well-being" (p. 48). If the staff of a CTC intervenes immediately after a traumatic event, the emphasis is primarily on safety building, self-regulation, limitation of retraumatization, and stabilization. It is only later in the treatment process that working through all aspects of a traumatic event can occur.

Van der Kolk, McFarlane, and van der Hart (1996) wrote that all treatment must be paced. It also must be phase based: moving from stabilization/education to deconditioning of the traumatic event and its memories and responses, to restructuring of meaning and traumatic personal schemas (beliefs and expectations), to restitutive emotional experiences to establishing of secure social connections and meaningful activities.

Carlson (1997) describes Williams and Sommer's (1994) theory well when she writes:

> Williams and Sommer have proposed a four-stage model for treatment based on the techniques, methods, and strategies described ... in the *Handbook of Posttraumatic Therapy*. In stage one of the model, the goals are to establish a safe environment, a therapeutic relationship, and an initial diagnosis; to educate the client about trauma responses; and to begin to establish control over self-destructive behaviors and the symptoms of PTSD. Stage two includes working with traumatic memories and using adjunctive therapies including medications. The tasks of stage three involve restruc-

turing of maladaptive belief systems and working on social skills and emotional intimacy. The fourth and final stage of the model focuses on finding intellectual and spiritual meaning in the trauma, initiating social action relating to the trauma, making efforts toward preventing future distress, and terminating treatment. (p. 188)

As a therapeutic milieu, the comprehensive trauma center can serve as a safe haven for trauma survivors. Survivors ideally will find an entire range of therapeutic interventions within these centers and will be able to work with center staff members to create the most suitable range of interventions for themselves, within a cultural context.

The question of what "works" in a treatment of trauma in a CTC relates back to the question of what is "effective" PTSD treatment. CTCs have many possibilities and choices of treatment offered. These possibilities can range from using what is now called more "short-term" therapy, more innovative techniques of eye movement desensitization reprocessing (EMDR), traumatic incident reduction (TIR), and thought field therapy (TFT), as well as defusings and debriefings, individual therapy, group work, family work, and/or case management, among others (Mitchell, 1996). Controversies and discussions about the utility, applicability, and efficacy of each of these methods and techniques are in full force at the present time. Any approach to treatment, however, whether short term or of longer duration, needs to be phenomenologically driven and eclectic in nature.

Marmar, Weiss, and Pynoos (1995) have described five different posttraumatic syndromes, each of which leads to a different treatment approach:

1. The normal stress response of healthy individuals exposed to one/ single traumatic event. These persons recover either without intervention or with one single debriefing session.
2. Acute catastrophic stress reactions with aspects of panic, dissociation, insomnia, and incapacity to function in daily life. Treatment includes removal from the traumatic event, medication support to relieve symptoms of panic, anxiety, insomnia, and brief supportive psychotherapy in a crisis intervention context. Also important is the provision of immediate support.
3. Uncomplicated PTSD. This condition responds to a variety of treatment approaches including cognitive behavioral, psychodynamic, individual, group, or pharmacological interventions in a singular or combination approach. Treatment includes retelling of the event within the context of wellness and the aim of developing more effective coping mechanisms. Newer treatment methods also may be effective (TIR, EMDR, etc.).
4. PTSD comorbid with other Axis I disorders such as depression, substance abuse, panic disorder, and obsessive–compulsive disorder. Concurrent treatment of both the PTSD and the comorbid condition seems to be most appropriate.

5. Personality disorder or complicated PTSD of persons exposed to prolonged traumas over a period of time. These individuals may have dissociative identity disorder and/or features that seem to be similar to borderline personality disorder. Trauma-focused treatment for these individuals is not brief in nature. Instead, establishing safety and some modicum of control over behavioral acting out, emotional acting out, and cognitive "acting in" (dissociation, amnesia) is more important. Inpatient treatment may at times be necessary as well.

PREPARATION FOR THIS VOLUME

When the authors initially conceptualized this volume, the first task was to create a comprehensive research protocol using theory from both organizational development and traumatic stress arenas. That protocol is found in Appendix II. Questions were then taken from that protocol and presented to traumatologists at international conferences and on the Traumatic Stress Internet Forum before responses were gathered from representatives of the trauma centers described in the volume.

Today's world is one of constant disaster and violence as well as one of global connection and instant communication. For example, a disaster in Australia or Japan or India is reported almost instantaneously through the media, if not the Internet, in all parts of the globe. In the United States, countless numbers of emergency response teams are ready to respond to a disaster at local, state, national, and organizational levels. They include the APA Disaster Response Team, Red Cross teams, teams from the National Organization of Victim Assistance, and the Green Cross Team organized by Charles Figley. Certified trauma specialists (licensed professionals), certified trauma responders, and associates in trauma support are "at the ready." The Association of Traumatic Stress Specialists certifies persons who have met minimum standards of training and education.

Knowledge about trauma is still in a toddler stage of development. There is a constant need for researchers, theoreticians, and practitioners to "reality check" whether what they are doing is actually working, In light of this need, we present descriptions of over 60 trauma centers. It is not our aim to critique the efficacy of each of them, nor is it our aim to critique the effectiveness or general merits of the trauma treatment strategies and methods they use. We do aim to familiarize the reader with their programs with two purposes in mind: as examples and models for the creation of additional centers and as resources for those in need of intervention. Already, we have received feedback that the research protocol for the interviews has served as a template for development of programs in the American West, in Canada, and in Europe.

3

Privately Developed Trauma Centers in the United States

The next ten chapters present descriptions of centers throughout the world. Each description was condensed from a personal, face-to-face or phone interview that was then summarized. The summary was sent to the interviewee, who reviewed its content and style and made corrections and additions when appropriate. Several descriptions were revised many times, as circumstances in the organizations changed; others were accepted "as is." Many of the centers also sent descriptive brochures, forms, and assessment materials.

TRAUMATIC STRESS INSTITUTE/CENTER FOR ADULT AND ADOLESCENT PSYCHOTHERAPY, SOUTH WINDSOR, CONNECTICUT

The Traumatic Stress Institute/Center for Adult and Adolescent Psychotherapy (TSI/CAAP), founded in 1987, is a limited liability company utilizing a Boulder staff model of organization design. In this model, clinical intervention and research inform and complement one another. This for-profit, independent mental health organization specializes in the provision of clinical service, professional training, consultation, community education, research, forensics, assessment, and critical incident stress debriefings.. It is staffed by individuals with doctoral training in clinical psychology. TSI/CAAP recently created a new organization, Trauma Research, Education, and Training Institute (TREATI). The purpose of TREATI, through grants, workshop fees, and outside collaboration, is to conduct trauma research and offer trauma community education and professional training. It will not offer clinical services nor rely on client fees for its existence.

Mission

The first part of the mission of the TSI/CAAP is to strive to increase understanding of the psychological impact of trauma at individual, community, and professional levels. In addition, TSI/CAAP seeks to help victims of traumatic events restore a sense of meaning to their lives. TSI/CAAP promotes this mission by providing professional training, consultation, and community education and conducting research. The institute is dedicated to making contributions to the "field of traumatic stress in order to ameliorate the destructive impact of violence and trauma." A second mission is to promote psychology as an autonomous profession.

The mission of TREATI is to increase the abilities of therapists and other mental health and social service professionals to provide "effective, ethical treatment for survivors of traumatic life experiences." This mission will be accomplished through the provision of professional training and community education programs as well as through research on the psychological impact of trauma on survivors and of the work of trauma therapy on therapists, as well as research on effective interventions with therapists and clients. The ethical base of the work of the organization is the American Psychological Association's ethical principles.

Funding

The staff of the institute is salaried. Eighty percent of the monies needed to support TSI/CAAP comes from client funds, and 20% from royalties, forensic fees, professional speaking fees, psychotherapy consultation fees, and other sources of income. Managed care and limited sessions authorized by insurance companies necessitate "creative responsibility" in response to the pressure for short-term treatment.

Staffing

The staff of the TSI/CAAP does not work in isolation. One major goal is to build a community of professionals within the workplace. Therefore, as the organization strives to provide effective and ethical service, staff communicate among themselves about the way the organization operates and about services provided.

Eleven doctoral-level clinicians, of whom two are postdoctoral fellows, comprise the staff of TSI/CAAP. Nine psychologists (3 males, 6 females) serve as the permanent clinical staff. Eight of the psychologists work full time and one part time; all are licensed.. Staff also include a part-time research assistant, two full-time administrative staff, and one part-time administrative support staff member. Volunteers provide additional administrative and research assistance. The institute has a relationship with psychiatrists in the community to whom clients are referred when medication consultations are indicated.

Clinical Services

The institute provides a variety of clinical services to its clientele. Among these services are psychotherapy for individuals, couples, families, and groups and forensic assessment. Initial sessions with the client(s) and the assessments described below provide information to form a picture of the client. Components of that picture include the understanding of the client about trauma and the readiness of the client to tolerate strong affect as he or she works through traumatic experiences (as well as resources and beliefs of the client that can provide support). Any diagnosis is shared and discussed with the client(s).

Treatment goals vary with the client being served. Populations served include war veterans, victims of crime/accidents, and childhood trauma survivors. The institute has treated only a handful of Holocaust survivors. Each clinical staff member is expected to work 27 hours per week with clients or fill the financial equivalent of 27 hours (e.g., through forensic work, training, etc.). The type of cases given to clinicians vary with their skills and interests and to lessen the impact of vicarious traumatization and/or burnout.

Training, Professional Education, and Community Outreach

TSI offers a variety of professional training and education services to staff, other professionals, and community groups. TSI also offers a formal postdoctoral program that includes clinical training, research, teaching, professional development and community service. TSI provides workshops to professionals outside of the organization. Between April 27 and May 2, 1997, for example, a week-long intensive training program in trauma theory and psychotherapy was offered to clinicians for a cost of $975. Staff of TSI train other professionals on a wide range of trauma-related topics as well as do pro bono community work in areas of child abuse prevention, crisis education, and community education. Senior clinical staff of the TSI also offer clinical supervision and consultation to staff and to other professionals. TSI/CAAP also collaborates with a variety of community agencies including local veterans outreach center, victim services organizations, sexual assault crisis center, and battered women's shelters.

Research

Research at TSI/CAAP is clinical in nature. Postdoctoral fellows design and complete a research study during their tenure at TSI/CAAP. When their studies involve TSI clients, their questionnaires are included in the questionnaire packet to be completed by each client after the third session. Clients are requested to take the battery home to complete the instruments, some of which have been created and tested by the institute. Often the instruments utilized are not standardized psychological tests. All staff engaged in research meet for 1½ hours a week to discuss their studies.

Forensic Evaluations and Testimony

Staff of the TSI/CAAP offer a variety of forensic services including evaluation, expert testimony, and consultation for both plaintiffs and defendants. Staff conduct competency assessments for criminal defendants who are about to stand trial and also serve as expert witnesses in trauma cases or about standards of care.

Theory Base of TSI/CAAP

Present and former staff of the organization have developed a theoretical model designed to understand the complex aftermath of traumatic life events in an individual's development and adaptation. This theory, constructivist self-development theory (CSDT), is a relational psychotherapy model based on clients' strengths and resilience; it also is an integrative theory that helps clients make meaning of the events that have happened to them. The core of CSDT is the *self*: the individual's identity, self-esteem, inner experience, and worldview. Aspects of the self include frame of reference, self-capacities, ego resources, and psychological needs for safety, trust, control, esteem, and intimacy. The frame of reference includes identity (sense of oneself), worldview (beliefs about others in the world, moral principles, view of causality, life philosophy), and spirituality (meaning, hope, connection with something beyond oneself, awareness of a nonmaterial aspect of life). Self-capacities include those inner abilities that allow an individual to maintain a sense of self- and self worth. Ego resources are the inner abilities that allow an individual to meet psychological needs and manage interpersonal relationships. They include will power, sense of humor, empathy, limit setting, intelligence, introspection, and self-awareness. This theory is described in detail in *Psychological Trauma and the Adult Survivor* (McCann & Pearlman, 1990, p. 491) and *Trauma and the Therapist* (Pearlman & Saakvitne, 1995). A workbook to help trauma survivors examine and test their belief systems is available (Rosenbloom & Williams, 1999, p. 496) as is a workbook for trauma professionals, *Transforming the Pain* (Saakvitne, Pearlman, and the staff of the Traumatic Stress Institute, 1996).

Services to Staff

TSI/CAAP as an organization recognizes and attempts to lessen the impact of vicarious traumatization on staff members. Therefore, anyone who does clinical work will receive adequate training and supervision through individual, small group, case conference, seminar, and informal consultation venues. Supervision of staff is done in an atmosphere of safety, trust, and respect. This atmosphere stresses positive self-esteem of staff and places control over the supervisory process and content in the hands of clinicians. Thus, supervision of staff is an integral part of TSI/CAAP. Each staff member receives 1–2 hours of supervision weekly on an individual basis; post doctoral fellows receive 2 hours weekly. Group supervision occurs every other week in a case conference. One hour a week is spent dealing with vicarious traumatization issues. In this hour, staff members are encouraged to express and process feelings related to vicarious traumatization. Group meetings also are a way to address group crises, to debrief staff formally, to provide factual information, and to help one another manage work-related stress.

Every other week for 1 hour, clinical and administrative directors meet to discuss internal organizational issues. Supervisors also meet every other week for 1 hour to deal with clinical issues. Staff meetings on Tuesdays take place over lunch. This meeting is of a more practical nature. Every other week, psychotherapy staff members meet for 1 hour to discuss articles read, alternating with a meeting to discuss nonclinical projects. Staff also participates in two all-day retreats; one is held in spring and one is in fall.

Staff members with fewer than 5 years of service are given 3 weeks of vacation; those with 5 or more years of service receive 4 weeks vacation. Each staff member is on call once every 11 weekends. The staff has a holiday party in the winter and a summer family picnic as well. The leadership of TSI/CAAP encourages staff and one another to take adequate vacations and time off for illness. The institute offers a good health insurance policy to its staff.

THE INTERNATIONAL TRAUMA RECOVERY INSTITUTE, MESA, ARIZONA

The International Trauma Recovery Institute (ITRI), under the leadership of Janet L. Bell, PhD, ACSW, and Sang-Hoon Yoo, MSW, serves both the American and the international community. ITRI provides practice, consultation, and research in the field and at various centers; conducts international seminars and conducts training programs; organizes community trauma management teams; provides information exchange; and serves primary, secondary, and tertiary victims.

The president and vice president worked together in various capacities prior to the creation of the organization. They developed and participated in critical incident stress management teams, established a crisis response program teaming social workers and emergency medical technicians (EMTs), and worked together on a longitudinal study of local village people involved in a Korean airplane crash. After recognizing the urgent need for professional help to initiate culturally sensitized community trauma management, ITRI was created.

ITRI began to do research with a 3-year pilot project on the worst domestic airplane crash in South Korean history. In 1995, ITRI initiated the first US program to team graduate-level social workers and EMTs in a response to psychosocial–behavioral 911 calls.

Mission Statement

ITRI is dedicated to the prevention and amelioration of the effects of traumatic stress in individuals, families, the workplace, and community settings. ITRI also is committed to assisting communities, regions, and countries who are in the midst of positive events including rapid development, industrialization, and improvement in the general quality of life, events containing seeds of trauma and turmoil resulting from relocation and reunification.

The mission of ITRI is to offer consultation, development, and implementation of specific reaction-reducing plans, and appropriate treatment options. Their services are designed to aid assessment and recovery in a prompt, knowledgeable, skillful manner, while taking into account culturally differing world views, expectations, relationship dynamics, religious practices, and historical factors. Central to a successful recovery is the goodness-of-fit between the social–cultural–community context of the trauma and the selection and delivery of any and all services.

Staffing

ITRI is staffed by one American PhD social worker who also is a full-time university professor, a Korean MSW, four part-time female MSWs (two are fluent in Spanish), and two BA computer/statistics professionals utilized for large-scale projects. ITRI also utilizes trained lay caregivers and volunteers as peers in debriefings or to provide assistance with training seminars, workshops, conferences, and research activities. Staff of ITRI network with medical care professionals and facilities for referrals. The organization is funded by grants, private contracts, and individual payments.

Theoretical Orientation

The models of trauma on which ITRI is based include contextualistic cognitive–behavioral, cultural relativism, and symbolic interaction models. Staff view trauma responses as diverse, influenced by ethnicity, location, and culture. These response impact client and system(s).

Service Provision

ITRI serves an international community through provision of macrolevel training, education, skills building, program development, research, and consultation to private practitioners, workplaces including social services and other governmental agencies, emergency services, and academia. ITRI also provides micro- and other services to individuals, families, and groups who have been exposed to traumatic events or are experiencing crisis. Microlevel services include assessment, counseling, and information and referral to concrete services. Treatment offered is generally brief and short term with prompt assessment and referral as appropriate. Brief psychotherapy tends to be cognitive humanistic and behavioral and is primarily task centered.

One macrolevel service is the Regional Trauma Management Program (RTM). This program provides cutting edge leadership to develop regionally and culturally appropriate traumatic stress management services. Consultation with and training of leaders of area indigenous governments, academia, and community agencies leads to the design and development of regionally specific rapid trauma response plans that facilitate the mobilization of subsequent services for victims, families, rescuers, and others in the community. These services take into account the community's culture, traditions and geography. RTMs can form networks to exchange information and provide support when large-scale catastrophes occur.

While ITRI provides traditional trauma services, it also is dedicated to help areas that do not have good trauma resources improve their responses to traumatic events. Central to successful recovery from trauma is a goodness-of-fit between the social–cultural–community context of trauma and selection and delivery of all trauma-related services. All activities conducted on behalf of those traumatized by an event must be culturally appropriate. ITRI staff specialize in program planning, on-scene services, and services for acute intervention (the first 3 months posttrauma). Interventions generally are time-limited and brief, with the possibility of recontracting for further sessions or referral.

Community Interventions

The Crisis Amelioration Response Effort (CARE) is a service delivery system that assists fire, emergency service, and law enforcement to provide for the social–behavioral aspects of crisis responses. Persons who are evidencing suicidality, who have been assaulted or raped, or who are agitated or anxious frequently need a different type of crisis response than that which fire and rescue normally provide. ITRI has assisted the Phoenix, Arizona, fire department in the development of CARE units comprising an EMT and a social worker. The CARE unit responds to a crisis in the fire department van and relieves rescue personnel. ITRI has helped the fire department design an appropriate model and has assisted with training, data collection, and record keeping.

ITRI offers training to community members to train traumatic event debriefing teams as well as workshops designed to train the trainer of TED teams. ITRI has trained National Association of Social Workers chapters in Michigan and Arizona, as well as staffs of various medical and psychiatric hospitals and social service agencies.

ITRI also is committed to developing a wide range of social work services and research in health care systems. Among the services offered by ITRI are information exchange, case conferences, seminars, technical support, consulting, referral, and research development. ITRI, since 1995, has worked with the Samsung Medical Center in Seoul, Korea, orienting staff to health care organizations and providing a seminar dealing with crisis intervention and discharge planning. The model developed for the hospital was consistent with Korean culture and tradition.

Debriefing and Critical Incident Stress Management

ITRI provides on-site debriefings after a catastrophic event. Traumatic event debriefings (TEDs) are typically held within the first week after an event, although some have taken place years later. TEDs have been used with aircraft crashes, mine collapses, mass deaths, line-of-duty deaths, industrial accidents, fires, and mass casualty auto accidents, among others. The model of debriefing upon which ITRI interventions is based is the Mitchell model (Mitchell, 1996; Everly & Mitchell, 1997). ITRI develops teams that meet specific needs of organizations, governments or communities within a variety of locations.

Research

ITRI has conducted a 3-year longitudinal study in South Korea investigating the responses of survivors and local villagers who rescued them in a domestic airplane crash. Instruments were modified to fit into Korean values and norms and symptomatology demonstrated are unique to a non-Western world. ITRI is in the process of developing alternative instruments that are designed to capture the trauma experience of the Korean people.

PORTER & PORTER CENTER FOR STRESS AND TRAUMA, MUNCIE, INDIANA

The Porter & Porter Center for Stress and Trauma offers comprehensive services for persons who have experienced trauma including individuals, couples, families, businesses, and those who work with them. The center is operated by Porter & Porter, Inc. and is staffed with trained, certified clinicians. It offers outpatient services and a comprehensive assessment program for war-related posttraumatic stress disorder on a fee-for-service basis. Therapy provided is based on a holistic view of the individual, keeping the patient informed and encouraging the patient to have influence over the eclectic treatment process. Porter & Porter also provide legal teams with support services as those teams prepare for the use of PTSD as a factor in the litigation process. Another service of Porter & Porter is critical incident stress debriefing following violence or disasters.

An additional component of Porter & Porter is the Reluctant Warrior program. This program has developed an informational video focusing on Vietnam veterans and their older children. "Walking in the Shadow of a Warrior: War Babies" describes what it is like to live with PTSD and grow up in a PTSD environment. Porter & Porter has brought attention to and raised public awareness about trauma and trauma survivors and the need for treatment in "their little area of the world," Muncie, Indiana.

The for-profit component is funded primarily by third-party reimbursements. The not-for-profit component is funded by donations, fund raisers, and the profits from a secondhand clothing store. The organization was created in 1992.

Mission

The mission is to provide respectful services to the traumatized population in a safe environment. The overall treatment goal is to allow the survivor to return to a level of functioning that enables him or her to be productive, reach goals, experience joy in life, and have positive feelings.

Staffing

The only employee of Porter & Porter is Pamela Porter who works with organizations and a local hospital program. That program is predominantly female and includes three psychiatrists, psychologists, social workers, nurses, physical therapists, and art therapists. Lay caregivers and volunteers are also used, particularly for advocacy and peer support for veterans who are making claims for benefits. In addition, wives and children of veterans run support groups. A major component of the program is based on the theory that only the wounded healer heals. Medical care is not provided directly by the Center for Stress and Trauma, but direct referrals to medical care are made. At the hospital, staff are formally supervised weekly in psychiatrist run staffings and informally in staff cases between trauma specialists. Consultation is provided by trauma experts as needed and debriefings for serious situations are mandatory.

Clientele

The Center for Stress and Trauma serves primary victims of a variety of traumas ranging from child sexual abuse, rape, and war; to secondary victims including wives, significant others, and children of trauma survivors; to tertiary victims to a limited degree including law enforcement officers and fire and rescue personnel. Clients who could benefit from services but are not presently treated in great numbers are emergency room workers and specialists who counsel the traumatized. Services are prioritized for those at risk for suicide and/or homicide.

Services

Individual treatment, trauma theme-specific groups, generic trauma groups, and dual diagnosis groups are among the services provided. Porter & Porter, through the Center for Stress and Trauma and the Reluctant Warrior program, provide advocacy but not political action. When a client enters the program, a psychosocial assessment is done as well as an educational and job history assessment. Referrals for medication are made when needed. The assessment process takes three sessions and uses instruments such as the Penn Inventory, the Mississippi Trauma Scale for Veterans, the Impact of Event Scale, the Beck Depression Inventory, and the Combat Exposure Scale. All testing is documented, but confidentiality is absolute unless there is a written release or the client expresses suicidality, threats of violence, homicidality, or perpetration of abuse. Many evaluations are conducted for social security and Veterans Administration disability claims.

Short-term treatment includes critical incident stress debriefing (CISD) (using a combined model), desensitization (10 sessions or less), education for substance abuse treatment, and stabilization for suicidality. The CISD model is primarily a Mitchell model without the use of a peer during debriefings and defusings (Everly & Mitchell, 1997).

During the late 1950s and early 1960s, young males were raised in "warrior" training. A warrior is a person engaged in or experienced in warfare. However, the only choice for many Vietnam veterans was to serve, even if reluctantly or unknowingly, in the pursuit of honor. These considerations are part of the foundation for an aggressive treatment approach for war trauma veterans. The veteran is led to explore his early influences in "warrior training" through a basic psychoeducational format. Establishing the base of who they were may lead to understanding what happened and who they are today.

Forensics

Ms. Porter has worked extensively on capital murder cases at both trial and postconviction levels providing PTSD evaluations. This population receives no treatment during years of imprisonment. Ms. Porter spends a minimum of 25 hours of direct contact with a client for a forensics evaluation.

Community

Porter & Porter, Inc. offers training using educational and experiential methods in a combined format. Ms. Porter has developed training programs for assessment and treatment of PTSD, assessment of emotional damage (forensics), assessment of the impact of domestic violence, and rape crisis intervention strategies. Materials and curricula are copyrighted. Porter & Porter,

Inc. staff provide educational seminars and breakfast networking sessions at the local hospital.

POST TRAUMA RESOURCES, COLUMBIA, SOUTH CAROLINA

In 1979, after completing a dissertation examining the impact of a veteran's PTSD on family members, the director of this organization went into partnership, obtained grants, and by 1982 founded the organization to work with Vietnam veterans and their families. In 1984, their funding was cut, and between March and September, after losing most of its clientele, the center changed to a trauma center. Also in 1984, the crime victims movement began and the center marketed its services to victims of crime. By 1987, the center had four clinicians on staff and subsequently has expanded further as it has become both a trauma center and a short-term psychotherapy center. In its latter role, the center provides services to numerous employee assistance program (EAP) contracted personnel. As a posttrauma treatment center, it provides specialized services after personal, work, and duty-related trauma. Post Trauma Resources (PTR) focuses its efforts also in the private sector and has developed program and intervention models to fit business and industry needs. The center is a private business and therefore cannot apply for grants directly, although it may subcontract with other grant recipients. It is the second-oldest private free-standing trauma group in the United States.

Mission

The goal of the center is to help survivors learn to cope with their experiences and prevent long term posttrauma consequences for themselves and their families.

Staffing

The center has seven employees who are clinicians. Dr. Bergman has a PhD in counseling; the other employees include three social workers and a licensed counselor. A psychiatrist comes to the center once weekly and functions as medical director. Each clinician has a caseload of between 40 and 50 people. The center also has a full-time receptionist, a full-time insurance filer, a part-time clerical employee, and a full-time practice manager. Staff meet together once weekly to discuss issues and Dr. Bergman provides clinical supervision weekly or biweekly. Each employee is licensed and Dr. Bergman is a certified trauma specialist (CTS) through the Association of Traumatic Stress Specialists.

Theoretical Model

The treatment provided generally is similar to a managed care model that is crisis oriented, directive, and short term. PTR has developed a debriefing model that provides information about trauma response, builds cohesion among survivor groups, promotes a thorough understanding of the traumatic incident, offers coping skills for management, and assesses debriefing participants. Debriefing is one component of an overall approach; a debriefing session generally lasts 90 minutes and after introductions includes each participant telling their story; looking at consequences of survival; providing information about posttraumatic stress and coping skills; and a closing statement. Survivors who are most impacted also receive psychological debriefings.

PTR has developed a trauma response model that includes:

- Immediate response focusing on provision of basic needs
- Support services planning including identification of survivor groups, assessment of humanitarian and psychological support needs, and scheduling/communication of support services
- Provision of humanitarian and support services including management meetings, debriefings, counseling, and return-to-work programs
- Follow-up services including individual follow up of high-risk survivors, on-site interventions, follow-up debriefings, management meetings, and case management
- Evaluation and long-term follow-up

Clientele

Approximately 30% of the clients are EAP referrals and managed care referrals. Other clients are referred by health maintenance organizations (HMOs) and practitioners. The State Accident Fund and other organizations refer clients for psychological injury and chronic stress evaluations. Center staff do a great deal of court work including personal injury work and testifying on behalf of children in Department of Social Services cases. Staff respond to duty-related trauma and hostage incidents for the Department of Corrections and other state agencies. Only approximately 10% of the clientele are long-term trauma survivors.

Treatment and Services

Staff utilizes the initial interview with a client to determine the diagnosis and to assess whether what brings the client to the center actually is a traumatic event. The average length of treatment is 12 sessions or 3 months. A major stressor for the operation of the center as well as a challenge to provision of treatment is how to do PTSD work in the context of managed care limitations.

Each staff travels 2 days/week to satellite offices in rural areas. Generally these offices are donated and appointments are scheduled. In turn, staff provided negotiated fees and train local personnel to go out and offer services themselves. Most of the staff are cognitive–behavioral in orientation.

Organizationally, PTR staff work with organizational managers to prepare appropriate responses to work-related traumas. Staff train supervisors and managers about the psychological consequences of traumatic events so that they can provide on-site support until trauma specialists arrive. PTR staff provide consultation immediately after a traumatic event and conduct debriefings after an incident. Individual recovery plans are developed and brief posttrauma counseling is provided if needed. These components (training, peer support by organizational staff, posttrauma debriefings, posttrauma counseling, organizational development, cultural change) constitute the trauma response program of PTR.

When a traumatic event occurs within an organization, PTR begins planning the response to the event by phone immediately. Staff are on site within 24 hours of the incident to ensure provision of effective services and brief managers and to provide ongoing contact and consultation in the weeks following an incident.

PTR has developed a client-information manual based on the premise that clients with information about what happened and what to expect in treatment make a more successful recovery. The manual describes the organization and its mission, its history, and its staff. It includes a primer about psychological trauma and describes the various types of treatments offered (posttrauma family and relationships counseling, posttrauma counseling for children), fees, attendance policies, and confidentiality restrictions.

Community Services Provided

PTR provides trauma response services to organizations, not just to a group from an organization. PTR helps a company develop and implement trauma response plans, train its staff, develop return-to-work programs, and design models that are organizationally specific.

Staff offer trainings on a variety of topics including trauma response, violence prevention, stress and conflict resolution, problem solving, and public safety. They also go into schools and make themselves available to the media for trauma-related informative interviews. Dr. Bergman and colleagues have developed a variety of materials and curricula, including training outlines. Those outlines are available on the website.

PTR also has trained organizations in violence prevention issues including developing a zero-tolerance policy and creating a threat assessment team. On short notice, team members investigate and make decisions about the most appropriate action to manage potentially violent situations. The organization may split into two separate parts of a whole. PTR, Inc. would provide therapy and other resources to managed care clients. Post Trauma Resources would do the posttrauma work.

THE NORTHEAST CENTER FOR TRAUMA RECOVERY, GREENWICH, CONNECTICUT

The Northeast Center for Trauma Recovery (NECTR) specializes in working with individuals, couples, and families who have problems relating to physical, psychological, and sexual trauma. Founded and directed by Charles H. Rousell, MD, Director of Psychiatry at Greenwich Hospital, this outpatient treatment center for victims of traumatic experiences seeks to repair a victim's sense of self and to restore the ability to trust. Located across the street from Greenwich Hospital, the center helps people access services and receive help. NECTR was founded in October 1993 and offers most services at its primary location. Services also are provided at NECTR offices in neighboring communities. While the center offers a broad-based practice for treating trauma, most of the clients have endured sexual abuse. The center also does some workplace-related intervention. Dr. Rousell and staff members specialize in hypnotherapy. This for-profit facility offers non-center-based services through a network of outside consultants who are paid on a case-by-case basis (consultants receive 60% of the assessed fees). Services are covered in part by many insurance plans. All 12 therapists are licensed or board-certified and are multidisciplinary in training and education. They are connected through the center and receive monthly peer group supervision. As they work with individuals, couples, and other family members, they cover the full spectrum of psychiatric care including treatment of depression and anxiety, alcohol and drug abuse, sexual dysfunction, eating disorders, sexual identity issues, and adolescent and family issues.

Mission

Many people understand the importance of taking care of their bodies but neglect the care and healing of the mind. NECTR helps people confront and overcome stresses and events in their lives that have caused them pain and impair their overall functioning.

A multidisciplinary outpatient treatment center, NECTR provides a total approach to psychological assessment and treatment. Traumatic stresses and events occur throughout the life cycle for everyone. Psychological trauma can be as subtle as occupational burnout or as dramatic as child abuse, sudden loss of a loved one, or acute life-threatening medical illness. Learning and integrating skills to manage the unavoidable stresses of life can enhance physical, social, and psychological functioning and well-being.

The staff of NECTR believes that joining awareness of the delicate interplay between mind and body creates resilience in dealing with physical disorders and emotional disturbances. Their team of licensed and certified professionals offers complete and coordinated psychological services for adolescents, adults, couples, and families in a sensitive and supportive environment. NECTR's services include psychotherapy, specialized trauma treatment, hypnosis, behavioral medicine, addictions/substance abuse intervention, art and other expressive therapies, preventive care, and stress management.

Staffing

The staff who work for and consult with NECTR are multidisciplinary. Included in the staff are two psychiatrists, social workers, an art therapist, marriage and family therapists, a psychiatric nurse, psychologists, and an art therapists. Members of the staff are trained in eye movement desensitization and reprocessing (EMDR) and hypnotherapy. At the present time, no staff members do forensic evaluations or provide critical incident stress management and debriefing. All are trained in trauma, frequently by Dr. Rousell who teaches workshops and courses. Staff participates in monthly peer group supervision and there is a pragmatic mandatory monthly staff meeting. Staff members also are available for consultation in addition to doing individual, group, and couples work as well as some workplace intervention.

Dr. Rousell also is a lecturer in psychiatry at Yale University School of Medicine. Devra Braun, MD, is the Assistant Medical Director of NECTR. She also is a clinical assistant professor of psychiatry at Cornell University Medical College and specializes in the treatment of eating disorders and bright-light therapy for winter depression.

Theoretical Bases

Traumatic memories are encoded and processed in a different part of the brain than are nontraumatic memories. While the gist of the traumatic action gets recalled, some extraneous details may be remembered differently. Complete recovery from a trauma requires dealing with the traumatic origins of the events. This process is a four-stage process that begins with (1) denial and a vague awareness of the event with substantial covering, and moves to (2) awareness of the event, which leads to (3) resolution as different parts of the person negotiate and integrate the traumatic experience, and concludes with (4) emergence when the past is left behind as the past and the survivor renews a sense of energy as a whole self. The goals of trauma-focused therapy are to process and integrate the trauma experience, to decrease distressing symptoms, and to change emotional expression to a more positive, adaptive form.

Clientele

NECTR clients range in age from 13 to 80. Most clients have experienced sexual, physical, or emotional trauma (or all three types of trauma) at some point in their lives.

Diagnosis and Assessment

All clients have an initial intake evaluation by a psychiatrist. NECTR uses the Structured Clinical Interview for DSM-IV Dissociative Disorders (SCID-D), a structured clinical interview, as a diagnostic tool as well as the Dissociative Experiences Scale and Beck's Depression Scale. Diagnosis takes place over time. Treatment is overseen by a psychiatrist. Psychiatric assessment and psychopharmacological interventions are integrated into the treatment program when indicated.

Service Provision

The center presents clients a means to understand their traumatic pasts objectively and scientifically in individual or group therapy using trauma-focused therapeutic techniques. In this practice, memories come forth in an uncontaminated form through a process of unbiased free recall enhanced by competent use of hypnosis. One technique utilized is cognitive restructuring, which helps persons see the way they perceive the stressful events in their lives and then helps them reframe those events in a different way. Additionally, a short-term, three-session format begins with education; sessions 2 and 3 teach a self-hypnotic exercise to prevent problematic consequences.

Treatment goals include helping clients function within their environments while putting their traumas somewhat behind. This is particularly difficult for trauma survivors who have a long-term history of traumatic events spanning 15 years or more. The repressed memory controversy has had a profound effect on the work done by center staff. Staff members are more careful and do not go in to "grab memories." Instead, they proceed cautiously with any type of memory work.

The center offers specific behavioral and psychiatric evaluations, individual treatment, and therapy groups. Treatment is presented utilizing a structured team-based approach that includes many methods ranging from hypnotherapy to art therapy. Much of the treatment is cognitive–behavioral in orientation and supportive in nature. Clients frequently describe their lives in narrative format. Much of the actual work deals with safety and containment. Dr. Rousell and Dr. Braun prescribe medication for symptom alleviation and for treatment of underlying depression and anxiety. Groups include a stress visualization group, a self-esteem group for women, and a group for overweight women with binge-eating disorder.

Training and Community Intervention

NECTR has developed a trauma prevention and management plan to help organizations deal with violence and other traumas in the workplace. The trainings teach organizational managers to be aware of the early warning signs of violence and help management plan and create a crisis management team. NECTR provides consultation and brief trauma-focused group therapy for survivors of trauma, witnesses, and secondary victims, including families, as well as individual sessions that are held at NECTR's offices.

The staff of NECTR in general, and Dr. Rousell in particular, offer a variety of courses including:

1. Psychodynamic and hypnotherapeutic treatment of trauma disorders: A stage-specific model
2. Dissociation and eating disorders with interviewing techniques based on a modified SCID-D format
3. Ego state therapy of the trauma survivor with methods to activate covert ego states hypnotically and techniques to achieve conflict resolution among ego states
4. PTSD: diagnosis and implications for treatment
5. Principles of art therapy for the mental health professional
6. The workplace at risk: crisis prevention and management

THE CENTER FOR THE TREATMENT OF TRAUMATIC LIFE SITUATIONS, STATEN ISLAND, NEW YORK

The center, located on Staten Island, New York, serves war veterans, persons diagnosed with PTSD, dissociative disorders including dissociative identity disorder, near and actual transportation accident survivors, persons struggling with life-threatening diseases, the bereaved, adolescents caught up in gang violence, and children. Clients range in age from 2 to 96. Families of these primary victims generally are seen in collateral sessions. Tertiary victims are group survivors seen in consultations or educational meetings (e.g., veterans groups or bereavement groups). The Center is designed to be a state-of-the-art treatment program as well as a training center for clinicians and trainees. The center is in its infancy, and Ms. Cosentino, director and founder, puts in a 75- to 80-hour week. The for-profit 4-year-old program, as a viable center, also encourages volunteer work.

Staffing

Ms. Cosentino is assisted by two full-time staff therapists and one part-time office staff who gathers basic information and insurance information. Ms. Cosentino does the majority of treatment with patients. Referrals are made to psychiatrists for clients who need medication. Therapists and trainees receive free supervisory sessions and training. Therapists who work with the center are licensed. At the present time, lay caregivers and volunteers work on the center's proposed children's journal as well as do other work where needed.

Services

Ms. Cosentino initially speaks with new referrals on the phone for 15–20 minutes at no charge to assess "what is doable." Appointments are given during the daytime or in the evenings or weekends. Services are available for individuals, couples, families or groups. Clients have a say in the pacing of their care from the onset. The center does not provide direct medical care but refers to psychiatrists, hospitals, and substance abuse programs. The office setting is secure and is equipped with a speaker system and a button system should trouble occur.

Treatment is designed to help clients integrate the problem situation (crisis, trauma) into their lives while managing their lives and living through and beyond the traumas. Provisional diagnoses are made through the initial consultation, but in-depth psychological testing is referred out. Within the first few weeks of therapy, Ms. Cosentino conducts a major assessment and uses the SCID and Dissociative Experience Scale (DES). Ms. Cosentino uses EMDR extensively as well as hypnotherapy and pet therapy; her pet dog is a transitional object for clients to hold and utilize as a feelings barometer.

Funding

Services are funded through insurance and self-pay. Clients may work out a payment plan and defer payment with no interest or collection fees until therapy terminates.

Theory Base

The model of trauma on which treatment is based is eclectic and includes Adlerian psychoanalytic methods, which are humanistic and existential, systems approaches, material gathered at International Society for Traumatic Stress Studies (ISTSS), EMDR, hypnotherapy, and memory theories based on the work of van der Kolk. When Ms. Cosentino is called on to assist in a debriefing, she uses the Mitchell model (Everly & Mitchell, 1997; Van der Kolk & McFarlane, 1996).

Community Services

Ms. Cosentino is developing a journal for children in which children may submit drawings, writings, and art work. Volunteers will work on the journal and a grant is available for startup funds. Training in treatment of dissociative identity disorder, PTSD, and dissociative disorders is based on sessions attended at various professional meetings as well as clinical experience, tapes of sessions, and prior Adlerian training. Ms. Cosentino has appeared on cable television and has presented at local schools and in other settings.

THE TRAUMA RECOVERY INSTITUTE, MORGANTOWN, WEST VIRGINIA

The Trauma Recovery Institute (TRI), a private, free-standing institute directed by Louis Tinnin, MD, aims to reverse regression and stabilize traumatic individuals as well as provide definite diagnoses. The institute's program also provides medical care directly and indirectly through referral. The institute developed as an outgrowth of the trauma program developed to train therapists to work with an increasing number of traumatized persons in the rural state of West Virginia. Established in November 1995 as a not-for-profit organization, the institute's status changed in 1996.

Mission

The TRI is dedicated to providing care for traumatized persons and training for trauma therapists through innovate trauma-related treatment not available in a traditional medical program. Treatment uses a dissociative model through nonabreactive trauma work using video therapy and brief therapy techniques.

Clients

Children and adults of any age with symptoms related to trauma, who are not abusing drugs or alcohol, are suitable for treatment. Primary survivors of sexual assault, sexual abuse, child abuse, domestic violence, traumatic accidents, combat stress, and acute or chronic stress are clients. Secondary victims served are family members of primary patients and tertiary victims are survivors of community disasters who receive debriefing.

Staffing

The treatment team is led by Louis W. Tinnin, MD and Linda Gantt; it includes psychiatrists, psychiatric nurses, psychologists, art therapists, counselors, and social workers. Family members are therapeutic assistants in some phases of treatment. Case managers are assigned to patients to monitor responses to treatment and to evaluate evidence of regression. The program does not utilize lay caregivers or volunteers. An advisory board consisting of consumers, community members, and staff from other centers helps offer direction to the program. Dr. Tinnin provides clinical supervision; however, the institute also has peer review and peer supervision. Staff meet regularly in a trauma study group. Therapists are certified by their local training programs at the therapist (MA, MSW) or psychotraumatologist (doctoral) levels.

Treatment

The majority of procedures used in the TRI program were pioneered by Dr. Tinnin. They include time-limited therapy, group art therapy, and video dialogue therapy (see Fig. 3.1). The approaches help to resolve traumatic memories without painful emotional reliving. TRI staff also provide psychiatric evaluation and consultation as well as Gestalt therapy. Individual and group therapies average 10 hours weekly (4 days/week) for 6–10 weeks; a longer course of treatment is for persons diagnosed with dissociative identity disorder (DID). If regression in scores on testing occurs posttreatment, the case manager activates an antiregressive treatment regimen and enlists family participation. A variety of groups are included in the treatment program including art therapy trauma-processing group, dissociative containment group, recovery process group, victim mythology group, and medication group.

Video technology allows patients to concentrate the therapeutic process in active "homework" review of videotaped therapy sessions. The sessions include recursive anamnesis interviews and face-to-face sessions. Review of some of these sessions at a later date helps prevent relapse. Treatment has three phases: resolving traumatic memories, addressing trauma-related behavior patterns, and promoting reconnection to others and preventing relapse through self-help measures. Treatment is not designed to change characteristic traits of personality disorders or the dissociative defenses of DID. Fees for these treatments are program and procedure specific with discounts for training cases.

Diagnosis/Assessment

The psychotraumatology evaluation includes a psychiatric interview, a CAPS (Clinician Administer PTSD Scale), self-administered trauma specific [e.g., Impact of Event Scale (IES)] and related instruments including the Dissociative Experiences Scale (DES): [20–35 is suggestive of PTSD; 35–50 dissociative disorder not otherwise specified (DDNOS); 50–75+, DID]; the Symptom Check List-45 (SCL-45), which measures global symptoms; the Toronto Alexithymia Scale (TAS) (a score of 74+ is indicative, but this scale does not respond to treatment in changes in scores); and the Dissociative Regression Scale (DRS). Each patient is given an individual treatment plan with appropriate therapy tracks and specific criteria for response and recovery.

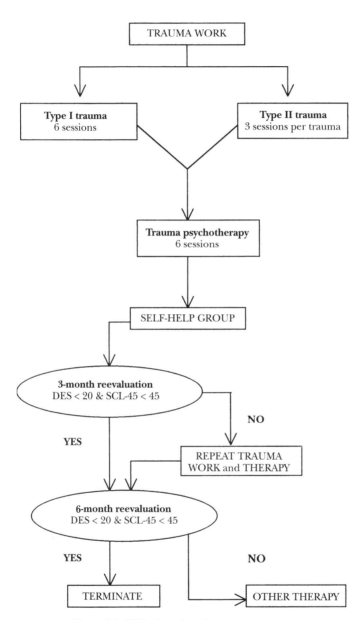

Figure 3.1. TRI's flow chart for trauma therapy.

Progress is assessed and monitored through repeated assessments using DRS and IES during the course of treatment, 1 week after termination, and 3 and 6 months posttermination (measuring extended outcome). A 50% reduction in IES and DRS scores usually indicates secure stabilization; cure occurs when the patient no longer has amnesia and dissociative symptoms and the DES is <20; TAS is <70; and the SCL-45 is <80.

The program uses an outpatient antiregressive regimen to reduce suicidal threats, addictive reenactment and dissociative regression. The program:

- Provides a stimulus barrier with psychotropic medications and behavioral management
- Reduces ambiguity of roles and boundaries
- Provides auxiliary ego functioning through volunteer task masters and helpers of the family
- Supports autonomous ego functioning (identity, volition) through a team approach of physician, nurse, and family members

The goals of treatment are to resolve dissociated traumatic memories and the influences of those memories on core symptoms. The changes that result include eliminating intrusive symptoms; diminishing avoidant behaviors, thoughts, and memories; and reducing arousal symptoms through 6 sessions of trauma work (phase I).

Theory

The theoretical approach of TRI is based on the concept of traumatic dissociation as described by Janet (1889) and van der Hart (1992). Treatment of PTSD does not result in cure if memories are sealed off from consciousness. Recursive anamnesis uses video recording technology and hypnosis to gain access to dissociated fragments and unites those fragments into a trauma narrative. Three types of fragments may recur intrusively as flashbacks:

- Fixed idea: a suspended intentional state interrupted by the onset of the traumatic event and the accompanying altered state
- Altered state itself, which may disrupt consciousness as a depressed or dissociated state
- Aftermath fragment included as grief or emotionless

The three fragments, as unfinished experiences, seek completion and closure to take them from present time to past experience and finished memories. Controlled altered states of consciousness gain access to fragments and reunite them into a narrative history of closure.

Dissociative anamnesis does not require a profound trance; it can be accomplished through a minor alteration of attention produced by assisted relaxation. Patients shift from verbal recollection to imagery through use of the "observer" mode: viewing memories as if they were outsiders watching themselves in the scenes. Use of the observer self allows for recovery of preverbal, sublimated, or implicit nonfully coded, nonverbal memories. Patients describe the traumatic experiences from before the point of danger to aftermath beyond the danger to the end point of the experience in their observer mode. The patient also is helped to identify the fixed idea/experience that occurred immediately before the traumatic event began and might include an intention to flee, fight, surrender, or freeze.

The anamnesis looks at subjective experiences of time distortion, depersonalization, out-of-body retreat to fantasized safe places, and/or substitution of an alter self to bear the pain as well as external, objective events. The session places the event into historical memory and then reintroduces the patient to the present. An ideal anamnesis is a detached recitation without emotional involvement or reliving.

Single-event traumas require two cycles of anamnesis (dissociation and recursive review plus review at home) for four sessions. The fifth and sixth session draw a graphic narrative of the traumatic experience in realistic and abstract forms which includes the aftermath and end point of the trauma. Recursive procedures are necessary for each primary trauma of the multiplicity of traumas and may occur over time with supportive therapy occurring between.

The theory base of phase 2 trauma psychotherapy notes that the patient's conscious experiences of the trauma were helplessly suspended in timelessness as vulnerability to victimization by others. After resolution of dissociated memories, patients yearn for illusions of restored invulnerability, security, and promises of just rewards. However, these illusions are just that—illusions—and must be grieved so that the patient can empower him- or herself and become more responsible for personal safety and reconnection.

Phase 3 trauma psychotherapy is designed to resolve the mythology of self as victim in a hostile and unmanageable world (Foa & Riggs, 1993). It increases a patient's sense of independent self-determination, awareness of choices and coping methods, adaptation of strategy to ensure reasonable safety, and connection with others. A different therapist conducts the third-stage work and begins by reviewing the trauma history. Work quickly shifts to exploring losses accompanying the trauma and examining the patient's philosophy of life as well as victim mythology (within three sessions). After the myth is formulated, the patient's task is to acknowledge and relinquish previously held illusions of invulnerability, entitlement to protection, future reward for injury, and the need and wish to be rescued (three sessions).

Community Services

The TRI networks with West Virginia University, Chestnut Ridge Hospital, the Center for Independent Living, the VA Hospital, and other facilities. It markets itself through mailings, public service announcements, and a teleconference system of educational seminars. Providing training to professionals is part of the mission of TRI and the training uses a "see one, do one, teach one" model. The staff has developed a training video and training curricula. Consultation is offered through video teleconferencing as outreach through the states' hospital program. A 3-day annual conference also offers information and training to those in attendance.

ROBERT H. MOORE, PhD AND ASSOCIATES, CLEARWATER, FLORIDA

This outpatient counseling practice has a strong trauma focus. As a for-profit agency, it operates on a sliding fee scale and receives funding from clients and third-party payers. State certification and listing of the program has made marketing less necessary. The organization is growing with relatively little effort, given Florida's mandatory arrest and referral of perpetrators of domestic violence.

Staffing

The practice is staffed by a full-time director and four part-time therapists. Three of the staff are masters-level counselors; two hold doctorates. One is female; four are male. Staff licensures include clinical social work, school psychology, marriage and family therapy, and mental health counseling. Clinical certifications include traumatic incident reduction, eye movement desensitization and reprocessing, thought field therapy, the Duluth model, and rational–emotive behavior therapy. Two staff members are certified trauma specialists through the Association of Traumatic Stress Specialists (ATSS).

Clientele

The clientele represent the demographics of the geographic area. Since Dr. Moore has been in the community for over 20 years, he is known and agencies refer to his program. Many referrals come from both victim and perpetrator populations in the domestic violence arena. Approximately 210 persons a week are seen in 14 groups. In addition, each clinician sees 5–10 individual clients weekly.

Theory Base

The theory base of the program began with Ellis and rational–emotive behavior therapy (REBT). However, the primary theoretical underpinnings are the Duluth model (Moore, 1993a,b), critical incident stress management (CISM) utilizing the Mitchell model (Everly & Mitchell, 1997), and traumatic incident reduction (TIR) as developed by Gerbode and colleagues (Gerbode & Moore, 1994). Dr. Moore has written about the use of TIR for resolution of PTSD.

The REBT model maintains that events and circumstances do not directly cause the feelings people have about them. In fact, certain beliefs about events determine one's emotional reactions. These beliefs (shoulds, oughts, and musts) and predications (awfuls and terribles) include imperative statements and identity statements. TIR is used as a means to achieve the resolution of known traumatic incidents and/or to resolve specific irrational feelings, attitudes, and emotions.

A guided cognitive imagery procedure, TIR requires the client to "view" a trauma internally in accord with a standard protocol in order to bring it to resolution. The procedure requires a high degree of client concentration in a safe space. By the completion of the protocol, the client has depleted the emotional charge on the incident, revised its embedded cognitions as needed, and feels completely free of its negative influence on his or her life. TIR is not dependent on the personality of the therapist. The therapist does not interpret or evaluate for the viewer.

This theoretical stance recognizes that the PTSD reaction is most easily distinguishable by the involuntary flashback that can be triggered by many cognitive and perceptual cues. PTSD is diverse in its symptomatic expression, often including extremely volatile memories of trauma. The memory of a traumatic incident, however, sometimes is substantially suppressed and/or repressed. In order to deal with past traumas in an effective way, the client must achieve a resolution through imagery and revise errant cognitions associated with the primary pain that is a residual aspect of the trauma.

Treatment

Dr. Moore believes that treatment should "cut to the chase" and do its job in a few months, not over a period of years. Staff work with psychiatrists to help clients get off extensive medications and process their traumata more thoroughly than chemical controls permit. The program tries to avoid forensic work. Many clients receive group counseling. The state has mandated a 26-week treatment of domestic violence for its involved offenders.

Training and Community Involvement

Dr. Moore and associates have offered TIR training to professionals. They also offer continuing education training for health professionals with continuing education units (CEUs) at the state level.

THE TRAUMA CENTER, BROOKLINE, MASSACHUSETTS

Over the past decade, the Trauma Center has been in the forefront of treatment, teaching, and research in trauma-related psychology and biological problems. The diagnosis of acute stress or posttraumatic stress is probably one of the most common psychiatric diagnoses. The center's nine locations throughout Massachusetts offer services for children or adults with recent or chronic acute trauma histories. Clinic locations range from Boston to suburban to rural. The center is actively involved in research to evaluate effectiveness of interventions and trains clinicians in highly specialized treatment skills.

The organization receives for-profit and non-profit funding, with an executive director for outpatient services, a CEO and a medical director, a program director (Dr. Becker), a clinical director, a training director, and a child coordinator. This arm is funded primarily by third-party payers (private insurance, Medicaid, Medicare) and some federal funds administered by the state. The clinical director of the program is Dr. Bessel van der Kolk, one of the founding fathers of the trauma movement. His research into the need for specialized treatment for survivors of sexual abuse and battering led to the creation of the center.

The 12-year history of the organization has been fraught with great funding troubles. The organization has been part of several different organizations. Presently, the center is a program of Arbour Health System, the largest private mental health and substance abuse system in Massachusetts. It includes a variety of hospitals and counseling centers. The center also receives partial funding from the Massachusetts Office for Victim Assistance. The center publicizes and markets itself through brochures and a weekly lecture series open to the public. The center also conducts a number of yearly conferences, which serve as a marketing and education tool.

Mission

The mission of the Trauma Center is to help trauma survivors reestablish a sense of safety and predictability in the world and to provide them with state-of-the-art therapeutic care during the process of reconstructing their lives.

Philosophy

The philosophy of the Trauma Center is that traumatic experiences disrupt adults and children on every level of functioning, from memory and concentration to neurochemistry and physiology, to emotional, social, relational, and spiritual functioning. The treatment model therefore has to be broad enough to touch all these areas as a psychosocial–biological model. Biological intervention, social intervention, and psychological intervention are equally important. Timing is everything and what needs to be done at what given moment is the focus of intervention.

Staffing

Staff members are two-thirds female and primarily psychologists; other staff members include psychiatrists, social workers, licensed marriage and family therapists, predoctoral trainees, postdoctoral students, and a movement therapist. These pre- and postdoctoral students receive extensive training in the treatment of traumatized populations as well as in the center's model of trauma, way of thinking about trauma, and understanding about trauma. Most staff members are licensed and certified by the State of Massachusetts. A volunteer development director is helping with fund raising. Approximately 30 therapists serve the nine clinics. The clinical director oversees clinical functions of programs and staff.

Attempts are made to balance caseloads as a means of self-care of the therapists. There are extensive shared consultations and good supervision. Regular, weekly staff meetings and treatment team meetings, birthday celebrations, and several yearly parties help add to this support.

Clinicians function primarily in a fee-for-service structure, that is, all the clinicians except for four administrators are paid by the hour for patients seen. The pay rate is fairly low and there is an increasing demand to lower overhead and increase productivity. The limits imposed by managed care insurance also have affected the quality of care, primarily in a negative fashion.

Trauma Model

The model of trauma is completely biopsychosocial and uses an eclectic range of interventions and strategies. The debriefing model utilized is a seven-stage modified Mitchell model (Everly & Mitchell, 1997) that is more process oriented. It includes sharing of coping strategies and generation of new coping strategies as well as education about acute distress and PTSD. The view of memory at the Trauma Center is that traumatic memories are processed differently in the brain. They have seen instances where it is known that persons have been traumatized yet the individuals have no particular memories of the traumatic events that happened years ago. Suddenly the memory surfaces in a way that they can understand and explain, perhaps in visual pictures or sounds that previously they were not consciously aware of.

Clientele

Clientele are from the approximately 7% of the general population who suffer from PTSD and related problems. The majority of adult clients have sexual abuse histories; child clients are primarily of school age and also have sexual abuse histories. The program also sees parents of abused children and family members. The community crisis team of the center work with various community groups and organizations. Additional clients are crime victims, survivors of fires and explosions, and those injured in work-related accidents. Persons with acute stress disorder are underrepresented. Clients give input into and state preferences as to gender of therapist, scheduling, and group participation.

Assessment

Assessment includes taking a trauma history and doing a mental status exam. The center has a computerized assessment program that generates a PTSD score, a disorders of extreme stress, not otherwise specified (DESNOS) or complex PTSD score and a DES score. The assessment was designed by Dr. van der Kolk. The assessment is conducted over the course of four or five sessions. Other instruments used include the CAPS and the Rorschach. The computerized assessment is a useful tool and is supplemented by a clinical interview that assesses the extent of the trauma, at least the small part that clients initially reveal. The assessment is done by any of the clinicians and is used to plan for treatment.

Service Provision

An initial screening determines whether the primary presenting problem is trauma related. There is some capacity for free care for persons with limited resources. A four-session evaluation process culminates in a treatment-planning meeting. In that meeting, information about the trauma history, preferences, and needs of the client are discussed and the team makes treatment recommendations. The clinic has a psychopharmacology program for both children and adults. Services offered to children include individual therapy, family intervention, consultation and specialized evaluation, cognitive–behavioral treatments, groups for parents and children, and forensic consultations as well as psychopharmacology. Services offered to adults include individual therapy, family intervention, group psychotherapy, psychoeducation groups, stabilization groups, cognitive–behavioral therapies, psychopharmacology, EMDR, and mind–body approaches. Crisis services and partial hospitalization are available in conjunction with Arbour Health System Hospitals.

The basic treatment goals are to help survivors reestablish a sense of safety and predictability and to help survivors improve their psychological, biological, and social functioning. The overall goal is to help people live their lives in the present, rather than continuing to experience the present day as a mere extension of the traumatic past. The treatment plan determines priorities, sets short-term and long-term goals, and focuses on areas of safety and self-regulation, understanding and integrating of traumatic memories, and making connections with others in a give-and-take manner. Some clients need services for an acute incident of trauma (e.g., an assault, witnessing of a violent crime); others need treatment for complex PTSD.

Community crisis interventions include debriefings, preparedness planning, and team training and development. The center has someone on call 24 hours a day. Additionally, staff members do limited forensic work when asked to do so. Several staff members are qualified as expert witnesses primarily in child and adult trauma. Dr. van der Kolk has testified specifically around repressed memory.

Training

The center has a 9-month certificate program to train licensed clinicians on the spectrum of trauma-related issues. Participants attend seminars, lectures, and supervision groups one day per week and also take individual elective courses in this postgraduate program. This weekly lecture series also is open to professionals not enrolled in the program. The center provides specialized training and consultation to persons from the community in the assessment and treatment of both children and adults. In the past 10 years, the center has trained over 60 psychologists and psychiatrists. The center has created brochures and publishes a newsletter, has a website, and also serves as a teaching clinic for Boston University School of Medicine. Center staff members have contributed many published articles and conducted many conferences. They also have produced several videotapes.

THE COPIN FOUNDATION, BUFFALO, NEW YORK

The COPIN Foundation (Caring of Persons in Need) was designed and conceptualized in 1983 and opened its doors July 3, 1985, to serve veterans as primary victims and their families as secondary victims. The foundation has had a 17-bed residence for veterans, the COPIN House, the first such facility in the United States. The foundation also has an outpatient service that treats between 200 and 300 veterans yearly. Treatment is given to all who come and includes medication management, psychiatric consultation, crisis intervention, and counseling. The foundation received financial support from the Agent Orange Class Assistance Program. Under that grant, the COPIN Foundation, Inc. served 2739 veterans, 672 children, and 833 family members for a total of 4244 persons. The foundation maintained a 24-hour crisis hot line, provided temporary, transitional shelter to veterans and (often) to members of their families. It set in place an internship program with students from local universities and provided mobile outreach services to Mohawk, Seneca, and Tuscarora Native American Nations. COPIN House became a safe place for many veterans. However, that funding ended and four staff members were laid off in May 1996.

The COPIN Foundation relies on external funding sources for much of its financial support. It is difficult to work otherwise because the organization does not take Medicare or Medicaid payments. Marketing is done by word of mouth. The foundation is a private, not-for-profit facility that has been applying for various grants, although there is no funding to pay professional grant writers. A 12 member Board of Directors oversees the foundation.

In June 1995, Executive Director McGrath was one of 64/5000 nominees to earn the Jefferson Award. The American Institute of Public Service, founded by Jacqueline Kennedy Onassis and Robert Taft, Sr. presented this award.

Mission and Philosophy

The foundation "really does not have a philosophy" other than "just do it." Ms. McGrath stated, "If we can't do it, then we will find someone who will."

Staffing

The COPIN Foundation had a psychiatric nurse, mental health trauma therapists, a social worker, and a part-time family counselor. Four staff members were laid off because of funding cutbacks. There is no doctor on staff and clients who need medication are referred for consultation. None of the staff is licensed so it is not possible to get third-party insurance reimbursement. However, all staff members are experienced in the field. Clinic Director McGrath gets supervision from external consultants and then she, in turn, supervises those on the staff. Ms. McGrath is a former VA nurse. The staff is "like a family" and those who are laid off will come back once funding is available.

The office is staffed 7 days a week by a group of consultants who generally are veterans. Veterans man the crisis office and field phone calls. These veterans collect information, filter information, and then make referrals. They are astute and have knowledge that is invaluable.

Theory

There are many basic physiological changes that occur when a client is traumatized, because trauma impacts neurotransmitters including adrenalin. Many clients have anxiety, depression, and hyperactivity. If clients do not have diagnosable medical problems, then it is important to "go for neurotransmitters." Prescribing Ritalin in small doses calms survivors. Executive Director McGrath questions why clients become addicted and why they relapse. She looks at the neurotransmitters to understand what clients are missing. The most important consideration is not the model of trauma treatment but the phenomenology. However, the model to which the foundation adheres is one of optimal wellness and health.

Clientele

Clients often walk in to the foundation as well as being referrals from other agencies. Approximately 50 clients are seen weekly. Many of the clients seen through the Foundation have diagnosable attention deficit hyperactivity disorder (ADHD). Many others have a dual diagnosis; approximately 90% have a substance abuse disorder. Total and permanent abstinence is a goal. The majority of the clients need long-term care.

Treatment

Treatment at the COPIN Foundation includes doing "whatever needs to be done." Much of the work done with veterans is educationally oriented. Veterans are taught relaxation strategies such as breathing. They learn to "go to the alpha state" within a couple of minutes so that reprogramming can begin. Veterans are empowered shortly after treatment begins and then are educated about brain physiology, anxiety, medications, and the limbic system.

A formal assessment includes taking a psychosocial history and completion of minimal paper–pencil instruments to measure ADHD. Assessment may lead to a medication referral and also is frequently utilized to substantiate disability claims. If the veteran is hospitalized in the inpatient program, the general inpatient stay is 60 to 90 days.

A significant percentage of treatment occurs in a group setting. The group looks at "what happened then, what coping mechanisms were used then, why those coping strategies do not work now, and what is happening in the here and now." In the groups, veterans (and some generic trauma survivors) learn about triggers and anniversary dates. Generally four psychoeducational, ongoing groups meet weekly. Groups are free in cost and most veterans who use them have minimal to no funds. The foundation also provides a number of social services including meals and clothing collection.

Community Services

The COPIN Foundation provides debriefing when requested. Through the American Red Cross, staff members have provided debriefing on site for hostage situations and to witnesses of attacks. Members are Red Cross volunteers. They utilize the Mitchell model (Everly & Mitchell, 1997) of debriefing and also educate those debriefed about basic physiology. Ms. McGrath is a qualified expert witness about the impacts of trauma.

POST TRAUMATIC STRESS CENTER, NEW HAVEN, CONNECTICUT

The Post Traumatic Stress Center is a private group practice that treats children and adults who have suffered psychological trauma, as well as their families. The center offers a variety of services ranging from individual, group, and family psychotherapy to creative arts therapies and symptom reduction treatment methodologies such as EMDR, prolonged exposure (Foa & Rothbaum, 1998) and the counting method (Ochberg, 1996). It also offers specialized services including the Women's Trauma Program, Women in the Workplace Program, the Family Program, and the Veterans Project.

Codirectors and comanagers of the program are Haddar Lubin, MD and

David Read Johnson, PhD. The center was created in 1994 as an extension of the directors' work with men at the VA Medical Center and women at the Women's Trauma Program of Yale Psychiatric Institute. The center became a full-time private practice in Fall 1996. Approximately 50% of the caseload is fee-for-service (private insurance, managed care) and 50% of the caseload participates in entitlement programs (Medicaid, general assistance, Medicare). The staff of the center are highly trained professionals deeply committed to the treatment of posttraumatic stress disorder and related conditions.

Staffing

An interdisciplinary staff at the center includes psychiatrist Lubin, psychologists (Johnson and two others), a social worker, and two PhD candidate researchers who are conducting a treatment outcome study to evaluate training. Several creative arts therapists have a collaborative relationship with the center. Weekly staff processing and peer supervision meetings help to maintain good work relationships, prevent burnout, and sustain excitement about work for the staff. All staff are licensed in their respective fields by the State of Connecticut.

Clientele

The predominant number of survivors seen by the staff in the clinic are survivors of sexual assault/sexual abuse. However, the categories of victims seen are widening. The center primarily sees adults up to age 80.

Program Services

The Post Traumatic Stress Center offers individual, group, and family psychotherapy. It offers creative arts therapies, psychoeducation, and symptom reduction therapies including EMDR, prolonged exposure, and the counting method. The center provides medication and can hospitalize patients when needed. Other services provided include evaluation for PTSD, including presence of, degree of severity, and functional impairment caused by the condition within life context; education for professionals, survivors, and others; and supervision.

The Women's Trauma Program provides trauma-focused therapy for victims of sexual assault, childhood sexual abuse, physical and emotional abuse, domestic violence, motor vehicle and other injuries, and natural disasters. The program utilizes a three-phase trauma-focused group that is 16 weeks in length. The group uses the interactive psychoeducational group therapy model (Lubin & Johnson, 1997), which views clients as "students" of recovery. Treatment is guided by the assumptions that some changes after trauma are unique to women and isolation and disconnection are at the core of the posttraumatic experience. Goals of the group model include (1) educating women about how traumatic experiences have impacted their lives; (2) facilitating a differentiation between the illness and unimpaired characteristics of the person; and (3) reducing symptoms.

The Women in the Workforce Program provides psychoeducation and psychotherapy to professional women who want to explore workplace issues in depth. Some of the issues include work-related stress resulting from gender-specific stressors and discrimination. The Family Program offers a wide range of services to traumatized families. Among these services are family therapy, multiple family therapy groups, play therapy for the children, and a psychoeducational lecture series about family issues.

The Veterans Project offers specialized services for Vietnam veterans. It focuses on their experience of the homecoming as it has impacted their lives, families, work, and social relationships. The program includes ceremony-based interventions and expressive therapies.

Staff conduct standard assessments with most new clients. Among the measurements utilized are the Clinician Administered PTSD Scale (CAPS), the Mississippi PTSD Scale (combat-related or civilian), the Combat Exposure Scale, the Homecoming Stress Scale, the Brief Symptom Inventory, and the Beck Depression Inventory Additional information is gathered through clinical interviews and personal medical histories. The program does not do debriefing.

The intensive psychoeducational group therapy helps survivors differentiate self-representations from traumatic schemas that the survivor may have assimilated since the event. This assimilation may lead to shame, social isolation, distorted body image, and sense of meaninglessness. The group utilizes cognitive distancing techniques, corrective interpersonal enactments, and specifically designed ceremonies to alter the survivor's relationship to the traumatic event(s) and PTSD.

Community Services

Staff from the Post Traumatic Stress Center consult with schools and social agencies. They serve as expert witnesses. Staff offer a variety of formal courses and workshops on PTSD within the local community. These trainings are generally for professionals and offer CEUs. Staff also supervise other mental health professionals in other agencies about PTSD cases. The center networks with community action agencies in the trauma arenas.

Theory Base

The orientation of the center is prosurvivor, treating the client as a person within a historical, social, and spiritual context. The steps of this process involve:

1. Telling the trauma story
2. Delinking traumatic events from clients' self schemas
3. Exploring the nature of the homecoming (the response of the family and social networks to the traumatic experience of the client
4. Facilitating coming to terms with the current social network
5. Encouraging "coming out" as a trauma survivor
6. Respecting the deep and long-standing effects of the traumatic experience
7. Approaching the existential issues that the trauma has raised

The center aims to empower the client through psychoeducation, speaking out against trauma as a means to prevent trauma, the use of creative and expressive media for communication about the trauma and engaging the client with family and society in productive ways.

Center staff members have written a number of articles outlining their theoretical positions. For example, the psychoeducation group therapy model (Lubin & Johnson, 1997; Lubin, Johnson, & Southwick, 1997) is a brief group therapy program that invites the client to engage in the therapeutic process in an active and dynamic way. The client is encouraged to use internal resources that have not been damaged irreparably by the trauma (intellect, resourcefulness, humanity). The model uses psychoeducation to educate victims about the effects of trauma on themselves, offers a structure to facilitate differentiation of the individual from the illness, and aims to reduce symptoms. An educational format provides emotional distance and creates a safe therapeutic environment wherein the client can lower defenses and heal. The group has three phases over its 16-week course: (1) the trauma and the self—fragmentation; interpersonal relationships; (2) reframing; and (3) being in the world—reintegration. Group sessions begin with an educational minilecture. The group itself becomes a laboratory for interaction in which members help one another in a competent manner. The group ends with a graduation ceremony and a public storytelling of the trauma story.

Another theoretical conceptualization is ordering clinical data through an adaptational, hierarchical framework of strategies hypothesized to be used by a traumatized individual (Johnson, 1997; Johnson, Feldman, & Lubin, 1995). These adaptations result in progressively greater damage to a survivor's personality, interpersonal relatedness, and behavior. The primary adaptation to trauma is dissociation, particularly if the trauma occurs during childhood when the memory traces of trauma are split off from representations of self. If the trauma occurs later in age, more transient dissociative responses may occur, including flashbacks or nightmares. A secondary adaptation to trauma manifests itself in defense mechanisms that dampen, avoid, or contain the traumatic experience. Among these are projection, reaction formation, denial, obsessive defenses, and avoidant behaviors. These defenses may permanently alter personality style. If these alterations become autonomous and separate from the context of the original trauma, they may develop into a personality disorder, for example, what manifests itself as borderline. Tertiary adaptations, the most generalized effects of trauma, include impairments in regulatory functioning (arousal, mood, cognition), poor impulse control, anger, anxiety, hopelessness, cognitive distortions, and others. The symptoms, if they become more prominent, can lead to posttraumatic decline.

Center staff members are particularly interested in conceptualizing the homecoming experience and believe that social attributions may be critical influences in the etiology of PTSD (Johnson et al., 1997). Many clients reveal deeply felt wounds stemming from their families' or authorities' negative reactions upon learning of their traumas. Often these "secondary wounds" become important foci of treatment, particularly when these negative assumptions or misperceptions can still be corrected.

Research

The center is engaged in a variety of research projects generally dealing with treatment outcome. Among them are a comparative study of various brief treatment methods (EMDR vs. prolonged exposure vs. counting method); the development of a Homecoming Scale that measures the impact of the homecoming experience on etiology of PTSD development; treatment outcome of the psychoeducational group therapy program for women survivors; pre- and post-self-report measures of treatment outcome; and the measurement of alexithymia as well its treatment through the use of creative arts therapies.

STANLEY STREET TREATMENT AND RESOURCES, FALL RIVER, MASSACHUSETTS

Stanley Street Treatment and Resources, Inc. (SSTAR) is a nonprofit, private, large, multiservice organization headed by a woman executive director, a woman director of operations, and a volunteer board of directors. SSTAR, in its two buildings, provides an inpatient detox facility and an ambulatory service center with a community health care facility on site. SSTAR staff also refers uninsured clients to providers through the Robert Wood Johnson-funded medical organization.

SSTAR originally was created in 1977 as the Fall River/New Bedford Center for Alcohol Problems, a nonprofit, public-sector inpatient detoxification center. Outpatient services were added, as were programs to meet the special needs of women. This change in focus led to the development of a woman center providing domestic violence and rape crisis services as well as the development of pregnant addict services in a women's center. Current treatment at SSTAR has a trauma focus because many clients have a severe trauma history.

Mission

The mission of SSTAR is to provide the highest quality health care and social services in the most cost-efficient manner and least restrictive setting to those individuals most in need, without regard to ability to pay.

Philosophy

SSTAR believes in a holistic philosophy of treatment that helps clients attain physical, mental, social, and spiritual well-being. The agency recognizes that clients with multiple traumas often replay that trauma over and over. These clients often have difficulty accessing appropriate services. SSTAR's "one-stop shopping" model aims to eliminate those obstacles. The substance abuse treatment provided by SSTAR is based on an abstinence model.

Theoretical Model

Healing must include biopsychosocial interventions. Treatment is based on a staged model (Herman, 1992) of safety and stabilization, memory processing and grief work, and self-development. Treatment of women clientele is also based on a relational model (Gilligan, Miller). Most therapists at SSTAR use a cognitive–behavioral approach. Female therapists generally have a feminist orientation. Empowerment and emotional growth are goals of treatment as client and therapist work together as a cooperative team. SSTAR acknowledges that traumatized individuals sometimes suffer from severe memory impairment and recognize that those individuals may recover memories of trauma in a fragmented fashion, over time.

Clientele

About half of the clientele at SSTAR are male; many of them are substance abusers. A high percentage of the other 50% of the clients, females, have a history of trauma and substance abuse.

Assessment

SSTAR has a lengthy, structured intake interview. This interview asks about a history of and present circumstances related to domestic violence, verbal abuse, emotional abuse, physical abuse, and/or sexual abuse as well as lingering problems related to any of those abusive experiences. The intake interview includes a questionnaire designed to identify posttraumatic symptoms (including DSM-IV criteria for PTSD) and asks questions about drug history. When indicated, at a later date, clients may be able to complete the Dissociative Experiences Scale, the Dissociative Disorders Interview Schedule, and Somatoform Dissociation Scale. They may be given a taped interview, the

SCID, when confirmation of a dissociative disorder is sought. This intake assessment packet is specific to SSTAR. The clinician assigned at intake begins this assessment and may or may not keep the case, depending on expertise and appropriateness of the client–therapist match. Clinical assessment reveals that SSTAR's trauma clients have a gamut of Axis II disorders. Among the most prevalent are Antisocial Personality Disorder, Narcissistic Personality Disorder, Borderline Personality Disorder, and Histrionic Personality Disorder.

Services Provided

SSTAR provides a variety of services to its clientele. Among these are domestic violence services, inpatient detoxification and short-term rehabilitation to pregnant women, rape crisis services, outpatient substance abuse services and mental health counseling, and family medical care. Clients in crisis can speak with a clinician immediately. If a client comes to the center without an appointment, that client is seen as soon, as is possible without a formal intake interview between 8:30 AM and 8:30 PM Monday through Thursday and 8:30 AM to 4:30 PM on Friday. If the situation is not an emergency, then an appointment is scheduled within 3 business days. All noncrisis new clientele receive an intake interview from clinical staff. Counseling staff members are available on an on-call basis during nonbusiness hours. The on-call service is only available for clients who are SSTAR's clientele.

Additional services provided include home-based outreach case management and a program for "children who witness." SSTAR also offers testing, counseling, and support for HIV, inpatient detoxification, and primary health care through SSTAR's Family Health Agency.

SSTAR staff has a variety of qualifications and credentials. One is trained in EMDR; another has advanced training in dissociative disorders. Staff provide individual counseling and psychotherapy, lead support and/or therapy groups, lead advocacy groups, provide medications, do court advocacy for victims of domestic violence and/or assault, participate in system intervention in schools (e.g., substance abuse prevention), and facilitate linkages with community supports.

Many of the clients of SSTAR are dually diagnosed. Some of them are dually diagnosed with substance abuse and dissociative disorder. In this instance, the timing and coordination of interventions is important. Clients are first connected with chemical dependency treatment. Then they begin the diagnostic process for DID. During this phase, panic and relapse often occur and the theme of safety unifies all areas of treatment. The transmission of hope is crucial in the treatment of DID/substance abuse. Clinicians who work with this population need specialized training. Clients are connected to a peer group of others in chemical dependency recovery to ensure a more positive outcome. An abstinence model of treatment for addictions and an empowerment model guide treatment.

Another service provided by the center is a domestic violence and rape crisis hotline. This hotline is manned at night and on weekends. Intensive case management services are available to some clients who are covered under Medicaid.

Staff does rape crisis counseling, domestic violence counseling, and substance abuse counseling. Methods include intensive psychoeducation, cognitive–behavioral interventions, confrontation, hypnosis, imagery for safe place work, contracting, expressive therapy and sand tray therapy, and fractionated abreaction and EMDR for some memory processing.

Long-term treatment may include continuous (ongoing) or continual (long term with some spaces between) treatment periods. Emphasis in long-term treatment is development of trust, establishing the therapeutic relationship, stabilization-oriented trauma work, processing of memories by some clinicians, posttrauma-stage self-development. Techniques for memory processing include hypnosis, hypnoprojective work (symbolic processing of memories first), split screen or screen viewing of traumatic events, and others.

Strengths of SSTAR's physical environment include a large, appealing playroom with a window through which parents can observe and check on the babysitter; three waiting rooms (substance abuse, women's center/AIDS counseling, medical center areas); and a nicely decorated outpatient center with soothing colors, appealing artwork, and private offices for therapists. Weaknesses include small offices with large desks (and no sofas or room to do and set up sand trays easily), closeness to a well-trafficked hallway, overhead paging, and other safety and concentration-inhibiting features.

Funding

Insurance reimbursement, Medicaid, Medicare, and other funding sources fund SSTAR. Government contracts of outpatient substance abuse and domestic violence programs also help provide financing. The center has some state contracts and federal substance abuse grants. SSTAR, serving southeastern Massachusetts and Rhode Island, has a 9 million dollar budget.

Staffing

SSTAR employs a variety of clinicians, medical personnel, and also utilizes volunteers to man the domestic violence and rape crisis hotline. Alcoholics Anonymous (AA) members visit in the detox unit and run AA meetings. SSTAR has female physicians, persons with bachelor's degrees to do some addiction and domestic violence counseling, licensed clinicians with specialized certifications, one staff psychologist, and three part-time psychiatrists.

Staff receive in-house individual and group supervision and consultation. Staff also receive informal consultation, participate in once or twice monthly in-service presentations, and can attend weekly Yoga sessions and/or potluck lunches.

Community Services

Once a year, staff of SSTAR offer free lectures and seminars on topics related to women and substance abuse. The center also offers a 36-hour training program for volunteers and local professionals on domestic violence and rape. Among the topics included in this training series are why women stay, the denial of incest and current backlash, teen dating violence, children who witness, and assisting the survivor in the medical setting. Staff also offer in-service trainings to professionals on trauma-related and trauma treatment-related topics. Staff have written sections of a new rape crisis manual, *Supporting Survivors of Sexual Assault*, for the Massachusetts Department of Public Health. Additional services to the community provided by SSTAR include consultation to the Department of Social Services through service on a multidisciplinary assessment team, prevention work in public schools in substance abuse and teen violence, and. informative interviews with media about domestic violence. Staff also network and cooperate with a variety of community mental health and social service agencies, as well as the courts.

SUMMARY

One of the most striking conclusions to reach about the centers described in this chapter is that the creation of a trauma center takes the dream of an individual or small group of individuals to bring that dream to reality. No matter the type of services provided or the population served, without that dream, the center would not exist. All these centers are dedicated to furthering the field through building public awareness as well as other professionals as to the impact, diagnosis, and treatment of PTSD, through increasing the knowledge base and abilities of staff members, and through providing competent care.

Each center described in this chapter provides a variety of services for a variety of populations Several of the centers began by professing the objective of providing treatment to specific populations (e.g., veterans or sexual abuse victims). Yet, over time, the provision of those services has changed to meet the changing demands and climate. The centers are committed to designing, implementing, and reporting on clinical research. Each center works within a biopsychosocial–cultural–spiritual–community context that examines the goodness of fit between client(s) and organization. As these services evolve, the centers develop and attempt to utilize models of trauma treatment. They view the ideal method of treatment as multidisciplinary, eclectic, and inclusionary rather than exclusionary. Treatment modalities and orientation are multiple and arrange from the use of contextualistic theory (Trauma Stress Institute) to ego state therapy (Northeast Center for Trauma Recovery) to recursive anamnesis (Trauma Recovery Institute).

Many of the centers described in this chapter are beginning to utilize "power therapy" methods such as eye movement desensitization reprocessing, traumatic incident reduction, thought field therapy, rational–emotive behavior therapy, and others. The hope of the authors of this volume is that the directors of these centers will commit themselves to investigating the efficacy of these methods through sound, empirically developed research projects. Other centers are looking at the role and conceptualization of traumatic memories and how those memories are processed by the human brain.

No matter the model employed by these centers, it differs greatly from the refugee-treatment-oriented model. None of the centers uses a case management approach to treatment that involves and networks with other agencies (courts, family services, health department, court services, and others), particularly in the treatment of children. It is the recommendation of the authors of this volume that such a model be examined and when appropriate implemented. Finally, these centers recognize the necessity of providing a safe environment for clients to "do the work" of trauma recovery. If that basic sense of safety cannot be provided, then any work done with survivors is in vain. In other words, developing safety-based plans and techniques is the key to good service provision.

4

Centers with Affiliations and Centers in Progress

Not all American centers are run by private individuals or groups of individuals. Some centers, while headed by an individual or a group, are affiliated with institutions or organizations. The institution generally is a university or college, hospital, or insurance company. The following centers are illustrative of this grouping.

CENTER FOR STRESS AND TRAUMA, CLEVELAND, OHIO

The Center for Stress and Trauma was created to help people who experience traumatic stress, a need that was not effectively addressed prior to the center's creation. The center offers specialized, comprehensive services to help victims, their families, and those who work with them. The center was created and is operated by Behavior Management Associates (BMA), a firm specializing in comprehensive programs addressing specific psychological needs of individuals and organizations. BMA offers customized programs designed to maximize effectiveness of helping.

The organization began in 1990 and has expanded from its original conceptualization as a women's resource center. Services offered do not have a specific end point and professionals in the center "do whatever they have to" to treat whomever comes to them. The center accepts pro bono cases to a reasonable degree, based on staff assessment.

Staffing

John P. Wilson, internationally known scholar, researcher, and clinician, is program director of the center. Dr. Joel Gecht and Dr. Robert Kaplan, principals of BMA, are psychologists who specialize in health psychology, corporate health promotion, and stress management. They develop and conduct employee assistance and specialized programs for a variety of corporate settings. Staff of the center include psychiatrists, psychologists, social workers, a secretary, and an administrative assistant. The organization does not utilize lay caregivers or voluntary professionals. The center has developed good working relationships with physicians who are educated about PTSD. The State of Ohio does not permit non-PhDs to provide psychological services; masters-level clinicians must be supervised as well as licensed. The center is very aware of countertransference reactions to working with traumatized individuals. There is an open-door policy for staff to come to the director (Dr. Wilson) or senior staff should they feel fatigued, burned out, or have any types of ongoing problems or concerns.

Services

Services provided by the center include:

1. Evaluation and treatment utilizing specialized assessment and treatment techniques designed to help victims deal with traumatic stress quickly and correctly. Assessment is done at beginning, middle, and end of treatment using structured protocols, projective measures, standardized psychological instruments, and vocational assessments. Dr. Wilson has created a Vietnam Eustress Inventory (VEST), a Traumatic Stress Inventory (for Pearl Harbor survivors), a specialized intake form based on DSM-IV, and other instruments. Assessment includes a clinical and psychosocial history, case conferences, and assessment of comorbid diagnoses and posttraumatic personality change. All staff do assessments using a common approach. Assessment also may involve conversations with extended family members who knew the person both before and after the traumatic event occurred. Some of this assessment material has contributed to the recent book by Wilson and Keane (1997). Treatment options are a judgment call made by the provider and range from short-term crisis intervention and management, brief psychotherapy, and desensitization for phobias to long-term treatment for survivors of rape or child sexual abuse, or for veterans.
2. On-site critical incident stress management for victims, their families, and co-workers in industrial accidents, traumatic work events, criminal and domestic violence, or catastrophe is provided through an on-call team trained to do psychological first aid. The Mitchell model (Everly & Mitchell, 1995) has been adapted as necessary to fit corporations and also to incorporate the center's theory. The model presently used is a modified crisis intervention model with three phases. Phase 1 looks at adaptation, normalizing, and understanding what has happened;

phase 2 helps clients to understand the reactions and responses they are having; and phase 3 examines behaviors that have resulted.

3. Claims and compensation consultation wherein experts assist attorneys and claims representatives settle claims faster, at less expense.

4. Expert witness services to evaluate cases, increasing the probability of proving or disproving claimed emotional damages in personal injury or workers' compensation cases.

Services are given based on an eclectic model in which "no one is pure anything" but all staff are trained in the principles of posttraumatic therapy.

Training

The center offers training programs to legal, medical, and claims professionals. Trainings offered include proving and disproving emotional damages; dealing with victims of catastrophic loss; evaluating and treating severe stress and trauma; and using stress to your advantage. Dr. Wilson recognizes that there is a broader need to implement programs and train staff systematically in ways more targeted to different trauma populations and to develop trauma networks. The center and its staff have developed a myriad of training materials that are given at routine training sessions. Information and brochures are mailed on request. Both trainings and mailings are ways to generate referrals. The center offers continuing education credit for training sessions as well as consultation to a variety of agencies, individuals, and settings. Prevention-oriented seminars at schools and other agencies are also provided.

Theory Base

Dr. Wilson has contributed extensively to the literature of trauma, particularly in areas of assessment, models of trauma transmission, countertransference, and multicultural intervention (e.g., use of the sweat lodge and other Native American rituals in healing). He has noted that psychological trauma and the events that lead to PTSD are not unidimensional or equivalent in their effect. Conceptualization of prevention paradigms, a first step to risk reduction, is difficult. Differing degrees of symptom presentation (in duration, frequency, and severity), combined with the cyclical or episodic presentation as well as potential delayed onset, must be taken into consideration when conceptualizing PTSD. Recognition that PTSD is not unidimensional in nature, has a variety of potential long-term effects, and has variable rates of appearance has led to the conceptualization of complex PTSD as a way to view victims who have experienced prolonged or repeated trauma.

The etiology of PTSD is not well understood, nor are the role of personality moderators, coping resource moderators, and social support moderators.

However, PTSD is an expectable reaction to abnormally stressful life events, a concept that can be taught at all levels of education. If prevention for PTSD is to occur and the theory base of PTSD is to continue to grow, international cooperation to address primary, secondary, and tertiary intervention is essential. Dr. Wilson notes that the International Society for Traumatic Stress Studies (ISTSS) could be the central networking organization to interface internationally to establish comparative epidemiological studies of prevalence rates and comorbidity; to design and study psychotherapy outcome; to conduct clinical trials for medications; to study culturally specific forms of recovery or coping; to develop culturally specific rituals for healing; to develop acute intervention strategies; and to assist in the creation of regional centers for the treatment of refugees and others victimized by natural disasters or those of human origin.

FORENSIC CENTER FOR TRAUMATIC STRESS

Dr. Wilson also founded the Forensic Center for Traumatic Stress (FCTS). Created in 1997, this center provides evaluation, assessment, and consulting services to individual and organizational victims of trauma. This forensic service is dedicated to ensuring the proper application of concepts of traumatic stress and PTSD in civil and criminal actions. FCTS provides a broad range of services to mental health and legal professionals as well as state and federal agencies, corporations, and international organizations.

FCTS promotes the highest scientific standards possible for those involved in litigation of trauma and PTSD. Prominent attorneys and international scholars form the organization's advisory board. The Forensic Center has developed trauma-related symposia for law schools and universities and detailed seminars for attorneys, legal scholars, and mental health professionals. The organization plans to produce a reference book for litigation concerning traumatic stress and publish *The Forensic Journal of Traumatic Stress* in the future.

NATIONAL INSTITUTE FOR THE PREVENTION OF TRAUMATIC STRESS DISORDER, SALT LAKE CITY, UTAH

The National Institute for the Prevention of Post-Traumatic Stress Disorder recognizes that recreational accidents occur every 4 seconds and workplace accidents every 18 seconds in America. Up to 20% of injured workers have a consistent pattern of prolonged injury recovery. Taking a proactive approach to help survivors "accept" altered physical abilities and diminished earning potentials helps to minimize prolonged disability. Emotional wounds often are neglected during the healing process and may lead to complicated, delayed, and problematic physical injury healing. Learning self-help strategies for lessening suffering and chronic pain is one of the most important factors in the overall healing process. When both physical and emotional wounds are attended to simultaneously, survivors become thrivers.

The organization has been in continuous existence since 1981. It serves Salt Lake City, Utah and its surrounding communities (11 metropolitan towns and cities) with a population of 1,152,000. The organization is a private corporation and a private for-profit practice. The treatment goal of the organization is work resumption and other meaningful activity as soon as possible.

Effective psychological (traumatology) ergonomics may effectively prevent long-term disability (Richards, 1990). When disabling injury survivors ruminate about injuries and losses for long periods of time, they become blind to options for wellness. Holding onto impractical expectations about the injury recovery process also can be problematic for all involved.

Wound and Injury Recovery Center of America (WIRC/America) is a subsidiary of the institute (NIP/PTSD). It targets casualty claims insurance providers and workers compensations carriers, businesses that provide insurance coverage for medical/health care services to respective claimants/ patients. Information provided by WIRC/America (injury recovery orientation education) significantly reduces the need for long-term treatment and expensive disability. Education provided through WIRC/America is proactive, wellness focused, participant involved, nonstigmatizing, time-specific, simple, nontechnical, and duplicative. The organization was founded because of inadequate/nonexistent educational information for injury survivors and caregivers about what to expect during the aftermath of work-related accidents and what to do (problem prevention strategies).

Mission

The institute is a private corporation dedicated to wellness after an injury and/or traumatic experience; it is also dedicated to preventing PTSD and reducing the need for expensive long-term treatment. The four objectives of the institute are

1. To help injury and trauma survivors and their loved ones anticipate normal emotional ups and downs and PTSD problems and know how to provide the sensitive, understanding, nurturing support the recoverees need to return to a meaningful, productive lifestyle.
2. To help health care practitioners provide early PTSD symptom relief simultaneous with initial medical treatment for trauma.
3. To help employers understand how they can assist an injured or traumatized employee return to work more quickly and in a positive, productive manner.
4. To educate the insurance industry about the cost-containment benefits of psychological–traumatology ergonomics in order to avoid a far

greater expense in medical and psychological treatments later for diagnosed PTSD.

The specific goal of the institute is to prevent the impact of unresponded-to emotional and psychological upheaval, which often accompanies job-related injury trauma and disability.

The mission of the WIRC/America is to assist individual survivors of injury, accidents, and traumatic upheaval learn how to optimize their recovery potential. To this end, WIRC/America seeks to enable survivors to resume preinjury activities with resiliency ad awareness of how to thrive versus merely survive, thereby enhancing their overall personal functioning, efficiency, and productivity in all spheres of their individual lives. The philosophy of the organization is that healing from physical injury and emotional wounds must be undertaken simultaneously as a combined effort between survivor and personal caregivers.

Staffing

Staff of the WIRC/America includes a clinical traumatologist, an occupational health nurse case manager, a rehabilitation nurse, an industrial medicine physician, consulting psychologists, social workers, physiatrists, psychiatrists, and physical therapists. Staff has masters level or above education, medical or educational certification, and a minimum of 3 years experience in the field.

Theoretical Basis

The trauma model on which the organization is based is an educational ergonomics model that is essentially cognitive–behavioral. Theoretical principles utilized come from a variety of theoreticians and models including casework relationship principles (Biestek), stress response syndromes (Horowitz, 1976), disability management (Fordyce), crisis intervention (Everly & Mitchell, 1997), critical incident stress debriefing (Everly & Mitchell, 1997), SPICE model, and Thriving after Surviving (Richards, 1990). Several factors substantially improve the potential for a more problem-free recovery from injury. They include early assessment of the survivor's coping capacities, adequate emotional support from family and close friends, educational information provided by qualified professionals, facilitation of injury-related thoughts and feelings without reinforcing denial and numbing or minimizing or invalidating the experience, and appropriate pacing of empathetic responses toward the survivor prior to the reintegration into preinjury activities. The primary concepts that permeate the strategy include:

1. Paradigm shifting to a prudent and realistic response toward needs and expectations.

2. Being proactive to prevent reactive consequences; involving survivors in their own healing.
3. Win–win thinking including sensitivity to needs of the survivor and allegiance to the cooperative concept of interdependence.
4. Seeking first to understand, then to be understood, including exchanging crucial information, so that mutual agreements can be reached more easily between all parties invested in the survivor's recovery (Covey, 1989).
5. Synergizing through teamwork in response to mutual expectations in the process of creative cooperation.

The SPICE model of treatment has five key components to provide proactive attention to the well-known needs of a work-injury survivor. The STEPS strategy (see Treatment section) is a catalyst to make the SPICE model more effective as a macromodel. The SPICE model consists of *s*implicity, *p*roximity, *i*mmediacy, *c*entrality, and *e*xpectancy. Another key to healing is planning, whether for acquisition of knowledge for the occurrence of steady and continual progress. Survivors are encouraged to plan on periods of roller coaster emotions and a steady resumption of physical activity as soon as medically permitted.

Prevention

Effective PTSD prevention within an organization must involve a commitment to a well-coordinated education and prevention strategy. Priorities for that program include:

1. Prioritization of the importance of an employee's well-being over completion of productivity and work-related tasks.
2. Commitment of adequate financial resources to training and education of all employees about PTSD.
3. Top-down management education about PTSD prevention ergonomics preceding the occurrence of a worksite accident or disabling injury.
4. Official recognition of all programs or assistance to an injured employee and introduction of a standardized response to *individual* needs.
5. Provision of a qualified employee assistance program with certified personnel to identify the earliest PTSD symptoms and then respond appropriately to them via referral of the employees to qualified traumatologists.
6. Provision for temporary absence of employees with work-related trauma by a "special leave of absence" without a "sick leave" label.
7. Development of a written document that conveys these provisions in a clear, succinct form and is available to all employees and has been developed in conjunction with employee input.

Assessment

The injury adjustment assessment (IAA) focuses attention on the patient's realistic potential for progress throughout stages of medical recovery. Assessment begins with clear, informative directions to allow patients to participate actively in their own healing process. An IAA documents what is most stressful to the patient, identifies the greatest concern, finds out how a survivor perceives the situation, and determines what frustrates the patient. It utilizes the Trauma Recovery SPEED scoring instrument. This assessment is conducted shortly after acute medical care of the patient. It identifies what needs to be known, reassures the patient that she or he will be heard and understood correctly and adequately, and emphasizes "how to" ways to avoid problems and delayed recovery. The IAA is a collaborative tool used between the injury/ accident survivor and all medical and health care providers. The survivor acknowledges the accuracy and acceptance of the assessment and provides copies to those in need of its contents. An IAA is a simple and straightforward format that provides baseline information about multiple variables likely to impact the recovery experience of the survivor.

Key factors ascertained by the IAA include the following:

- How close is the employee to retirement?
- How "accident prone" is the employee?
- Were other workers killed or seriously injured in the traumatic event?
- Could the traumatic experience have been prevented according to the employee?
- How strong is the employee's social support system?
- Has the employee contacted an attorney?
- What is the employee's perception of management's response to the event?
- How secure is the employee about returning to work and keeping her or his job through the recovery experience?
- What does the employee expect from management?
- The Trauma Recovery SPEED scoring instrument.

Assessment occurs promptly, after the individual is medically stable, and uses a standardized format with recorded verbatim comments. This strategy uses (at least) two separate 90-minute assessment interviews. Assessment balances information gathering and information giving. It documents a clinically precise summary of findings as they impact and affect healing. Information about the employee's previous exposure to traumatic events associated with employment, records of military experience, marital status, employment status of spouse, sources of social support, and baseline personality traits of the employee also are included in the assessment protocol.

Treatment

The program identifies and uses specific person-centered strategies to meet the traumatized employee's immediate needs, including:

- Critical incident debriefing
- Organized grief resolution procedures
- A "celebration of life" ceremony in support of survivors
- Death response teams
- Dissection of information
- On-site professionals to respond to individual needs and provide trauma incident reduction (TIR) defusings
- Peer support groups
- Empowerment orientation sessions

These strategies were explained in Covey (1989). STEPS is a pragmatic response influenced by the work of Stephen R. Covey (1988) that corresponds to survivors' primary concerns after temporary or permanent disabling injuries. STEPS provides prompt and specific directions to enable survivors to minimize after injury problems and stop impractical expectations as well as prevent negative consequences; it also is a potent remedy for delayed injury recovery, unforeseen difficulties, and excessive medical bills. The injury recovery STEPS orientation (IRO-STEPS) educational procedures have been used since 1991 to help injury survivors improve recovery as they undergo medical treatment and the healing process. The key elements include:

- *S*timulate positive thinking and initiate proactive directions.
- *T*ackle unrealistic fears through developing clear perspectives and appropriate reassurances.
- *E*ducate about options to identify realistic alternatives and make decisions.
- *P*lan for the future through coordination of medical, health care, and other community resources.
- *S*top impractical expectations; injury recoverees need concrete, specific directions to accept realities of insurance coverage and future capabilities and limitations and/or loss.

IRO-STEPS work is implemented quickly and begins with the end in mind, that is, the visualization of overall functioning coordinated with the emotional supPort of personal caregivers; educational support of professional clinicians, and encouragement and support from other survivors of similar injury or trauma. Self-help incentives and personal determination are prioritized versus "fix me" expectations.

Survivors learn to question common impractical expectations through the strategy. A few of the impractical expectations include:

1. Legal action will remedy delayed injury recovery.
2. Any/all medical and health care clinicians have traumatology expertise.
3. Injury survivors all recover the same way.
4. Optimal recovery is possible without emotional healing

Publications and Research

Dr. Richards has written *Thriving after Surviving* (1990) to help the layperson understand PTSD prevention strategies and promote efficient healing.

The institute commissions research in order to identify successful treatments for PTSD prevention.

Training and Consultation

Corporate management and supervisory personnel are routinely provided instructive education about strategies and procedures. Extensive training materials have been developed. The organization routinely participates in public service educational presentations via all types of media. Through these educational efforts, WIRC/America endeavors to bring about a change in the way accident and injury survivors are treated (responded to vs. reacted to).

THE CAMBRIDGE HOSPITAL VICTIMS OF VIOLENCE PROGRAM, CAMBRIDGE, MASSACHUSETTS

The Cambridge Hospital Victims of Violence (VOV) Program was co-founded by Mary Harvey, PhD (Director) and Judith Herman, MD (Director of Training) in 1984. It was established as a clinical training program of Cambridge hospital's Harvard-affiliated Department of Psychiatry in 1985, and was awarded its first Victims of Crime Act (VOCA) funding in 1986. Since 1986, VOV has developed new and needed services for crime victims and crime victimized communities. Victims include economically disenfranchised women whose lives have been punctuated by violence from exposure to physical and sexual violence in childhood to lives in or on the run from dangerous homes in their present lives.

In 1988, VOV received the American Psychiatric Association's Gold Award for Innovative Hospital and Community Service. VOV then initiated the first publicly funded Community Crisis Response Team (CCRT). The CCRT recognizes that entire communities can be traumatized by violence suffered by community members. VOV serves as a unique clinical resource for victims, a training center for graduate and postgraduate clinical trainees, a consultation and training resource of national and international significance, and is an originator of and participant in various efforts to prevent domestic and community violence. Research conducted by VOV assesses recovery and resiliency in trauma survivors and evaluates the benefits of VOV care through treatment outcome research (VOV Brochure).

Mission Statement

The Victims of Violence Program recognizes the prevalence and psychological harmfulness of violence and crime victimization in American society, the value of community-based social action to prevent violence, and the importance of competence building and empowering care for those who have been harmed. VOV's mission within the hospital and larger community is to develop comprehensive mental health services for crime victims and crime-victimized communities. VOV emphasizes clinical care that facilitates mastery, mobilizes resiliency, and promotes renewed hope and restored self-esteem. Group treatment offers the promise of reduced isolation, opportunities to form new attachments and new avenues to community. Through the CCRT, VOV initiates community interventions that mobilize the healing, health-promoting capacities of affected communities. (VOV Mission Statement)

Clientele

Clients of the program are primarily crime victims, including rape victims, victims of childhood trauma, battered women, men and women who have been exposed to violence, homicide survivors, and mothers of sexually victimized children. Through the CCRT, VOV also serves communities that have been traumatized by violent crime. The program treats secondary victims who are members of households in which someone was murdered as well as families of sexually victimized children and partners of rape victims. VOV clients represent ethnically and racially diverse populations, though predominantly Caucasian, including recent immigrants. It is the economically disenfranchised who need the organization most.

Clients range in age from 15 to 76 years of age and are about 70% female and 30% male. The program serves over 500 clients a year, whether for a one-time crisis appointment or for a more lengthy individual or group therapy. A substantial portion of VOV clients (50–70%) have histories of childhood abuse.

Funding

Support for the clinical and community services of VOV is provided by VOCA funding, program generated income, and support from the Cambridge Public Health Commission. Community-oriented policing and Violence Against Women Act funds from the Commonwealth of Massachusetts as well as various foundation and small grant awards and donations also provide support. This support enables VOV to extend assistance to refugees of political violence and survivors of war-related trauma, for example, and to initiate and participate in communitywide efforts to address and reduce domestic violence in the City of Cambridge. Other non-VOCA funds enable VOV to conduct research on recovery and resiliency in trauma survivors.

Theory Base

VOV services are guided by a feminist understanding of violence in the lives of women and girls and by an ecological view of the interrelationship of individual and community and of the role that community plays in shaping human identity (Harvey, 1996; Harvey & Harvey, 1995; Koss & Harvey, 1991). An ecological view of psychological trauma and trauma recovery (Harvey, 1996) takes for granted the possibility of resilience in the face of harm and wellness in its aftermath. This view is interested in the origins of resilience and the pathways to wellness that individual trauma survivors force and make use of.

Within this theoretical framework, violent and traumatic events are viewed as ecological threats not only to the adaptive capacities of individuals but also to the ability of human communities to foster health and resiliency among affected community members (Harvey, 1996). While violent events can tax and overwhelm community resources, community values, beliefs, resources, and traditions can support victims' resilience in the wake of violence. This perspective reminds everyone that the origins of violence and victimization lie not only in the pathology of the offender but in the quality of community life and community resource afforded to the victim.

Harvey (1996) draws on this perspective and the role of environmental factors as they influence traumatic outcomes and make resilient outcome possible to propose a multidimensional view of trauma impact, recovery, and resiliency. These are expressed across eight interrelated domains of psychological experience. Criteria for each domain can be used to assess the recovery status of individuals, to plan appropriate treatment, and to assess treatment outcome. The criteria for recovery, defined by Harvey (1996), are authority over memory, integration of memory and affect, affect tolerance, symptom mastery, self-esteem, self-cohesion, safe attachment, and meaning.

Event factors are the salient attributes of the traumatic event. They include the frequency, severity, duration, degree of violence (if any); details that are assigned significance by the survivor; what the victim considers to be the most traumatizing part of the experience; and others.

Environmental factors include the ecological context within which the event(s) was experienced (home, school, work, neighborhood), the support system that is or is not available to the victim, the ability of the support system to assist adaptive coping, prevailing community attitudes and values about trauma, cultural constructs related to race and gender, political and economic factors relating to access to care, and services available. There are goals of treatment that include:

1. Developing authority over the remembering process to recall and make use of personal history
2. Integration of memory and affect, joining remembrance of the past with feelings from the past and feelings bout the past
3. Affect tolerance so that feelings no longer overwhelm or threaten to overwhelm the survivor
4. Mastery of symptoms to make them more manageable or to anticipate or even avoid them by use of healthful routines

5. Repair and mastery of self-esteem and self-cohesion with mastery of self-injurious behaviors and impulses through self-exploration of guilt, shame, and self-blame
6. Safe attachment with safe and stable connectedness to others replacing isolation and detachment
7. Assignment of new meaning to the trauma and to the self as trauma survivor (Harvey, 1996)

Internal and external individual resources and ecological circumstances accompanying traumatic exposure and recovery impact may or may not lead to impact from a traumatic event. Resiliency is evident when one or more domains are relatively unaffected by the trauma and when one domain mobilizes to lead to repair in another. These domains describe a multifaceted definition of the outcome of psychological trauma that offers a set of benchmarks against which individual recovery from trauma can be assessed.

Herman (1991b) describes the process of recovery from trauma as unfolding in three broad stages. Early recovery issues center around securing safety and stabilizing symptoms. The work of trauma recovery begins only after safety is established. The second stage of recovery therefore involves the in-depth exploration of the individual's traumatic past. The final stage of recovery focuses on expanding and revitalizing the relational world of the survivor (Leibowitz, Harvey, & Herman, 1993).

Staffing

The staff of the VOV program is multidisciplinary. The staff is primarily female from psychiatry, psychology, social work, and nursing. Because the setting is a training facility and part of Harvard Medical School, staff need to be licensed mental health professionals. The program's Community Crisis Response Team has 58 members, professionals, and paraprofessionals including street workers and gang violence workers as well as Harvard psychologists and psychiatrists. It is administered by CCRT coordinator and her two community liaison staff. The 58 CCRT volunteer members come from all sectors of the community.

The clinical staff of VOV pattern is well balanced and there is at least one core staff member for each trainee. At the time of the interview, VOV had 11 full- and part-time staff members and about 8 trainees. The VOV program has used honors undergraduates to manage intake activities. They also have had volunteers to help with office tasks and research.

Each week clinical trainees of VOV participate in a clinical team meeting, trauma seminar, crisis seminar, and theory–practice integration seminar and receive 2 hours of individual case supervision and 1 hour of group supervision. Staff have a weekly staff meeting and staff seminar as well as periodic retreats. Program director Mary Harvey, PhD, evaluates staff performance.

Staff members work well together and collaboratively have developed group models.

Assessment

Staff members complete an initial assessment that is fairly comprehensive. They review all cases at the end of every year and assess progress in treatment. Urgent assessments can be done during weekly team meetings or at a patient risk meeting. Time-limited groups have pre- and postgroup assessments. Assessment utilizes a PTSD measure, a behavioral inventory, a depression inventory, the Dissociative Experiences Scale (DES), and the Multidimensional Trauma Recovery and Resiliency Interview Likert scale. Assessments are done by clinical staff and trainees; staff takes responsibility for the assessment. This assessment takes 90 minutes. Information then is brought to a clinical team meeting where an initial disposition is made. The disposition may include assignment of a therapist, assignment to a group, and/or a request for a medication evaluation.

Clinical Services

Clinical services of the VOV include crisis response (emergency room liaison, crisis assessment, crisis counseling) to acutely traumatized crime victims, longer-term clinical care (psychological assessment, treatment planning, psychotherapy) for adult survivors of physical and sexual violence, and a wide array of groups. VOV extends clinical and support services to witnesses, family members, and others affected by crime victimization.

Treatment goals are to treat patients respectfully and with dignity and to engage with patients in a treatment-planning process that recognizes resiliency and viability of their resources outside of therapy. The program offers patients interventions that make sense according to the safe setting with safe boundaries. Staff see psychotherapy as an instrument to help patients mobilize the capacity to recover.

Short-term treatment includes some cognitive–behavioral work. Crisis work includes 12 sessions within a year's time. At times, treatment may be episodic if an individual cannot participate in regular, ongoing therapy. Individual therapy is organized primarily around the stages of recovery model. Work changes over time, may become more relational in orientation, and may involve other family members.

Community initiatives of the VOV include the multiagency CCRT and leadership of or participation in numerous city- and statewide efforts to reduce and respond to sexual and domestic violence against women. CCRT services include consultation to assist local resources in their own crisis response planning, traumatic stress debriefings for affected community groups, and training. The CCRT's role in a community crisis is to help the client community mobilize its own response to trauma. CCRT members therefore function primarily in a consulting role. The CCRT model of intervention is the community empowerment model. The staff wait to be called and maintains confidentiality about that call. The staff do not deal with the media and do not publicize interactions with communities in distress. They try to listen to what the community wants and also ask questions. Any debriefing done tends to be educational.

Training

Any trainee participating in the clinical work of the VOV program has dyadic support and receives crisis training and supervision of individual and group psychotherapy. VOV training also occurs at the site of service delivery. Trainees observe staff doing the work and staff members participate with trainees. Training emphasizes a theoretical frame as well as technical training that focuses on how to use the theoretical frame in clinical practice. There are usually about eight training spots each year. Of the places, two are reserved for social work interns; at least three for psychology interns or externs, and the remaining two or three for psychology postdoctorates and psychiatry residents.

The program also provides specialty training in interpersonal violence, intrafamilial and domestic violence, sexual abuse, battery, and how to work with adult survivors of childhood trauma. They participate yearly at a conference at Harvard Medical School and have developed training materials and curricula.

VOV staff offers consultation to area clinicians, clinics, and treatment centers, as well as grassroots providers and researchers. Staff members who are assigned to the consultation service receive a request and bring it to the staff. The program is a member of the Domestic Violence Free Zone Task Force of Cambridge. Some staff members do forensic work.

Research

The vast majority of current measures for assessment of traumatic exposure and its impact generally fail to assess complex, multidimensional response to traumatic exposure. They also do not attend to expressions of trauma recovery and resiliency. Over the past 5 years, a research group within VOV has been working to translate their ecological perspective (with its emphasis on resiliency and recovery) into assessment instruments for use in both clinical and community research. VOV is interested in learning how awareness of individuals' strengths and how articulation of clear recovery goals inform treatment planning, help shape more effective clinical interventions, and provide groundwork to undertake theoretically informed treatment outcome research. VOV is also interested in discovering nonclinical sources of resilience and the varied pathways that survivors may travel on their road to recovery.

TRAUMA RECOVERY INSTITUTE AND RESOURCE CENTER, SAN FRANCISCO, CALIFORNIA

Trauma Recovery Institute and Resource Center (TRIARC) is a community-based nonprofit organization designed to assist trauma survivors achieve optimal recovery, reduce suffering, reduce utilization of the health care system, and thereby reduce costs. Executive director Kate Garay, RN, MS, defines "trauma" as physical injury significant enough to require immediate attention from a specialized surgical team; therefore the organization is designed to work with survivors who have been physically injured through traumatic events. Half of those who survive traumatic injury develop severe psychological and/or social difficulties unless they are given effective therapy. Their injuries result in lost time at work and cost the economy between $75 and 100 billion yearly. Injury also is the leading cause of death for individuals up to 44 years of age in the United States.

In one year, over 2.5 million Americans are hospitalized due to traumatic injuries from automobile accidents, fires, falls, physical assaults, and assaults with weapons. Their traumas also impact their families, communities, and the professionals who treat them. The legacy of these injuries often is a life of chronic pain, depression, physical disability, financial difficulty, and family stress. As a societal problem, traumatic injury is largely unrecognized by the public. However, aggressive attention to secondary prevention in trauma centers will reduce societal costs and reduce human misery.

Mission

TRIARC is dedicated to assisting trauma survivors achieve optimal physical, mental, and emotional healing and to recreate the lifestyle of their choice. TRIARC focuses on policy and program innovations in trauma care delivery systems and the development and promotion of prototype trauma centers that emphasize secondary prevention as an integrative approach to care along the continuum from resuscitation to return to the community.

Clientele

The average trauma patient in the hospital is between 15 and 35 years old and is likely to have a record of multiple injuries. This is a disease of urban youth. TRIARC serves the San Francisco Bay, CA area.

Services

TRIARC researches trauma issues, disseminates information, builds collaboration, and inspires innovation when advocating program and policy change. In 1996, TRIARC sponsored focus groups of former trauma patients from San Francisco General Hospital and their families. These individuals reviewed the process of recovery and the proceedings were audiotaped and transcribed. Key trauma staff and administrators attended the focus groups behind a two-way mirror. The results of the groups were disseminated within the hospital.

TRIARC sponsored an invitational conference for key trauma-related staff and administrators at San Francisco General Hospital in 1996. The objectives of the conference were to develop collaboration between disciplines involved in trauma care delivery, to define key elements of an integrated delivery system, and to focus on a preventive approach for recovery. This new model of care will be implemented once funding (through grants) is obtained.

TRIARC has produced and published a resource directory for survivors of traumatic injury, their caregivers and professional care providers. The directory lists counseling services, government agencies, and contacts for housing and food, rehabilitation centers, job training, and educational services. It also contains support groups, advocacy contacts, and others and is available as "Finding Empowerment after Trauma" Resource Directory for $12.00.

TRIARC holds 1-day courses at the University of California. In January 1998, the course "Recovery from Traumatic Injury—A Psychosocial Perspective" was held and participants learned to describe a three-risk factor model that predicts poor psychosocial recovery from traumatic injury, to perform a self-assessment for secondary traumatization, to assess patients for common symptoms of PTSD, to list self-care measures for trauma survivors and phases of recovery from traumatic injuries, and to assess patients for depression.

THE CENTER FOR THE STUDY OF GENOCIDE, VIOLENCE AND TRAUMA, NEW HAVEN, CONNECTICUT

There is a growing international awareness of the political and personal effects of violence. The field of traumatology and research provides a key to analyze and categorize these events in the present and from the past. The concept of trauma has disrupted and challenged fundamental ideas of what constitutes pathology. To study trauma is to study both the external events as well as the internal experiences of "woundedness" or "wounding" in individuals and groups. The study of trauma is a new tool to explain and treat violence in the fields of historical and psychotherapeutic inquiry.

Interest in activities that led to the development of the concept of the Center began in the late 1970s with the Holocaust Survivor Film Project. This was probably the first video testimony project. The project started a video archive from 30 centers around the world that had collected survivors' stories. These 4000 testimonies need to be examined in detail to see what they say socially, historically, and in any other manner so that intervention strategies can be developed. In 1987, the project became part of Yale University.

The center proposes an interdisciplinary effort to address the problem of trauma and to develop preventive strategies. No one discipline can attempt either to comprehend or respond to trauma in isolation. Traumatic events, in the past, have evaded knowing, witnessing, and assimilation; research has pointed backward to what occurred in the past but has never worked consistently on the present (or the future). Thus the center would provide a means for collaboration among individual specialists from different disciplines and institutions.

Major goals of the center are to provide support and continuity for collaboration; to allow for constant expansion of existing understanding; and to rediscover, rejuvenate, reappropriate, and refine knowledge both in historical record and the present. The center would offer consultation services and encourage exploration of and response to trauma among members of the community as well (welfare workers, urban planners, policymakers, legal professionals, school professionals, child care providers, correctional officers, and others). It would include study of the sociological aspects of trauma and examine how to meet trauma needs by historical thinking.

The center is unique in its scope and its use of an integrated interdisciplinary approach. It could become a national and international resource for humanitarian activist organizations such as Amnesty International, the Red Cross, Doctors Without Borders, and others. The center would offer consultation for the purpose of comprehensive analysis of newly emerging as well as refractory crisis situations. It intends to recommend policy decisions for innovative prevention, early intervention, and "treatment" of these situations. It will focus on the least understood and most urgent of issues in trauma research: the recognition of and intervention in contemporaneous traumatic events with particular attention (internationally) to genocide and (domestically) to urban violence.

Mission

The mission of the center is to promote and develop an integrated approach to study and research and strategies to respond to trauma, genocide, and violence and to prevent and treat the effects of trauma, genocide, and violence on humans. It also aims to do outreach, curricular development, advocacy, and scholarship with practitioners, scholars, and investigators.

Funding

Finding funding for the organization has been problematic. Originally, avenues for fund-raising through the Development Office of Yale University were explored. A private donor gave a grant as seed money, which funded some of the activities of the center. The center has had many letters of support from individuals (Elie Wiesel, Kai Erickson, Robert Lifton), organizations (the Holocaust Memorial Museum, Yale Law School, Yale School of Medicine), and others. Approximately $400,400 is needed for the initial start-up costs and the proposed annual budget is $750,000. In 1997, the International Trauma Center (ITC) was formed with an independent board of directors to assist in its further development and fund-raising.

Staffing

At the present time, the staff consists of Dr. Dori Laub, Director, and a part-time research assistant. The ITC organization has a board of directors and advisory board and there is a "Friends of the Center" organization. Ideally, the center would be run by a core steering committee from various disciplines as well as members of veterans organizations and other treatment facilities.

Clientele

The proposed clientele of the center include survivors of political persecution, inner-city violence, and perhaps child abuse. Child survivors and children and descendants of survivors of various traumatic events, as well as dependents of perpetrators also will be included to highlight the intergenerational transmission of the traumatic experience.

Theory Base

The art of trauma is limited not only to traditional literature, music, and sculpture; it also should include "imaginative acts" that occur spontaneously within the process of survival itself as the survivor attempts to "know" the traumatic events that confront that person. Videotaped oral testimony also is a form of art. Laub and Auerhahn (1993) have written on "Knowing and Not Knowing Massive Psychic Trauma: Forms of Traumatic Memory." In this article they propose a continuum of forms of knowing for survivors including not knowing, fugue states, fragments, transference phenomena, overpowering narratives, life themes, witnessed narratives, and metaphors. Remembering of fragments, for example, involves retention of parts of a lived experience in a decontextualized, isolated, meaningless way. Transference phenomena grafts isolated memory fragments of the past onto current relationships and life situations, thereby "coloring" those relationships and situations. At the witnessed narrative level, knowing takes on the form of a true memory while retaining the perspective of the observing ego. In other words, the person remembers and knows that he or she remembers. The variety of levels of remembering and preserving horror of traumatic events lead to targets of information gathering, research, and intervention in a trauma center. As the authors write, "Understanding the level of traumatic memory is crucial in knowing where therapeutic intervention must focus" (p. 300).

Services Proposed

The center has proposed numerous activities:

1. The organization and delivery of interdisciplinary seminars and courses on trauma-related topics
2. Interdisciplinary and interinstitutional research activities including coordination of efforts and assistance in grant writing
3. Intramural research using existing databases
4. The creation of further archival stories of testimonial collection from different areas of trauma including taping, the collection of written and audiotaped testimonies from other researchers' collections, oral history projects, and social media projects using video testimony and/ or oral histories for intervention in current crises. Testimonies from Bosnia and homeless persons or victims of inner-city violence might be included.
5. The creation of a library of trauma books and articles as a database to link with other trauma networks, including artistic and clinically oriented films and videos
6. A fellowship program for junior and accomplished scholars in research work from conceptualization and planning of interdisciplinary activities to personal research pursuits
7. Support and supervision for doctoral candidates in their dissertation work
8. Sponsorship of an annual international conference as well as ongoing study groups, seminars, and colloquia
9. Training groups on social, therapeutic, and legal intervention in ongoing crises and the treatment of secondary and vicarious PTSD
10. Publication of a newsletter that includes information about ongoing research and conferences

Among the disciplines that would work together would be history, philosophy, law, literature, psychiatry, psychology, neurobiology, sociology, communications, filmmaking, and others.

Previously Sponsored Activities

The center has applied for funding for several projects. Among them are a video testimony project in Israel for chronically hospitalized (up to 45 years) Holocaust survivors diagnosed as schizophrenic and the Intergenerational Testimony Project of fathers and sons including World War II victims living in the United States and in Germany as well as perpetrators or bystanders living in

Germany. Another study to be funded is the study of intergenerational transmission of trauma in children of Holocaust survivors in collaboration with Jewish Family Services. The Bosnian Refugee Trauma Program offered mental health services for 50 refugees and their families and conducted research in the years 1993–1995.

The center held a retreat for 30 trauma professionals in July 1995, entitled "Coming Home from Trauma: Transmission to the Next Generation, Muteness and the Search for a Voice." The retreat was in anticipation of the establishment of the International Trauma Center and was designed to discover directions for concerted efforts, generate ideas, and integrate ideas into a plan of action. One aim of the retreat was to produce a common language to form research hypotheses for interdisciplinary studies. Work groups in the United States and Europe prepared collaborative study proposals from the work done at this retreat and at a Bad Teinach, Germany, opening conference in November 1995. The International Study Group for Trauma, Violence, and Genocide attained legal status in Germany in April, 1996.

Training

One of the major objectives of the center is to serve as a training resource, particularly in areas of testimony and the application of testimony. The center already has offered some trainings in taking testimony and Dr. Laub has taught a course at Yale Law School.

SUMMARY

Obtaining funding is a major problem for trauma centers. When a center has an affiliation with a larger group, be that group a university, business venture, insurance company, or private corporation, funding is less of a problem. At times, affiliating means limited services to more specific populations (e.g., affiliation with WRIC/America leads to specialization in service provision to victims of injury and accidents). In other instances, affiliated centers have a mandate to build theory and develop new models of service provision and intervention strategies. This is particularly true of the Victims of Violence program.

And what of centers in progress or centers that are in the conceptualization stage? Since the initial conceptualization of this volume, Germain, Inc. has been created. It will be a residential trauma center for children over age 12, located in rural Virginia about 50 miles west of Washington D.C. This center, and others in formation, are seeking to embody many of the principles espoused in the final chapters of this volume. They seek to find innovative ways to help trauma survivors and are building interdisciplinary teams to achieve those goals. Jan Philip Reemtsma, through his Institute for Social Research, is

seeking to create a network of trauma centers primarily in Europe. An explora-
tory meeting of trauma experts and center directors was held in Hamburg,
Germany in December 1998. At that meeting, a new organization was founded.
It is through the efforts of groups and individuals that the work of trauma
prevention, education, treatment, and training will go forward.

5

Private and Not-for-Profit Centers around the World

The United States is not the only location for privately owned and operated trauma centers. There are centers located in other parts of the world, as well. This chapter describes the trauma centers found in other countries.

TRAUMATYS: CENTRE FOR TREATMENT AND RESEARCH OF PTSD, MONTREAL, CANADA

Traumatys is a private clinic and consulting firm with expertise in preventing, detecting, diagnosing, and treating psychological trauma related to work accidents, including on-site crisis intervention, as well as to physical assault and car accidents. Traumatys establishes and maintains administrative and clinical liaison with employees and insurance/compensation agencies.

Among the services offered to either individuals or organizations are the following:

- Assistance to develop organizational policies aimed at managing crises and their consequences
- Information to managers about trauma through lectures and pamphlets
- Tailored decisional process manual for crisis situations
- Diagnostic services leading to treatment and prognosis and employees with PTSD
- Ongoing telephone assistance
- Emergency intervention during crisis situations ("debriefing")
- Specialized individual or group psychotherapy that is short or longer term
- Complementing with psychotropic medication prescribed by an affiliated psychiatrist

103

- Personnel selection for high-risk jobs
- Training agency personnel who manage crisis situations
- An available team of specialists for major catastrophes

Dr. Gaston began her intense study of PTSD during her internship in San Francisco, California, with Horowitz, Marmar, and Weiss. After completing this internship, she founded her clinic in 1990 and began the trauma training in 1991. Traumatys has expertise that allows for a solid prognosis of the length of leave of absence an employee with PTSD will need, the type of specialized treatment needed, and the costs associated with treatment and salary reimbursement.

Mission

Traumatys offers to individuals and organizations a clinical expertise specialized in managing the aftermaths of work-related traumatic events.

Staff

Clinicians who work with Dr. Gaston in actuality are consultants with their own offices. The government sets a $65 fee for services; clinicians pay $15 per session to the organization and either earn the $50 or use it toward payment of training. Fifty-two consultants work part time 2–10 hours a week as clinicians. Training lasts 24 months. Generally they are all psychologists. Dr. Gaston spends most of her time doing training and supervision.

Clientele

Many clients have treatment paid by Workmen's Compensation; others, by the Quebec government after being victimized by criminal acts or experiencing car accidents. These clients can receive therapy twice a week for extended periods of time. Approximately 150 clients/year receive treatment. Referrals are made from physicians, victim witness organizations, and agencies. Seventy to eighty percent of the clientele treated experience resolution of PTSD at the end of the process; some clients may have specific avoidances and a few residual symptoms.

Theory Base

The model of treatment used by Gaston is a comprehensive dynamic approach that is brief in orientation and is based primarily on the work of Horowitz (1986), with the additions of cognitive–behavioral techniques along with hypnosis and eye movement desensitization reprocessing (EMDR). The approach focuses on trauma, associated conflicts, and the resolution of those conflicts. The duration of treatment depends on the severity of the trauma, the chronicity of the trauma, the client's ego structure, and the client's motivation for therapy. When intrusion and denial phases are out of the control of the trauma victim, when the oscillation between reexperiencing and avoidance is involuntary, when defense mechanisms and coping strategies interfere with the processing of the traumatic information, then a posttraumatic stress reaction (PTSR)/disorder is more likely to occur. Losses attached to the traumatic event also can maintain symptoms of PTSR/PTSD.

Dynamic psychotherapy aims at restoring the client's premorbid functioning and eliminating symptoms of PTSD. Gaston (1995) wrote that the goals "... are limited to ideational and emotional working-through of the stress response syndrome to a point of relative mastery ..." (p. 170). The therapist helps the client accept his or her traumatized self by viewing psychological distress as noninfantile; helps the client regain or develop a realistic sense of mastery over external and internal worlds, helps the client make his or her psychological structure accommodate the new information the trauma brought or at least assimilate some degree of information into the self, and assists the client to learn to view traumatic events as opportunities for growth.

Dynamic therapy requires an active stance by the therapist while giving control to the trauma survivor, within limits. The therapist guides the survivor into acknowledging the traumatized self and revising the traumatic event. The therapist also helps the survivor repair damaged self-esteem. The work of therapy is done in tolerable dosages, with nonjudgmental acceptance, expert understanding, and involvement.

Assessment

Traumatys diagnoses the presence of PTSD using a multidimensional approach with a structured interview and a battery of specialized psychological questionnaires. This assessment includes a variety of instruments including the Millon Clinical Multiaxial Inventory (MCMI-2), Structured Clinical Interview (SCID), Mississippi Trauma Scale, the Impact of Event Scale, the Minnesota Multiphasic Personality Inventory (MMPI), the Trauma Constellation Scale, and others. Dr. Gaston has conducted research utilizing the MMPI with civilians and has developed two MMPI scales for assessing acute and chronic PTSD. Traumatys has evaluated the presence/absence of PTSD in refugees.

Workplace Interventions

Traumatys intervenes in organizations in order to implement a standardized procedure at the time of a crisis situation (accident or violent event). The intervention strategy is adapted to the needs of the individual and/or organization. Traumatys trains managers to implement the crisis situation decisional process with on-site presentations and a clear, precise manual. Traumatys then intervenes on site and determines parameters of treatment depending on the severity of PTSD symptoms.

Services

Employees who have experienced a minor trauma keep working during their short-term psychotherapy. Employees who have experienced a major trauma temporarily stop working to prevent deterioration of their condition, especially if they work in high-risk jobs. Treatment is phase-oriented. The first phase establishes the treatment alliance, gathers information, completes the history, encourages seeking of emotional support, reduces anxiety baselines, and addresses avoidance mechanisms. The second phase involves a detailed inner and outer world revision of the event, addresses associated defense mechanisms and conflicts, and eliminates PTSD symptomatology as the traumatized self is accepted and as the traumatic information is integrated. The third and final phase encourages the survivor to practice new defensive, cognitive, and behavioral patterns until they become automatic. The duration of the therapy process varies from 3 months to 2 years, depending on motivation for change, severity of symptomatology, and premorbid ego functioning. The average length of treatment is 9 months.

Treatment utilizes a variety of techniques and interventions ranging from cognitive therapy, behavioral therapy, and existential therapy. Dr. Gaston believes that debriefing works in reducing acute stress, particularly when combining educational, experiential, and emotional components. However, it is not effective as a treatment for PTSD.

Ninety to ninety-five percent of clients have stopped working and many need medications. Dr. Gaston uses a psychiatrist and general practitioners to prescribe medications.

Training

Traumatys offers advanced training in PTSD. Among the topics covered in this training are diagnosis, epidemiology, etiology/risk factors, sequelae, treatment, and other issues including vicarious traumatization, transference, and countertransference. The complete 2-year training includes theoretical seminars and clinical supervision for at least 1 year and then biweekly theoretical seminars and supervision for the second year. Dr. Gaston has developed a formula for training that allows trainees to pay for their $8,000 training fee by giving their time not their money. Trainees pay by the number of hours they work. Generally, a group of 12 clinicians participates in the training at any one time. Ninety-five percent of them have had between 5 and 10 years experience.

ERGOS, GmbH: A PRIVATE INSTITUTE
FOR THE TRANSFORMATION AND INTEGRATION
OF THE CONSEQUENCES OF SHOCK AND TRAUMA, GmbH,
MUNICH, GERMANY

Tania Küchler and Amelia Küchler-Sanktjohanser are codirectors of this urban clinic that serves victims of trauma through psychological intervention. ERGOS, a private practice, is based on the trauma model of Dr. Peter Levine (Levine, 1997), somatic experiencing, and offers psychotherapy and system intervention. The institute gets referrals from a variety of sources and offers acute intervention during an incident, early postintervention, late postintervention, and very late intervention to World War II survivors. The institute also does crisis intervention and offers training to professionals.

Theoretical Orientation

Somatic experiencing (SE) is a body-psychotherapeutic method of healing, transformation and integration developed from the work of Dr. Levine in collaboration with Dr. Angwyn St. John. The chronic stress symptoms of physical and psychological trauma manifest themselves in the body and psyche in many complex ways. SE recognizes that the symptoms are individual responses of the nervous system that lead to psychological somatic illness, depression, and other systems for years after an event occurred. SE is a method to interpret these mechanisms; it sets free the energy connected with the symptoms so that energy can be used in healing. This process activates the healing vortex. The method is based on differing, varying psychotherapeutic changes, neurophysiological perceptions, as well as observations of comparable reactions of humans and animals under stressful circumstances.

The goal of SE is to release the consequences of traumas and symptoms by steps so that the person learns to deal with stress without attempting to relive the trauma. The method activates sources of strength as well as previous individual resources in order to integrate the experience.

Training

The directors of the clinic have developed an extensive series of trainings for professionals at a variety of levels. Initial, beginning level seminars last 3–4 days. Somatic experiencing courses are 2 days long and are designed for psychology professionals, doctors, and physiotherapists. Some seminars are given in English. Intermediate seminars are longer and look at differential work with different traumas, principles of "relative balance," and issues of supervision. "Skills and drills" sessions and trauma work for body workers also are part of the curriculum.

INSTITÜT FÜR TRAUMAPÄDAGOGIK UND THERAPIE, BERLIN, GERMANY

The institute was originally founded in 1990 when workshops for group home counselors and the needs of the populace revealed that there was no specific PTSD service for German clients in the city of Berlin. The institute has been at its present location since 1995. The organization serves as an umbrella for self-employed colleagues who offer trauma-related services to children, adolescents, and adults who have experienced a recent trauma, who are suffering from PTSD and related symptoms, or who are families of primary victims. Most Germans are underserved because they are not aware that help is available.

A good fourth of traumatized individuals (in the catchment area of the institute) develop a full-standing picture of a posttraumatic stress disorder. Decisions about the form and course of treatment are made in partnership between patient and caregiver. The patterns of posttraumatic reactions are as different as fingerprints. Traumatized individuals believe that their reactions and they themselves are no longer totally normal.

The institute is under the leadership of Oliver Schubbe and Michael Borbonus. Among the self-employed practitioners working under the umbrella of the institute are three male psychologists, three female psychologists, one female social worker, one female pedagogue, male pedagogue, and a female psychologist intern. Supervision is provided by two supervisors from outside the institute, but Mr. Schubbe, as clinical director, maintains quality control.

The theoretical model for treatment in the institute is a cognitive–behavioral model, accompanied by the techniques of EMDR, systemic work, and energy work. Staff do counseling, psychotherapy, advocacy, system intervention, and political action. Systemic work is based on Virginia Satir's theories. The primary treatment goal of therapy is the resolution of trauma. The institute also has sponsored the first website pages on trauma in Europe (http://www.is.in.berlin.de/~oli). Mr. Schubbe recognizes the existence of repressed memories, but these memories do not need to be questioned for the purpose of therapy as is necessary in legal procedures.

Assessments at the institute examine client history and problem history and include a genogram, the Impact of Event Scale (IES), the Dissociative Experiences Scale (DES), hand-dominance test, and others as needed. Assessment takes between two and five sessions, parallel to treatment. Treatment options include EMDR, pain treatment, client-centered treatment, systemic intervention with group homes and families, education, and supervision. Long-term treatment rarely is needed. Staff does crisis intervention immediately after a trauma but does not do debriefing.

Clientele

The individual clientele of the institute are 70% male and 80% adult. In workshops, clients are 70% female. Ninety percent of clients are German. Workshop clients/trainees constitute 20% of the clientele; 80% are in individual therapy. About 20% of clients receive government subsidies for therapy.

Theoretical Base

The patient has to take part in the decision-making process as to what type of therapy to use. It is important for patients to find their own strength and to take charge of their lives again. An important part of treatment is to give clients the chance to bring overwhelming emotional experiences and intrusive memories under control through what is called "Bifokal Traumatherapy," which looks at the here and now as well as the traumatic event(s). When words are not able to describe the experiences, then symbolic forms can be used; among them are metaphors, pictures, rituals, games, and others. Art is a form of expression of traumatic experiences. As the client goes deeper into the intrusive memories, it also is important to identify the themes that come through. Also, the client should not remain in a dissociated state or unsafe situation after the session; therefore it is important for the client to have a safe place and to use the light stream method. Bifokale Traumatherapy brings the intrusive memories into focus and to the attention of the client. One process is through a biographical anamnesis that takes an in-depth look at the history of the client's current problem. Functioning, social support, dissociative symptoms, and others are examined. Development of recognition of secondary symptoms and how to deal with those symptoms also is part of the treatment. The major phase, though, is the working through of the traumatic experiences.

Training

The institute offers various classes to professionals and laypersons about trauma therapy. Staff offers radio interviews and lectures. Information about PTSD and possible help (e.g., the institute's services) is given out by police personnel to each crime victim and victim of an auto accident. Institute staff do preventive work with group homes for children and through public education.

TRAUMA CENTERS, MARI-EL REPUBLIC, RUSSIA

Since 1993, Dr. David Niles, former director of the Trauma Recovery and Counseling Center of Alexandria, Virginia, a private trauma clinic, has assisted in the opening of numerous (over seven) trauma centers throughout the various Russian republics. Under the auspices of the Russian Surgeon General and the Medical Academy of Sciences, these centers provide services to traumatic stress reaction sufferers (clinical and nonclinical); substance abusers (e.g., alcohol), and a wide variety of survivors of family violence, sexual assault, and other crimes. Intervention is based on a holistic framework and recognizes the multidimensional levels of traumatic stress reactions.

Trauma centers in Russia are founded on a developmental, multidimensional, holistic model (i.e., biopsychosocial–spiritual). This model is in contrast to the nonholistic underpinning of interventions in America. Western therapeutic concepts incorporated into the model are reframed by the Russians into their own cultural contexts.

The uniqueness of the Russian Trauma Center is the integration of trauma counseling, Survivors Anonymous (SA) 12-step recovery programs; Alcoholics Anonymous (AA), traumatic incident debriefings, peer counseling, and Transcendental Meditation™. This integrative program provides a framework for centers dealing with family violence and battered wives as well.

Dr. Niles has helped to create the Russian National Psychotherapy Association (NRPA) to establish training, education, licensure, and certification standards for mental health professionals. Dr. Niles is director of the Program for Trauma Center Development and is also professor of psychology, Moscow Open Social University Branch in Mari-El Republic. Additionally he is an adjunct faculty member of the George Washington University, Washington, DC.

Russia's Traumatic Stress and Substance Abuse Crisis

Russia faces a crisis with traumatic stress reactions and alcoholism. It is the number one nation in the world for alcohol consumption and is the only industrialized nation with a decreasing life span. The average life span for a Russian man is 57; for a woman, 59.

Exacerbating the Russian situation is the relative nonexistence of trained professionals and paraprofessionals who are competent to deal with traumatic stress problems, such as family violence and sexual assault.. There is an urgent need for program development in trauma psychology as well as training and education using a human resource development focus within the republics of Russia. This is especially true in the large portion of unemployed adult learners who could be retrained and educated.

Traumatology training, education, and development is an integral part of the human resource development effort to establish comprehensive trauma centers in Russia. Training for professionals and paraprofessionals is designed to help victims of traumatic violence and substance abuse. The training is expected to be used immediately by the learners on the job as they work with victims of traumatic violence.

Education programs leading to academic degrees focusing on trauma psychology intervention now are being established at various universities. For example, the George Washington University is pursuing a human resource development masters degree program at the Russian Academy of Medical Science. This program trains and educates medical personnel in the field of trauma psychotherapy. Developmental programs designed to gain public awareness of traumatic stress and alcoholism also are being offered to businesses, television viewers, and other agencies such as police and fire departments.

From the human resource development perspective, programs are designed to provide for the mental health of staff members without direct financial return to the center. The focus of the programs is to help workers deal with stress associated with working in the traumatology field (i.e., compassion fatigue, vicarious traumatization, pseudogenerative burnout).

Each center meets the cultural needs of the republic in which it is located. Russia is an extremely diverse, multicultural nation. For example, Mari-El is a very small republic with a population of about 1 million. Half the republic speaks Russian; the other, Mari. Programs are community-based and designed to consider the unique cultural diversity of their populations.

The Trauma Critical Stage Intervention Model

The Russian trauma centers/clinics are built on the foundation of the trauma critical stage intervention model (TCSIM). This holistic progressive–curvilinear–regressive (PROCURE), multidimensional model was developed by Dr. Niles in the early 1900s. It is dynamic, cybernetic, and holistic and has broad applications for individuals, couples, families, and organizations. As a cybernetic model, it provides constant feedback analysis and evaluation at each stage of trauma center development (see Figure 5.1 for model). As a developmental model, it incorporates human resource development concepts as they relate to training, education, and development. TCSIM begins with a linear concept of trauma and stages of integration, disintegration, and reintegration. Each stage is expanded from a simple to complex analysis.

Integration is examined from a holistic (biopsychosocial–spiritual) conceptualization of human life span personality development. From a mental health perspective, this holistic, synergistic process leads to ever higher levels of competency-based skills in dealing with life. The process results from a healthy unification of body, mind, and spirit.

Disintegration occurs through traumatic violence. From this perspective, a more complex analysis emerges relating to personality disintegration at the time of acute or chronic trauma. At this time, the personality has limited possibilities of action and the individual can experience fight, flight, or freeze. Psychological reactions, on a nonclinical to clinical continuum, associated with physical reactions are deny–dissociation (freeze), anger–rage (fight), or bargain–beg (flight). In the moment of vulnerable disintegration, with limited possibilities for action, memory is encoded and stored for future reference and is related to behavior occurring at the time of trauma. Fundamentally, the memory is often distorted and lays the foundation for posttraumatic stress reactions.

Reintegration is the posttrauma stage of personality reaction to the trauma. Because of the traumatic disintegration of the body, mind, and spirit, the victim is separated from the core sense of self. Interventions must focus on the reestablishment of the sense of self to ensure their healthy reunification.

A traumatic reaction is the healthy reintegration of the victim. A traumatic stress reaction is the immediate shock reaction worked through by traumatic incident debriefings, which provide facilitative support rather than psychotherapy. Delayed reactions include posttraumatic stress reaction and posttraumatic stress disorder. PTSD is nonclinical and worked through with peer support, peer counseling, or nonclinical counseling intervention. PTSD is the clinical reaction most often seen in dual and differential diagnoses. Extensive clinical trauma training and education are necessary to work with and help victims appropriately.

Intervention is based on diagnosis of level of traumatic reaction as well as stage of personality reintegration. This diagnosis is based on the verbal communication (words) and nonverbal communication (body position, movement) the person uses to describe traumatic issues.

The general TSCIM stages relate to

1. Wisdom or level of consciousness (i.e., denial, rationalization, intellectualization)
2. Safety, trust, and mistrust issues (i.e., hypervigilance, startle response)
3. Fears of losing control (i.e., anger, rage)
4. Distorted guilt (i.e., behavior at the time of trauma, flashbacks)
5. Competency issues (i.e., self and others, job problems)
6. Commitment to goals and objectives (i.e., fidelity to self and others, lack of concentration)
7. Interpersonal relationships (i.e., fears of intimacy)
8. Caring for self and others (i.e., stagnation, existential anxieties, depression, sleep disturbances)

Each stage of personality development has specific intervention strategies to help a person reintegrate the traumatized personality. The survivor often moves forward, stabilizes, and then goes back to work on previous stages. However, the skilled traumatologist instantly recognizes the stage (issue) from a healthy to unhealthy continuum. A constant focus on diagnosing provides the path to appropriate intervention.

Mission

The mission of the centers is based on an organizational development model. A strong philosophy generates public and governmental support and overcomes the general cultural denial and resistance to problems related to traumatic stress. Fundamental to the philosophy is to avoid revictimization. This is the art of helping without hurting.

Specific goals for the center are based on the strong philosophical foundation of the center and state-specific prevention and intervention strategies that support each stated goal. The synergistic philosophical goals and objectives that relate to trust–mistrust issues are the scaffolding of a center. The organization's structure provides the framework for decision making to recruit personnel to fill jobs.

Staffing

Centers recruit highly motivated paraprofessionals, peer counselors, nonclinical counselors, and clinical psychology, social work, and medical staff personnel to deliver services. The director of each center may have a clinical, nonclinical, or paraprofessional background, depending on the needs assessment that has been completed. Frequently in Russia, staffing is based on the political and economic realities of the community in which it is based. There are weekly staff meetings that conduct case studies and case reviews.

Attracting staff that fit the goals of a center is important. Each staff member needs to be knowledgeable in a variety of modalities and methods aware of ethical standards in the field and to work within the framework of cultural influences and impacts. Also, since conflict and friction bring inefficiency and require greater effort leading to ineffective goal achievement at the least and revictimization at the worst, it is important to have staff who identify with the mission and philosophical goals of the center and are committed to the framework of services.

Each staff member has working knowledge of a variety of trauma treatment modalities and intervention methods, and is aware of ethical standards in the field of traumatology and works within the cultural contextual framework. Staff members work only at the level(s) for which they are trained and educated.

Directors/managers provide employee (staff) assistance programs (EAPs) to combat compassion fatigue or traumatic stress burnout caused by staff caring too much for others and not taking care of self. Through the EAP, program managers demonstrate an ability to have compassion for others. These concepts of commitment, love, and caring for workers are in contrast to the traditional Russian societal experience. Previously, workers were expected to show commitment, love, and caring externally to society through absolute self-sacrifice to the government.

Theory

The theory behind the Russian trauma center is a synergistic, cybernetic, constant process of feedback and evaluation of each critical stage of healthy organizational and personality mental health development. TCSIM combines critical stages of healthy development for both the individual and the trauma center, which include:

1. Philosophy (wisdom)
2. Goals and objectives (trust and safety)
3. Organization structure (self-control)
4. Human and economic resources (initiative and motivation)
5. Efficiency and teamwork (self-competency)
6. Management/director and staff mutual commitment (self-commitment and fidelity)
7. Human resource development training, education and development program (love)
8. Employee (staff) assistance programs (caring and compassion)

An Eastern perspective of this integrative model is based on natural law. Specifically, the following natural laws relate to TCSIM and trauma center development:

1. Philosophy (wisdom): law of unification
2. Goals and objectives (trust and safety): law of unlimited possibilities
3. Organizational structure (self-control): law of detachment
4. Human and economic resources (initiative and motivation): law of dharma, or doing the right thing
5. Efficiency and teamwork (conservation and cooperation): law of least effort
6. Commitment and fidelity: law of intention and desire
7. Human resource development (love): law of karma or doing the right thing
8. EAP (caring and commitment): law of giving

This integration of Western personality and organizational development concepts with Eastern natural law developmental perspectives helps to train and educate Russian traumatologists and managers. Integrating TCSIM personality reintegration concepts with the trauma center organizational development model and natural law helps the traumatologist to identify critical stages of development quickly. A healthy, dynamic, integrative organizational personality is important for trauma center development because, "You cannot do for others that which you cannot do for self." A traumatic stress reaction is the result of violating natural law. If the center follows natural law, healthy manifestations of integrated personality and organization development appear. If the center violates natural law, traumatic stress disintegration symptomatology manifests itself. This leads to revictimization by a center and by the victim to self.

Service Delivery

The specific job tasks of a trauma center relate to goals and objectives (see Fig. 5.1). Human resources are recruited to meet the tasks, and other resources

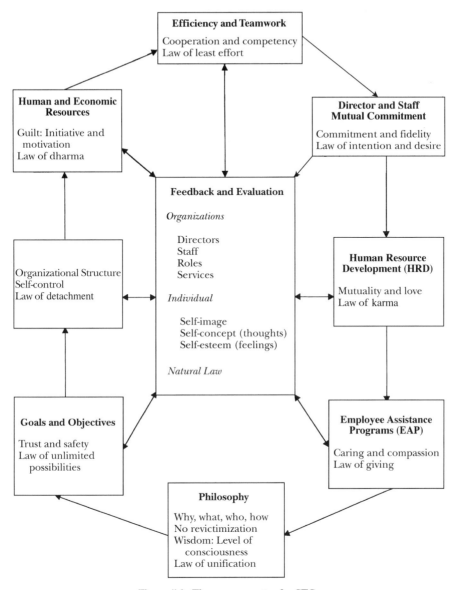

Figure 5.1. The components of a CTC.

(location, buildings, furniture, etc.) also are collected and evaluated. The center must commit its often very limited economic and human resources in a way to ensure the survival of the center as well as to provide for the needs that are identified by needs assessments. Services offered by these centers run along a multidimensional continuum ranging from:

1. Phone debriefings dealing with immediate, individual traumatic reactions through peer support (i.e., hotlines)
2. Traumatic incident debriefings for traumatic stress reactions provided through professional and paraprofessional facilitative support
3. Posttraumatic stress reactions with nonclinical counseling interventions, to include peer counseling
4. Posttraumatic stress disorder with clinical interventions associated with dual and differential diagnoses (i.e., PTSD, alcoholism, personality disorders).

Community Service Delivery

Since Russian trauma centers focus on prevention, assessment, and intervention, services relate to levels of traumatic stress and the population(s) served. Cultural considerations, needs assessment (e.g., surveys to determine cultural context), and resource development for community disaster response (e.g., Cherynoble) need to be taken into account. Other aspects that need to be taken into consideration relating to training in trauma intervention and posttraumatic stress include:

- Promotion of psychological individual rehabilitation
- Promotion of social rebuilding in the family
- Development of peer support through 12-step programs
- Primary prevention of psychological distress through stress management programs
- Traumatic incident debriefings offering facilitative support
- Peer counseling to law enforcement and fire departments
- Staff debriefings to combat compassion fatigue

Professional development programs for individual skill building and professional competency and research protocols based on needs assessment to determine the most appropriate delivery systems for services in an economically constrained environment are further community-oriented foci of the Russian trauma center. Community services also include hot lines, clinical and nonclinical counseling programs, 12-step programs, Transcendental Meditation™ (TM) programs, and services for children, youth, and families. A key component of the holistic intervention model is the use of TM. The 11th step of Alcoholics Anonymous (AA), Survivors Anonymous (SA), and other similar programs focuses on the use of prayer and meditation. TM leads to the emergence of spirituality in the self-recovery process. TM is simple, easy to learn, and cost-effective. It has over 35 years of empirical research with over 500 published research studies worldwide to document its effectiveness. It focuses directly on immediate empowerment and reestablishment of an internal sense of safety. TM also is a technique for dealing with stress. It is not a religion. It does not require a change in lifestyle or belief system. It transcends cultures and is a powerfully synergistic technique when used by both staff and survivors. TM helps to support the self-recovery intervention process at each critical stage. TM helps the survivor reestablish an internal sense of safety and trust in self that leads to a strong sense of self-control and supports the emergence of initiative, motivation, and cooperation. Two 20-minute sessions daily can help to resolve posttraumatic stress. Increased self-awareness gained through TM can decreases the suffering caused by the past trauma.

AA's 12 steps, books, and literature are already translated into Russian and AA groups are established in larger cities (e.g., Moscow, St. Petersburg). However, there is a general cultural denial as to the severity of alcoholism in Russia, and establishment of groups elsewhere is a slow process. The trauma center has zero tolerance for alcohol abuse at all levels from survivor clients to staff. Staff members are trained to recognize detoxification symptomatology as it relates to PTSR/PTSD; in fact, these symptoms are often the emerging traumatic stress symptoms and may be misdiagnosed.

Survivors Anonymous is a unique 12-step program developed by Dr. Niles in Russia (see Fig. 5.2). SA stresses healthy forgiveness and grieving. SA helps in the intervention process of empowerment. Sharing with others leads to understanding the impact of trauma on the survivor's current life situation. As the survivor learns to accept that she or he did the best he or she could at the moment of trauma, change occurs.

There are actual and/or perceived conflicts between AA and the post-trauma personality reintegration focus of TCSIM. SA focuses on an empowerment model, not a powerless position. AA focuses on the harm the individual has done to others; SA, with the victim as recipient of harm from others. A victim who understands these conflicts gains understanding of traumatic stress and the process of self-medication through alcohol. The focus of SA is upon self-recovery. Kazan University's Department of Psychology is currently teaching this SA model. Other community-oriented projects are pilot projects offering training in peer support, peer counseling and debriefing, and rehabilitation and vocational guidance projects.

The constraints of Russian reality mean that resources for the trauma center are often gathered by donations (e.g., furniture). The hardest procurement, though, often relates to obtaining a building for the trauma center. Since the government still owns most buildings, government support of the center is often primary. Limited economic resources also are a fundamental concern. The center must commit its limited resources carefully to ensure efficiency and effectiveness of service provision; this is mandatory, if the center is to survive. In addition, efficient internal integration of human resources measured by external effectiveness of the center on the population being served is critical. Inefficiency and ineffectiveness result in the quick demise of a trauma center.

Thus, therapists who work in centers in Russia have knowledge of AA, SA, trauma counseling, traumatic incident debriefing, peer counseling, and

1. Admitted we were powerless at the time of the trauma, but did the best we could as human beings. Since the trauma, the quality of our lives has diminished and become meaningless and purposeless.

2. Came to trust a power greater than ourselves can help empower us through understanding what impact past trauma is having upon our current life situation. Since we survived, we seek meaning and purpose for our survival through this empowerment process.

3. Made a personal decision, based upon trust in our self, to turn our will and lives over to the nurturing care of God, as we understand God. This helps regain self-control over our lives.

4. Based upon this personal decision to take self-control, we make a searching and fearless moral inventory of our guilty thoughts and feelings related to the trauma.

5. Take the initiative to admit to ourself, another human being and God, the exact truth of our reactions during the trauma, as we understand the truth. We also take the initiative to share any suicidal or homicidal thoughts.

6. Are entirely ready to have God remove these guilty thoughts and feelings that lead to rage, hate and fears of intimacy. This decision is based upon our emerging commitment to life and living it in a meaningful, purposeful and faithful manner.

7. Humbly ask God to remove our distorted guilty feelings and thoughts. Furthermore, we ask for empowerment over the trauma through understanding ourselves, others and the environment at the time of the trauma. This understanding emerges through the process of forgiving ourselves, others and God.

8. Make a list of all those who suffered or died during the trauma that we honestly knew and can grieve for in a healthy manner. This includes our loss of innocence as a result of the trauma.

9. Face our painful memories and experience healthy grieving for self, friends and loved ones by accepting their loss. Through healthy grieving, we begin to realize that we bring meaning and purpose to their memory through living life in a healthy manner.

10. Continue to take personal inventory and when distorted thoughts and feelings arise making us feel powerless, we immediately acknowledge them as distortions. We then release them and regain our empowerment in the self-recovery process.

11. Seeking through prayer and meditation to improve our conscious awareness of self, others and our contact with God. Through this process of prayer and meditation, we come to realize who "I am" and why I survived the trauma. This results in emerging self-responsibility to find meaning and purpose during this posttrauma period of my life.

12. Having had a truly spiritual awakening of empowerment as the result of these steps, I carry this message to other trauma survivors. This is the practice of loving-kindness and compassion through self-respect for myself and others in all aspects of life.

Figure 5.2. Survivor's Anonymous (SA): a twelve-step self-recovery program. Dr. David P. Niles, Trauma Education Consulting Center (TREK), Stillwaters Cottage, Sebago, NE 04029. Tel/Fax: (207) 787-2172.

TM. Interventions aim first to reestablish an internal sense of safety and trust. They allow for ventilation and validation, which leads to self-control while limiting fears of loosing control. The next stage is predicting possibilities that may emerge as the personality becomes integrated or in dealing with abreactive processes of PTSD. The focus then turns to reflection on resolutions, helping the survivor gain greater self-control and self-competency in his or her work.

THE CRISIS CONSULTATION AND EDUCATION CENTER, OULU, FINLAND

In 1987, the Finnish Suicide Prevention Research Project built a network of professionals in the Oulu, Finland area and brought the needs of crisis intervention into the daylight. One of the cofounders of the organization (Soili Poijula) was a field interviewer in this project. She envisioned developing a prototype organization for systematic early crisis intervention since there was no center for crisis/trauma psychology in the entire country. As the idea of utilizing early crisis intervention, crisis teams and psychological debriefing became accepted; the first crisis teams were established in 1989. Dr. Poijula started the team in Oulu in 1991. The network supported the idea of a specialized center to help trauma victims through provision of specialized treatment services.

In 1994, four volunteer organizations (the Mannerheim League, Federation of Mother and Child Homes and Shelters, the Red Cross, and the Finnish Association for Mental Health) and the city of Oulu met and formed a project team along with members from child guidance organizations, the health care and social welfare systems, the Evangelical Lutheran Church, the Oulu administration board, law enforcement agencies, and Oulu University. The end product of the team was the creation of the Crisis Consultation and Education Center.

Goals of the center are to provide psychosocial support to victims of trauma, to develop a systematic model to help victims of trauma, and to care for helpers who work with the traumatized. The center offers early crisis intervention, crisis therapy, and posttraumatic therapy; organizes training in diagnosis and treatment of PTSD as well as crisis intervention and innovative therapies; sponsors EMDR seminars and coordinates the Finnish EMDR network; informs the public and media about trauma and its impact; conducts research; and networks with professionals on an international basis.

The Crisis Consultation and Education Center serves a population of about 500,000 persons; as trainers, staff members serve the entire country of Finland, a population of about 5 million persons. The center is dependent on government funding. In the summer of 2000, the founding psychologist left the center to form her own organization, Oy Synolon, Ltd. (Center for Trauma Psychology).

Mission

The mission of the center is to help people learn as much as possible from a stressful event, to reduce their pain, help them heal, and help them grow through open communication, enlisting a person's social network for support. This crisis intervention is the free right of all citizens of Finland.

Staffing

Prior to the summer of 2000, the staff of the Crisis Consultation and Education Center consisted of two female psychologists, one psychiatric nurse–psychologist, and one part-time child psychiatrist. The center needs additional staff members to compose a multidisciplinary team: male and female psychologists, psychiatrists, social workers with psychotherapy training, all of whom are good trainers, and a secretary for office work. Translators are occasionally utilized. Staff of the center has trained 14 voluntary helpers who are mainly social and health care professionals for rape victims in acute crisis situations. One goal of the center is to develop more self-help groups and networking using ex-clients and survivor professionals. Supervision has been provided by a Finnish trainer of psychotherapists and international trauma experts. A project team consisting of multiorganizational and multiprofessional members meets regularly. An associate professor of psychiatry, a professor of child psychiatry, the director of the local child guidance clinic, and the director of the local university hospital's psychiatric clinic are included in this team. Staff participate in national and international meetings, networking, e-mail correspondence, and trainings, as well as by regular supervision and consultation.

Services

The three psychologists who comprised the staff of the center provided care to primary victims of trauma—persons who are the direct victims and who are most seriously impacted; to secondary victims—the helpers who work with them; and tertiary organizations. Several levels of service provision exist:

1. Early crisis intervention through emotional first aid/psychosocial support assistance in viewing of a body; defusing; and psychological debriefing between 25 and 72 hours posttraumatic event
2. Follow-up services
3. Crisis therapy that is focused
4. Posttrauma therapies
5. Help for helpers

Staff recognize that timing of support is crucial after a traumatic event. The center creates a caring climate for those who use its services.

Services are prioritized for clients who need special trauma and grief counseling and posttrauma therapy. Clients needing long-term psychotherapy are generally referred. When a client calls the center directly, he or she is interviewed by phone and then the client has three to five appointments for diagnosis and assessment. In times of acute need, the center turns to the network of locally trained professionals to help. Confidentiality is absolute and does not appear on primary health care records. Treatment generally has been free to clients, though some clients have insurance. Sessions for forensic purposes may be taped. Short term therapy may use EMDR. Long-term therapy is more psychoanalytically oriented individual therapy or solution-oriented individual therapy and systemic therapy. Persons served have input into the services that are provided. Clients give feedback to help staff members develop the work of the center. In some instances, specific groups of survivors complete questionnaires to evaluate treatment.

Theory

The model of trauma on which the organization is based is integrative and includes belief, affect, social, imaginative, cognitive, and physical components. Basic principles of posttraumatic therapy are followed. Initially, the center creates a safe, caring climate. Staff listen without interruption in an active manner to victims of trauma, maintaining eye contact, and relating in an honest and direct manner. Clients are encouraged to talk about the worst of their experiences and staff accepts the reactions as normal and nonpathological.

Debriefing of helpers is done as a planned, structured group activity that reviews the facts, thoughts, impressions, and reactions of helpers following critical incidents. Debriefing, based on the Mitchell (Mitchell & Everly, 1993), Dyregrov (Dyregrov & Mitchell, 1992), and Ayalon (Ayalon, 1992) models, aims to prevent unnecessary aftereffects of exposure to trauma, helps to accelerate normal recovery, stimulates group cohesion of the rescuers, normalizes their reactions, stimulates emotional ventilation, and promotes the gaining of a cognitive "grip" on a situation. The debriefing method used by the center has been shown through research to work effectively in early crisis intervention, compared with cases where there was no debriefing. The treatment goals of the organization relate to the theoretical stance.

Community Work

The center organizes seminars for professionals throughout Finland. The center markets the trainings in professional magazines, through press conferences held as part of seminar presentations, and through media interviews and articles. In September 1997, for example, Charles Figley presented a seminar on compassion fatigue and helping traumatized families.

Center staff have helped to train and supervise 45 crisis teams that now exist in central Finland. These teams meet four times a year. The center provides services to schools and workplaces and uses the media to inform the general population about psychological trauma, its consequences, and ways to heal.

The staff members of the center provide trainings themselves. Specialty areas include traumatic grief, children and trauma and grief, traumatic stress and PTSD, psychological debriefing, disaster management, contingency planning, helping the helpers, compassion stress and compassion fatigue, creative tools in helping, and group work with children of battered women. Staff members also provide phone consultation to professionals from the entire country.

TUNNECLIFFE AND ASSOCIATES: EMERGENCY SUPPORT CONSULTANTS, PALMYRA, WESTERN AUSTRALIA

This cooperative, professional group composed of three licensed clinical psychologists serves the state of Western Australia and its 2 million people. Working under the banner of the "emergency support network," this group aims to provide training and facilitate information sharing in areas of crisis intervention, peer support, crisis phone work and trauma response. The organization is a commercial venture but staff donate considerable time and energy to various groups including victims of crime and self-help organizations. Much of the emphasis is on training peer supporters who can meet the immediate needs of persons in times of stress and trauma, particularly in rural areas, and give them practical assistance. Peer support is the use of volunteers from the work area who are trained in appropriate methods of assistance to persons subjected to stressful critical incidents. Peer supporters provide short-term rapid intervention through stress defusings on a one-to-one basis or in small groups, arrange contact with family members when appropriate, promote normalization to reestablish control, provide information to assist an individual's coping process, encourage use of social supports in addition to the families, and encourage practical steps to reestablish personal power.

The emergency support network customizes professional development courses, staff trainings, employee education, and specialized consultancy services to address the needs of course participants and client organizations directly. The staff members provide materials and course follow-up to assist clients to translate educational content of programs into desired workplace practices. All staff and associates conduct themselves in ethical and responsible ways, thereby promoting professionalism of the industry.

Mission

The emergency support network aims to provide training, consultancy, and facilitate information sharing in the areas of crisis intervention, peer support, crisis phone work, trauma response, and managing violence in the workplace. This organization is committed to ensuring the delivery of high-quality educational programs.

Staffing

All members of the organization have done either postgraduate work of extensive in-service training in the trauma arena. All are state licensed and at minimum have a masters degree as a terminal degree. The staff members moved from hospital or organizational psychology into private practice and then into this organization. Staff functions in a specific resource role relating to emergency support work.

Theory

The theory base of the organization is cognitive–behavioral with recognition of a number of basic influence factors relating to trauma:

1. Trauma may well be a "normal" experience for a significant proportion of the human population.
2. Many addictive behaviors (alcoholism, drugs, medication, dependence, etc.) and their associated problems may interfere with efforts to cope with life trauma(s).
3. Problem reactions to traumatic events are normal and expected and should not be pathologized with an immediate call for medication or counseling.
4. The resilience of individuals and groups to cope with traumatic events can be increased by prior education and raising awareness.
5. The impact of a traumatic event is mediated by three major considerations: the individual involved, the nature of the event, and the environment in which it occurs. Within each area are a number of factors that determine what an event means to an individual involved.
6. Connective support procedures, delivered by collegial or community support programs, provide great assistance to people subjected to traumatic events.
7. Trauma counseling has a place in the trauma recovery process; however, it needs to be provided according to indicated needs, within an appropriate time frame, and by a professional with appropriate training.

Services

The organization does little direct intervention with trauma survivors and tends to refer individuals and families to other providers. Services are primarily training and consultation requested from the organization.

Training and Consultation

The training and consultation areas are the major foci of the organization. Training is given to both laypersons and professionals via public courses and upon request. Training standards are set "in house," based on the Australian Federal Government Accreditation System. The organization is a nationally recognized training provider and conducts a number of courses that include stress awareness, stress management, stress auditing, peer support skills, stress debriefing, crisis intervention, crisis phone answering, critical incident recovery, emergency response, management of aggression, and conflict mediation. The organization has produced the *Emergency Support Newsletter* and has developed extensive materials and workbooks for training; however, only some of these are available outside of the courses.

One book, *The Crisis Support First Aid Kit: What Everyone Should Know about Helping Others in Times of Emotional Stress* (Tunnecliffe, 1997) stresses that crisis intervention is the provision of immediate assistance to those undergoing intense stress to help with coping and situation management. It details the six steps of crisis intervention including rapid intervention, practical assistance and support, use of verbalization to defuse emotional tension, normalization of thoughts and emotions to reestablish personal control, engagement of social support networks, and encouragement of practical steps to reestablish personal power. Other training manuals, all of them by Tunnecliffe, are the *Crisis Intervention Course Manual* (1996); *Peer Support Training Manual* (1997); and *Emergency Phone Response Course Manual* (1996). In the latter book, the five keys to good phone management of a crisis are given: (1) provision of respect and courtesy to the caller; (2) patience while guiding the caller to the information; (3) provision of a sense of confidence and reassurance; (4) involvement with and explanations as to what is going on; and (5) empowerment through giving suggestions as to what the caller can do. Basic peer support training includes training on the theory, nature, and types of stress; principles of peer support; aims and objectives of peer support; role and process of support; practical, defusing, and debriefing levels of support; communication skills; referral skills; personal stress management skills; specific demands and needs of support; and role of professional guidance and advice.

In addition, the organization offers fee-based consultation to organizations. Although staff members have been requested to serve as expert witnesses on many occasions, they decline to do so because of the time it would take. One staff member provides mediation training for interpersonal conflict, workplace grievances, and harassment situations.

PSYCHOSOCIAL TRAUMA PROGRAM, ISTANBUL, TURKEY

This trauma program is part of the Istanbul University's medical/ psychiatric department and is led by Dr. Sahika Yüksel, also founded two nongovernmental organizations (NGOs): the Women's Shelter Project (an independent feminist organization) and the Turkish Human Rights Foundation for Torture Survivors. These organizations work together when necessary. The latter provides direct medial care. Dr. Yüksel provides supervision for the organizations. The needs of the country, torture survivors, domestic violence survivors, and others led to the creation of the center in 1994.

Staff

At the time of the interview, the center had two female staff members, a psychologist and psychiatrist. The center needs social workers as well as more psychologists and psychiatrists. Staff meet monthly to discuss their problems and needs and yearly in a grief work-oriented group. Employees of the NGOs were chosen because of personal history and clinical experience. Psychiatric residents also work with the programs. Employees of all three organizations cooperate together.

Clientele

Clients primarily are victims of domestic violence, childhood sexual abuse (adults and children, mostly female), and victims of torture as well as family members of these primary victims. Clients are primarily referred from other psychologists or medical services, for example, emergency rooms. Clients generally are between ages of 14 and 45 and have 5–10 years of education. They generally come from urban areas. The majority are sexual abuse survivors.

Theory

Dr. Yüksel's background is primarily etiological. Consultation and treatment generally uses a cognitive–behavioral therapy framework. PTSD treatment does not apply to all trauma survivors and must be adapted to fit the problems of survivors, including those with complex PTSD.

Assessment

A clinical interview generally takes between 1 and 2 hours and uses the Symptom Checklist-90, the IES, and a posttrauma assessment form (Post Trauma Scale) developed by Dr. Yüksel. Diagnosis is based on DSM-III-R and DSM-IV criteria. Dr. Yüksel also may use the SCID-D. Comorbid disorders most frequently presented include major depression and somatoform disorders.

Services

The center provides individual therapy and group therapy. The goal is to provide short-term counseling while helping victims with social and psychological needs. The goal also is to help clients become more independent. Clients generally come for help between a few months to years after a trauma or a suspected trauma has occurred. Treatment can occur for as long as clients need it and are living in Istanbul. The clinic also supplies medications. Cognitive and dynamic approaches are used for longer-term treatment. The center does not do debriefing. However, psychoeducation is offered as part of the treatment process.

Training

The center offers seminars, workshops, and conferences. The center offers a 20-hour training program to volunteers and laypersons who work with those who use the Women's Shelter Project. They offer training also to people who work with sexually abused survivors and battered women and have developed training materials. Staff members also offer consultations to the medical and psychiatric departments in the hospital of the university. They may give interviews to media and write papers for journals as well.

SUMMARY

Perhaps one of the most well-developed trauma centers outside the continental United States is the center in Oulu, Finland. During the fall of 1998 and the winter of 1999, codirectors of the center, Soili Poijula and Paivi Saarinen, with the assistance of Raili Rinne, developed and began to implement a 3-year trauma training program for therapists. In March 1999, participants in the training program met with Dr. Roger Solomon and Dr. Mary Beth Williams in a 3-day Internat. The Internat brought everyone together at a hotel in Lapland for study, work on self through exercises and EMDR, relaxation (e.g., dancing, dining, and listening to the fantastic music of Duo Mennen), and exercise (cross country and downhill skiing, sauna, swimming). The goals of the Internat were to build a safe therapeutic community for participants to work on and learn about themselves, to resolve pressing issues, and to learn the Internat model as well as theory and practical issues about trauma treatment. This Internat is only the first in a series and will be expanded in later sessions. It will be described in a variety of publications that can be incorporated into the training programs of other trauma centers.

The efforts of the individuals who have developed the center at Oulu as well as other centers are to be commended. They recognize the need for trained professionals who can intervene with trauma survivors at a variety of points of contact and levels of intervention. In spite of financial constraints, the centers described in this chapter are making valuable contributions to alleviating pain and suffering as well as contributing to the knowledge basis of the field of traumatic stress.

6
Nonresidential Affiliated Centers throughout the World

Centers have been established under the auspices of universities and hospitals in many countries. The majority of the centers described in this chapter are affiliated with universities. The populations they serve range from survivors of Stalinist persecution to automobile accident victims.

THE CENTER FOR TRAUMATIC STRESS
AT HADASSAH UNIVERSITY HOSPITAL, JERUSALEM, ISRAEL

This open clinic is designed to treat any individual who has been traumatized in any manner. The clinic is not designed specifically to treat secondary victims, although significant others, spouses, and relatives are welcome. Expenses of treatment in this outpatient clinic are covered by various Israeli insurance companies. Because the clinic is part of a larger hospital structure, it is not isolated or independent. Many of the survivors treated are also being treated within the larger framework of outpatient treatment; in fact, approximately one third of patients in the hospital are trauma patients.

Israel as a country and Hadassah University Hospital as an institution have experienced a number of traumatic events. The proposal to establish a trauma center in the hospital was initiated in 1989. Over the next 2 years, hospital staff trained themselves to treat trauma survivors. Staff then began to network with others for referrals.

The clinic is unique because it offers clients the opportunity to identify and help solve their own problems while being educated about the impacts of trauma and thereby reducing the impact of the problems that cannot be solved. In addition, the clinic offers staff and trainees the opportunity to do research that combines psychological and physiological impact studies. The program hopes to improve therapy for trauma survivors through publication of research results and through discussions and presentations. The clinic hosted the World Conference on Traumatic Stress in 1996. The majority of publications deal with the progression from acute trauma to prolonged PTSD.

Mission

The mission of the center is to treat trauma patients within the context of general care and the general framework of psychology and psychiatry. The mission also is to provide care to survivors of trauma and their relatives and to conduct research to improve knowledge.

Funding

Hadasseh Hospital has been funded since 1936. As Dr. Shalev stated, "the hospital is funded in part by medical insurance and miracles."

Staffing

Staffing of the clinic uses psychologists, social workers, and psychiatrists who specialize in the treatment of trauma. The clinic does not use lay caregivers and volunteers. The staff is embedded in a working department of Hadassah University Hospital and there is no specific psychosocial support for its employees. However, no staff member treats more trauma survivors than she or he can handle. Generally only one third of clients treated are trauma survivors. Cooperation among staff is good and staff members are very cohesive. Senior staff members have tenure within the framework of the larger medical health organization. New staff members who come to the institution need a year of training as they begin to see patients/clients before they can treat trauma survivors independently. This on-the-job training accompanies formal and informal teaching. Staff are licensed and certified by their own professional organizations (the Israel Association of Psychology, the State Social Work Organization, and others).

Clientele

Approximately one-third of clients referred to the clinic receive trauma-based treatment. These individuals are generally not in the acute stage of reactivity to trauma. Clients frequently have comorbid depression, anxiety disorder, and personality disorders related to personality changes following trauma. Some patients are experiencing acute grief; others, acute anxiety; still others are overwhelmed and unable to cope with the demands of life.

Clinical Services

The clinic provides individual psychodynamic and cognitive psychotherapy and some group therapy, primarily with persons with prolonged PTSD.

The clinic also offers psychopharmacological therapy, family and couples therapy, and short inpatient admissions. The needs of the individual determine treatment methodology and decision making, and clients have input into treatment choices with the professionals who treat them. Pharmacological treatment is accessible through the same outpatient unit. The clinic does not have enough resources to respond to all cases of acute trauma; however, the hospital constantly receives patients who are acutely traumatized. Staff also do crisis intervention and debriefing.

Assessment

The basic assessment of an individual is a clinical interview accompanied by rating scales and structured questions. Psychological testing may occur at a later date, as may psychophysiological testing. Assessment is done primarily at the beginning of treatment rather than at the end, as a means to assess treatment outcome. Rating scales utilized include the Impact of Event Scale (IES), Mississippi Scale, State-Trait Anxiety Inventory, and others. The clinic staff has developed a scale to assess immediate response to trauma and has modified trauma history questionnaires to fit the culture of Israel (e.g., terrorist acts in contrast to hurricanes or tornadoes as traumatic events). Staff is publishing research on assessment of acute response to trauma and physiological assessment of prolong response to trauma.

Theory

The clinic utilizes an eclectic model of treatment based on integration of different therapeutic approaches. The idealogy of the clinic is to match approaches to the needs of the patients at the given time.

In order to optimize and tailor treatment, it is necessary to be flexible and in tune with the needs of the patient. Different individuals in different stages need different treatments and different forms of therapies. A combination of behavior therapy, psychodynamic understanding, and medical intervention as a multidimensional intervention strategy is ideal. Staff of the clinic have developed their own theoretical models for multidimensional treatment of acute and prolonged traumatic stress.

Community Services

The clinic has created brochures and newsletters to provide to the community particularly in times of crisis. The clinic cooperates with welfare services, social services, and nursing services in the larger community as well as with institutions that provide insurance coverage for treatment (e.g., the Ministry of Defense). Clinic staff offer training in treatment of acute trauma and chronic (prolonged) PTSD to professionals and share the burden of training others. In addition, staff has developed curricula for basic training of new professionals who come to the clinic and offer consultation to other professionals, including emergency room nursing staff, as needed. Staff occasionally does forensic work in cases ranging from rape to road accident victimization. A few of the senior staff are expert witnesses.

THE POST TRAUMATIC STRESS DISORDER UNIT, UNIVERSITY OF NEW SOUTH WALES AND WESTMEAD HOSPITAL, NEW SOUTH WALES, SYDNEY, AUSTRALIA

This PTSD unit is based at Westmead Hospital at the University of New South Wales in Sydney, Australia. Funded by the Department of Health and the National Health and Medical Research Council, the unit is researching assessment and treatment of acute stress disorder (ASD) and PTSD following civilian traumas. Everyone who comes to the hospital with a trauma-related injury is looked at in terms of ASD and hospital staff has developed a structured clinical interview based on DSM-IV for assessment. The program has been operating since 1992 and receives little support from the hospital per se, except for the provision of free space. In return, the program offers a novel free service to the hospital and the two programs are on good terms. The organization was awarded the Gold Award, the National Award for Mental Health Services in Australia, in 1996.

The unit provides early treatment within 2 weeks of a trauma to persons who have experienced a traumatic injury. Over the past 5 years, 220 persons yearly have been seen. The general treatment methodology is a five-session cognitive–behavioral therapy program that begins while the patient is in the hospital and ends approximately 4 weeks after the traumatic event. Persons receiving treatment are divided into groups. Those who have received cognitive–behavioral therapy have a 10% follow-up rate of PTSD; persons who have been in a nondirective therapeutic control group have an 80% rate of PTSD at a 6-month follow-up. Thus the program serves to assess all traumatized patients admitted to the hospital, to identify those at risk of developing PTSD, and to provide early treatment as well as outpatient referral. It is the only program in Australia to provide a thorough assessment of stress reactions following traumatic injury admission to a public hospital. It is the first program in the world to demonstrate that early cognitive–behavioral intervention in trauma patients can prevent PTSD. The unit also has developed the first psychometrically sound diagnostic structured clinical interview of ASD.

Program Goals

The program has six main goals:

- To develop a comprehensive assessment program for trauma survivors
- To initiate a scientifically based treatment program for PTSD

- To conduct research into PTSD and its treatment
- To develop a center of excellence to provide consultancy services
- To promote prevention strategies to mitigate development of PTSD
- To develop international links between the unit and other centers.

Staffing

Dr. Bryant heads the program and supervises staff. He has a masters degree and doctorate in clinical psychology. At the time of the interview, program staff consisted of three full-time and one half-time clinical psychologists, all research trained, one with a PhD in acute stress. Staff meets weekly to discuss the unit's operation as well as individual cases. An independent clinician evaluates staff performance through outcome studies of treatment programs. Jobs are funded by research grants and therefore are not secure. Positions exist for 2 years at a time. Various consultant specialists also are available to the program.

Clientele

The program works with adults. The majority of clients are patients at the hospital. One major study has been examining PTSD in traumatic brain-injured patients to determine the rates of mild to moderate disorder. Other persons served are survivors of mass shootings, industrial accidents, assaults, disasters, and bush fires. Law enforcement officers have fliers about the program and distribute them to victims of criminal assault. The program has begun a child equivalent component at a nearby children's hospital. Every child with a traumatic injury will be tested at 1 and 6 months post-injury. Treatment protocols will use instruments from Pynoos (Pynoos & Nader, 1988, 1990), an anxiety measure, and the Child Behavior Checklist. Child sexual abuse survivors are not going to be included.

Treatment

The unit's early treatment program is one of the first in the world to provide a structured, objectively evaluated treatment of PTSD during the acute trauma phase as a means to prevent symptoms from becoming entrenched. Treatment interventions, all of them individual, are based on the work of Foa (Foa & Rothbaum) and incorporate prolonged exposure and cognitive restructuring. The emphasis is on early detection and prevention through resolution of traumatic memories before avoidance patterns become entrenched. Persons with identified traumatic responses participate in a five-session cognitive–behavioral therapy program. The program is directive and clients have a significantly lower rate of PTSD than individuals who receive a 6-week nondirective counseling program. In a separate study of community referrals (Bryant & Harvey, 1995, 1996), nondirective therapy, prolonged exposure without cognitive restructuring, and cognitive–behavioral therapy–restructuring plus exposure are being compared. Persons are assigned to treatment protocols in a purely random fashion. Psychiatric backup is available. Generally, the program provides services shortly after an incident; however, they have been instituted up to 5 years postevent.

The unit assessed the after-hours needs of Vietnam veterans and monitored the extent to which their PTSD was managed when other mental health agencies were not accessible to them. The unit also surveyed veterans, monitored crisis line calls, and evaluated performances of crisis phone responders. Recommendations made by the unit were adopted by the Department of Veterans Affairs in 1995.

Treatment contributions made by the unit include:

- A theory that outlines the PTSD response of individuals sustaining traumatic brain injuries and who have impaired memory for their trauma and also describes their PTSD profile
- Clarification of the relationship of ASD and PTSD, challenging the emphasis of dissociation in the diagnosis of ASD
- An early intervention program for ASD that effectively prevents PTSD by providing short-term cognitive–behavioral therapy
- Development of measures of ASD including a structured clinical interview, a self-report inventory based on DSM-IV, and a traumatic cognitions questionnaire

Community Services

The unit has acted as a consultant to various agencies and organizations, helping them develop policies on stress management, and has served as a center for expert resources during disasters, providing advice, referral information, media releases, and management strategies. The need for a coordinated structure for debriefing after major events also has led to the development of a three-tired system made up of (1) clinical psychologists doing diagnosis and treatment; (2) counseling psychologists trained in specialized techniques; and (3) general psychologists doing trauma management and debriefing. This organization discriminates between those doing debriefing and those who do therapy. Dr. Bryant, director of the program, hopes that a system of disaster management will reach the eye of the Australian government and was in place by Olympics 2000. There is concern that persons who provide debriefing are properly trained and ethically competent. Services for major disasters therefore need to be coordinated at the tactical level. The unit also has provided advice on policy and treatment development for agencies managing PTSD populations.

Staff of the program acts as consultant to the government on large forensic cases, for example, a test case looking at the impact of atomic testing in the

1950s on 30 soldiers and survivors of an aircraft carrier accident is one such case. Staff also has been hired by the Department of Veterans Affairs to run workshops for rural areas on assessment and treatment of PTSD. The unit also has provided training to rural psychologists in the form of workshops.

Research

Dr. Bryant and others have published numerous articles examining acute stress in victims of motor vehicle accidents, in head injury patients, and in victims of other traumatic incidents. Among their findings were that head-injured patients displayed fewer acute stress symptoms than non-head-injured patients. Intrusive symptoms, in particular, were more prevalent in non-head-injured patients (Bryant & Harvey, 1995). In another study (Bryant & Harvey, 1996), the authors found that a significant portion of motor vehicle accident victims experience disturbing levels of posttraumatic stress immediately after the accident, as well as state anxiety. The level of physical injury did not predict intrusive or avoidant symptoms, except for the absence of head injury. International journals have published 20 research papers and at least 8 more are in press.

CENTRE FOR THE STUDY OF VIOLENCE AND RECONCILIATION, JOHANNESBURG, SOUTH AFRICA

The Centre for the Study of Violence and Reconciliation (CSVR) was launched in January 1989 as the Project for the Study of Violence. The center has expanded and now is a multidisciplinary organization with a staff of 35 full-time employees and additional volunteers and interns. The trauma clinic was formed when a group of psychologists based at the University of the Witwatersrand saw the need for trauma work with groups of traumatized township youth. In 1991, the CSVR (then the Project for the Study of Violence) hired a social worker to run the trauma clinic. In the original target group were persons traumatized by political violence. The mission and staffing have since broadened to include victims of all types of violence. The trauma clinic receives most of its funding from international donors. Thus far, the clinic has not received any funding from the South African government.

The center translates its research into policy proposals and prioritizes intervention strategies, in particular, to the spheres of trauma management and counseling, education and training, institutional change management, and socioeconomic development. The center plays a central lobbying and advocacy role as it utilizes its expertise in building reconciliation, democracy, and a human rights culture within South Africa's governance and society. The center therefore is active in generating policy on violence and development, crime prevention, and work with the Truth and Reconciliation Commission.

The center has established contact and has developed working relationships with trade unions; resource, service, and professional organizations; legal and paralegal organizations; educational institutions; press and media organizations; and victim aid centers, peace structures, and policing institutions in South Africa and abroad. These contacts have ensured that the work of the center is tailored to the needs of the broad South African community. Through education an training programs, research, victim aid strategies, dialogue generation and capacity-building enterprises, the center has begun to make significant contributions toward engaging with the problem of violence in South Africa. These programs service the process of transition and help generate peace and reconciliation in order to assist sustainable socioeconomic development in South Africa.

Mission

The center is dedicated to making a meaningful contribution to peaceful and fundamental transformation in South Africa and is committed to helping South Africans better understand the effects of the past on the present, developing ways to prevent violence and combat its effects, overcoming intolerance, building a human rights culture in South Africa, facilitating the rebuilding of the "social fabric" and a civil society, managing and facilitating reconstruction and development initiatives, transforming and democratizing state institutions, and developing and transferring skills needed to build reconciliation and democracy. The CSVR vision is to service the processes of transition and democratization and to help generate peace and reconciliation, which is essential for long-term sustainable socioeconomic development. The primary goal of the CSVR is to utilize expertise to build reconciliation, democracy, and a human rights culture within South African governance and society.

Staffing

The CSVR has multidisciplinary professionals including sociologists, psychologists, criminologists, social workers, lawyers, historians, and educationalists under one roof. The expertise of these staff members include violence and conflict (including criminal, political, domestic, and gender violence; violence against children). Eight full-time staff members work in the trauma clinic. Mary Robertson is coordinator. The clinic needs more multidisciplinary staff members but are unable to recruit due to financial constraints. They need a pediatrician, psychiatrist, researcher, and more psychologists.

Volunteer counselors are trained over a 10-week period (two afternoons/week) and receive ongoing supervision and training. Although there is a relatively high turnover of these counselors, they provide significant help and expand the counseling capacity of the center. At the time of the interview, there were 40 volunteer lay counselors. These volunteers may be professionals (such as teachers, social workers), unemployed individuals, or university students. There is a preference for African-speaking volunteers. There is no medical director on staff. The clinic staff work with community psychiatrists for medication evaluations; there is a psychiatric nurse on staff.

The clinic staff cooperate together as a multidisciplinary team. They have regular supervision, variation in work hours, variation in work duties (to include training, research, community work), peer debriefing, and regular case conferences to prevent compassion fatigue. The organization is sensitive to the emotional demands of the work and accommodates time off and flexible working conditions. All staff members are trained in trauma counseling. They have other professional qualifications and board registry.

Theory

The theory base of the trauma clinic is cognitive–behavioral and psychodynamic. The model of counseling was developed by Wits University staff in a four-step model that incorporates cognitive–behavioral and humanistic principles. The model of debriefing is Mitchell and Bray's critical incident stress debriefing (CISD) model (Everly & Mitchell, 1997).

Funding

Many embassies, institutions, and foundations made contributions to support the activities, projects, and programs of the CSVR. Among them are the European Union, the Ford Foundation (USA), ICCO (the Netherlands), embassies of Ireland and Belgium, Save the Children Fund, the Royal Danish and Royal Netherlands embassies, and Justice and Transition, among others. The trauma clinic has had difficulty in raising a secure funding base. Since clinical services are free, if clients can afford those services, they are asked to give a donation.

Clientele

Clients of the trauma clinic of the CSVR include victims of political violence, victims of criminal violence, survivors of rape or domestic violence, victims of long-term imprisonment and torture, and political returnees and their family. Services are provided to all victims of violence across economic classes including adults and children. At the time of the interview, the clinic was receiving 120–140 new referrals monthly. At outreach clinics, staff may see 40 people a day. Clients are required at intake to give a description of their traumatic experiences.

Services

The CSVR engages in many direct services to meet its broad objectives. These include trauma counseling, conflict management, and prevention work.

The trauma clinic delivers free short-term trauma counseling to victims of violence including political violence, violent crime, and sexual and domestic violence. The clinic had 853 new referrals in 1995 for individual trauma counseling (759 adults and 94 children) and 1185 new referrals in 1996. The majority of the clients were seen for short-term counseling of four to six sessions. Many of these clients needed bereavement/grief counseling in addition to trauma counseling. The clinic also conducts group debriefings in stores, banks, mines, schools, emergency service groups, clinics, and security industry sectors. Companies have contracts with the clinic to provide services to their organizations (individual counseling and group debriefings) when needed.

One major goal of the individual intervention is to help clients retell their stories. Other interventions include working with their feelings and thoughts and helping them reframe what happened to them and having them find meaning. Volunteer counselors see many clients for individual trauma counseling. They also assist with debriefings, outreach work, and trainings (particularly in the schools). The goals of treatment are to assist clients to confront, explore, and cope with traumatic experience and the symptoms of trauma so they can function effectively in their lives. The counseling relationship helps clients verbalize the details of their traumas, experience empathy through the process of retelling, and look at ways to cope with trauma.

Interventions are made at various stages of traumatization. Clients are first seen for individual counseling as soon after the event as possible. Debriefings may occur a few days after an incident. Some clients get counseling years after the event occurred. Admission of the existence of trauma is necessary for treatment at the clinic. Many clients have experienced complex multiple traumas and require longer-term counseling.

Community Services

The CSVR engages in a variety of activities within the local, regional, and national communities. These include policy formation, advocacy, lobbying, education, training, curriculum design, development of multi-media educational materials, intervention and service delivery projects, and provision of national and international consultancy services. The CSRV works with many organizations, constituencies, and stakeholders at governmental and nongovernmental sectors including community organizations, government departments, nongovernmental organizations (NGOs), schools, prisons, police, political organizations, industry, and development agencies.

The resource center of the CSVR contains a library of articles, books, and policy documents on various aspects of violence, reconciliation, and human rights. These materials are utilized by researchers, NGOs, community groups and libraries, members of the press and electronic media, the public, and many individuals from abroad.

The trauma clinic provides numerous training programs ranging from introductory talks on trauma to 3- to 5-day training workshops. The training programs are offered to a wide range of interest groups including corporate clients, teachers, emergency personnel, medical and paramedical professionals, police, and others. Training is offered in various areas including identifying trauma, working with multiple areas of traumatic stress, vicarious traumatization, defusing and debriefing, child abuse, and trauma counseling, among others. Volunteer counselors who complete the training course receive certificates. The clinic has developed numerous training materials for sale and for sharing.

The trauma clinic works with various organizations involved in service delivery in South Africa. Among these organizations are the Red Cross, Childline, Compassionate Friends, the Cape Town Trauma Centre, and the National Institute for Crime Prevention and Rehabilitation of Offenders. The clinic also networks with international organizations such as Amnesty International and with international trauma counselors. The clinic makes referrals and has mutual visits, speaking engagements, and projects with these organizations. The networking is helping to build a service infrastructure.

The trauma clinic also has developed lobbying and advocacy activities, though these activities are secondary to service provision and training. However, the clinic recognizes the importance of helping develop public perception and state policy formation in the area of victim support. One goal is to build public awareness of service and policy priorities including child abuse and mental health issues.

The Truth and Reconciliation Department of the CSVR has worked to gather information on victims of gross human rights violations across South Africa. It also has developed mechanisms to provide counseling support for traumatized victims of human rights abuse under Apartheid. The department began to develop a partnership with several victims who wished to testify before the Truth and Reconciliation Commission (TRC). The department also has worked to inform and bring awareness to the South African population about the operations of the Commission. This process includes development of educational materials (including a video, trainer's manual, and radio program), creation of support groups that have helped shape the educational tools, and provision of workshops to NGOs, businesses, media, and others. The project on truth and reconciliation began in 1994 and contributed to the establishment of the TRC. The Khulumani Support Group is a victim and survivor support group established in 1995 as a response to the TRC. It encourages people to speak out about the political atrocities that have happened to them. Khulumani is nonpartisan; it networks with local victims and victim organizations and those in other countries. It helps victims form a collective voice and educates victims on the work of the TRC. IT also assists victims in getting to the TRC to make a submission and provides emotional support for those who testify. The Khulumani refers survivors, victims, and their families to psychological, social, legal, and support services.

The youth department of the CSVR aims to establish trauma units or support services in schools. It seeks to help children who have been traumatized by any type of political, criminal, or family violence as well as parents or families of victims of violence and teachers and other caregivers who work with victimized children. The program provides counseling to victims and next of kin, trains teachers to identify symptoms of trauma in children, empowers teachers with coping skills, educates parents and the community on the symptoms and effects of violence, and refers cases of trauma not related to violence.

Research

The Criminal Justice Policy Unit of the CSVR looks at policing policies and prisons and has helped to develop a national network of NGO agencies involved in policing policy formation and training. All departments in the CSVR have produced research related to their areas of expertise.

CENTER FOR VICTIMS OF POLITICAL PERSECUTIONS, KRAKOW, POLAND

The center was officially recognized in December 1994 and is the first in Poland to diagnose PTSD. The university also is the first educational setting to offer a short course in PTSD. The center continues the tradition of the scientific work of Polish psychiatrist A. Kepinski (1918–1972), a survivor of the Nazi concentration camps. The clinic is housed within the Department of Social Pathology as an outpatient department designed for victims of the totalitarian system of government that ruled Poland after World War II. It is the only rehabilitation center in the country. Within the current political milieu of Poland, fully independent centers are impossible to create and maintain (Gierowski & Heitzman, 1996; Heitzman & Rutkowski, 1996).

Staffing

The staff of the center includes one lawyer, one psychologist-professor, three psychiatrists (one professor and two assistants), and psychology students who work as volunteers to do testing at sessions subsequent to the first session. These students do not do therapy. The lawyer offers official opinions in court-related cases. The professors and assistants must teach at the university and work as therapists only during their work hours. Interns are doing diploma work.

Mission

The mission of the center is to provide therapy to victims of political persecution from the Stalin era, as well as other periods of persecution, and refugees.

Clientele

The patients who come to the clinic are survivors of political persecution in Poland from the Stalin period. After World War II, approximately 50,000 persons were suspected by the secret police, arrested, often tortured, and imprisoned as political prisoners in progress prisons. At present, 30,000 of them live in Poland. Many of them belong to the Political Prisoners of Stalin Period organization. Their average age is 65 and this is the first time they have sought or received help. They have carried a sense of shame with them should they seek psychiatric help. Consequently, they often come in secret to the clinic. These survivors do not trust and it is the first time they have begun to deal with their trauma. Since the election of a Communist president in Poland, many of these victims have returned to their earlier fears of loss of freedom, further persecution, and the secret police. Some of them also are victims of concentration camp imprisonment by the Nazis; others were transported and now are refugees from Russia and the other former Soviet republics. Approximately 3,000 survivors live in the Krakow area. Between 50 and 70 of them were seen at the clinic during its first year of operation.

Provision of Services

A variety of services are provided to clients within the university. Among them are free health care, family therapy, and admission to all university clinics.

Some of the clients were Siberian deportees who became prisoners. They tend to display a constant feeling of undefined fear and anxiety and specific fears of being imprisoned or deported. They gather provisions about them and do not throw things away. They are afraid of authority, uniforms, snow, and winter and have intensive stressor reactions to reminders of their slavery. They are sensitive, suspicious, and do not trust.

Other survivors who come for treatment are deportees who were not prisoners. Their symptoms are similar to survivors of a natural disaster. They frequently were helped by the Russians and do not hate their persecutors. Survivors receive pharmacological treatment and individual psychotherapy. Staff do not yet do crisis intervention or run groups. They do seek to establish a "trustful attitude" toward a patient and try to be understanding. Sometimes they find it difficult to imagine or understand what they hear from their clients/patients. However, they try to maximize responses of compassion and empathy and recognize that the compensation for these survivors lies in "making truth about them public, listening to their truth," and helping them with gaining money, should circumstances allow. It also includes providing them with emotional support.

Research

One hundred survivors of victimization by Stalin, former soldiers of underground movements, were included in a research study. They had been sentenced for acts against the Communist system and the country and frequently were sentenced by courts-martial. Most had been in prison or labor camps (63 had been in prison and others worked in mines, quarries, or industry). All had been persecuted and tortured. Ninety-two percent were men ranging in age from 60 to 83 years. Research revealed that they had been deported or in camps up to 18 years with an accompanying long duration of physical and mental stressors including believing their life was in danger and encountering threats to their physical integrity. They had been constantly exposed to death and had experienced constant suffering.

The study had four dimensions: documentary, historical (as a moral justification), diagnostic-therapeutic, and scientific (examining symptomatology and physiology of chronic PTSD). There were some difficulties in making a diagnosis in that psycho-organic disturbances were mixed with typical PTSD clinical symptoms. Thus both the International Classification of Diseases, 10th edition (ICD-10) diagnoses and diagnostic criteria adapted from DSM-III-R were utilized. Seventy-eight percent of the subjects had a depression–anxiety syndrome. Many of the subjects had had traumas to the head that might have precipitated organic disturbances. The diagnosis of PTSD was made in 71% of the subjects, although the criteria are not precise and not entirely applicable to this group. Diagnostic criteria were influenced by the age of the sufferers and biological aspects of PSTD were closely related to the psychophysical traumas experienced many years before many of the symptoms occurred. Some symptoms of mental disorder were present in almost all of the 100 subjects; only 2 were symptom free.

Community Intervention

Staff of the center have contacts with victim organizations throughout Poland. These organizations know about the services the center provides and introduces those services at meetings. Organizations provide referrals to the center. The organization also ran an ad on television.

In Poland, in general, students do not learn about the consequences of torture in their classes. In addition, a large number of doctors and lawyers do not know about torture or its consequences. The center staff is beginning to offer courses for students and doctors. At the undergraduate level, the courses are to be obligatory for students of medicine, psychology, and law. There is no push for legal reparation for these survivors. It is the hope of the center that education of lawyers will help to encourage reparation. However, the population soon will decrease significantly as its members continue to age. The center also hopes that it can assist in the development of units elsewhere in the country and in the creation of new laws and health policy regulations that will lead to the creation and implementation of a network of similar units (centers).

Theory

The theory base of the center is cognitive–behavioral. Additionally, center staff recognize and try to "get across" the intergenerational impacts of trauma, since many families do not understand the connections between persecutions of relatives and generational psychological problems.

Assessment

Assessment is a major component of the Clinic program. In the first 2-hour examination upon arrival, assessment is begun. Some of the tests given include the Beck Depression Scale, Kendall Psychogenic Changes Scale, the Mississippi Civilian PTSD Scale, and the State-Trait Anxiety Inventory. Thus rehabilitation is connected with scientific examination.

Funding

General funding comes from the university and the Department of Social Pathology. However, this money is limited and the economic situation is difficult. The clinic would benefit from governmental support and funding but the government does not give money for outpatient visits. Because of the limitations in service provision, directors note the need for money to fund further services, for governmental support of the program, and for cooperation with other areas of the country to build a network of similar services.

Training

Staff of the program want to train young people in traumatology. In addition, they want to develop a model that could be offered to other areas of the country so that a network of similar programs would exist.

THE SINAI CENTER: THE JEWISH MENTAL HEALTH SERVICE, AMSTERDAM, HOLLAND

The Jewish Mental Health Service was founded in 1897 in the Netherlands. Part of that service is the Sinai Center: The European Center for Jewish Mental Health Care and Psychotrauma Treatment. The center is particularly skilled in treating the consequences of war and violence on its Jewish clients. In fact, the Centre has expanded to treat Gentile victims of war as well, including former internees from the Dutch East Indies, victims of civil wars, and victims of man-made disasters.

The Sinai Klinick opened in Amersfoort, Holland in 1959 with 75 beds. An ambulatory service in Amsterdam was added to provided follow-up care. There are presently 57 ambulatory mental health institutions (RIAGGs) funded by the Dutch government. The Sinai Center's RIAGG in Amsterdam, with 25 staff, counsels over 1700 clients annually, many of them trauma survivors, SHOAH survivors, child survivors of war, their partners, and the so-called members of the second generation.

At the present time, the Sinai Center has evolved from an institution to a network organization, providing help to specific target groups. These programs eventually will determine the structure of the institution and its relationships with other institutions. One purpose is trauma treatment.

The newest facility combines efforts of the Sinai Center and Centrum 45, the Dutch center for treatment of members of the resistance and war victims. This cooperative effort will offer psychotherapy groups for the postwar generation of former Dutch East Indian descent, groups for the first generation of former Dutch East Indians, groups for part-time resocialization treatment for war victims, a group for the Jewish postwar generation, and groups for veterans and first generation war victims. A major focus will be child survivors of the war with single or multiple traumatizing experiences at a very early age, even preverbal. The objective of the program is symptom reduction and improvement of functioning, helping survivors place problems in a context from which new meaning may be derived. Treatment for these survivors will include individual therapy, group therapy, creative work (art), and social–psychiatric support. The service will be flexible, open, client-oriented, and allied with other institutions.

This information was gathered from a presentation given in June 1996 in Jerusalem given by H. I. Elzas, Director of Ambulatory Services, Sinai Ambulant Amsterdam. Assumburg 2, Van Nyenrodeweg 1081 GC Amsterdam.

BOND VOOR NEDERLANDSE MILITAIRE OBORLOGS (BNMO): ASSOCIATION OF DUTCH MILITARY WAR VICTIMS, GOUDA, HOLLAND

The BNMO historically has worked with Dutch veterans from World War II, the conflict in Indonesia, and the Korean War. Recently, the BNMO Veterans' Center opened its services to United Nations veterans. The strategy of the center is aimed at broadening its focus to begin to offer services to law enforcement, fire, and emergency medical service personnel. BNMO originally was created in 1945 as an association of members and was funded by private sources. It originally was created to provide assistance for veterans who were disabled and who felt they needed follow-up assistance after revalidation. The BNMO was created in 1983 and worked with veterans who had physical and/or psychological damage due to war experiences or experiences during service.

In 1993, the institute began to investigate and do research into the quality of the work of the center and a model for secondary prevention of traumatic stress as well as a health counseling model. The BNMO offers three levels of service to its clientele ranging from brief informational and educational group discussions and meetings up to 20-day programs for persons with readjustment and readaptation problems to fairly short-term residential programs to longer residential programs for persons with traumatic disorders. Funding for the programs might change somewhat in the future as governmental organizations are becoming more interested in the services that the BNMO offers.

Staffing

The BNMO has a fairly large staff of approximately 60 persons. Twenty of the staff are mental health professionals representing a broad range of disciplines (social work, activities therapists, creative arts therapists, sport instructors, physiotherapists, physician, psychologist, and minister). The center uses peers extensively in the initial marketing of services, in groups as corroborators of the need for and value of services, and as peer counselors. Peers try to build bridges with other veterans and service recipients. The staff of the BNMO did not have extensive training in trauma when the focus of the organization changed. However, a training program in basic psychotraumatology on a theoretical and practical level has been organized. By now, this basic training has been completed and a system for further education and staff supervision has been developed. Temporarily, for the duration of the government-sponsored quality project, additional staff members for consistency or quality, program development and health education are employed.

Clientele

In the past, the clientele of the BNMO were older veterans. Intervention with these older veterans was generally late intervention, while intervention with younger veterans can be given earlier in time. Another group of persons for whom the BNMO considers offering service is humanitarian workers or missionaries who may get some debriefing and treatment elsewhere, as well.

Theory

The primary theory base of the BNMO is a cognitive–behavioral model using eclectic methods of treatment. The model is adapted to individuals, couples, and groups. Much of the theory is provided to clients through educational group services.

Treatment Services

The first level of service helps clients cope with traumatic events through informational and educational means. The use of audiovisual materials, group discussions, brief meetings, and informal group sessions is of particular value.

The second level of service intervenes with persons who have problems of readjustment and readaptation. Among the services offered at this level are day programs and 1- or 2-week information and education programs that allow clients to stay in the center with partners and have a follow-up program 2–3 months later. Group sessions for the second level are cognitive and have a heavy training emphasis. The third level of service is provided to persons who are seeking to work through past experiences that are contributing to psychological disorders. Treatment for these clients is more elongated and includes an initial 10-day inpatient program, a 5-day program 6 months later, and another 5-day program at 1 year after initial participation. Some of these veterans have complex PTSD and need a different type of work for their serious problems; others have partial PTSD and also do not fit the specifics of the program.

In this program, treatment begins with the individual, moves to couples work, and then expands to group treatment and eventual mixed group treatment. The program includes some provisions for aftercare. The BNMO has a network of social workers who do outreach in the home areas of the clients. In the traditional model of service delivery, clients referred themselves through self-report. In the newer model of service delivery, clients also can be referred through a professional referral that institutes the intake procedure. Clients have an initial interview either at the center or in their homes before being admitted.

Community Services

Staff of the BNMO work with veterans organizations in the community. In addition, staff members are working with the Ministry of Defense of the Army. Staff members of the center offers consultation and supervision to humanitarian organizations such as Doctors without Borders and to other professionals. The center currently is planning to undertake research to measure outcome and effects of intervention.

TRAUMATIC STRESS CLINIC, LONDON, ENGLAND

The Traumatic Stress Clinic is a National Heath Services (NHS) resource and a national referral center for adults, children, and families. Affiliated with the University College, London, the clinic offers assessments, critical incident stress management, training programs in assessment and management of traumatic stress reactions, and treatment for survivors of traumatic events. The Adult Service, established November 1987, was awarded a national contract in 1991. It has been an NHS-funded facility since April 1994. The Child and Family Service was established in 1993 and joined the Adult Service in April 1995. The director of the clinic is Dr. Stuart Turner.

Clientele

The clientele of the clinic have been exposed to a range of traumatic stressors including assault, crimes of violence and extreme violence, domestic violence, and childhood sexual abuse. A large number of refugees and survivors of organized state violence and torture and a few combat veterans also were treated. Children with a primary stressor of long-term sexual abuse are generally not seen. Most clients meet the criterion A (DSM-IV) (American Psychiatric Association, 1994) requirements for PTSD, and many also exhibit symptoms of complex PTSD as well as evidence of enduring personality change. These enduring changes include distrust, emptiness, hopelessness, feelings of alienation, social withdrawal, feelings of humiliation, and changed attitudes toward the meaning of life. Clients are referred to the center by general practitioners, psychiatrists, or other medical specialists. They also may be referred by social service departments, attorneys, and guardians ad litem. Clinic staff also offers consultation to other agencies about clients.

Funding

The clinic is part of the British Health System and, as such, essentially is part of a trust (managed care system) with governmentally established budgets and contracts. Service contracts are applied for, for example, with a local health authority. There is a substantial opportunity for local contracts since services at that level have been limited. The budget of the clinic between 1994 and 1996 expanded from 75,000 pounds to 600,000 pounds. Events that led to receipt of funding for the clinic were the Kings Cross Fire, the 1991 Gulf War, and the homecoming of torture survivors from that war. Dr. Turner won a grant in 1992 to do research with those survivors and to begin the center. In order to provide treatment to patients now, approval from local health authorities is necessary before treatment may begin. The trust is given money on a case-by-case basis from national funds for those patients; however, staff are salaried.

Staffing

Dr. Stuart Turner, Medical Director of Camden and Islington Community Health Services NHS Trust, is also manager of the clinic. Dr. Dora Black joined part time to offer more child-oriented services. At the time of the interview, staff of the Adult Service included four full-time psychologists and psychology interns, three part-time psychologists, one half-time psychiatrist, a part-time physiotherapist, a child psychotherapist, a part-time family therapist, and a clinician/researcher. Recruiting for additional clinical (including a bicultural clinician to work with Bosnian refugees) and lecturer positions as well as a third administrator/secretary was envisioned. Administrative staff include a business manager and two full-time secretaries. The business manager function of Dr. Turner's role includes obtaining funding approval, completing administrative reports, recruiting, and training. Staff members are hired with permanent contracts for open-ended service. Dr. Turner does direct supervision with clinical staff members.

Clinical Services

Clinicians generally have 20–30 sessions weekly with direct individual client contacts. They do not do group work. Many clients also receive psychotropic medications. Dr. Turner does medication reviews for clients seen by the clinical psychologists. In the 1993–1994 year, services were given in 947 sessions; in 1994–1995, 1302 sessions. Clinicians take extensive notes during every session; these notes belong to the trust, not to the clinician. However, patients have access to their treatment files and the notes. Treatment for adult clients tends to be limited to approximately 20 sessions within the managed care system of health care. For some clinicians, one day a week is a research day and/or a mental health day. Four times a year, the entire clinic participates in a research week. Adults are screened with a variety of instruments including the Clinician Administered PTSD Scale (CAPS), General Health Questionnaire (GHQ), Symptom Check List (SCL-90), Impact of Event Scale (IES), Beck Depression Inventory, and Penn Inventory.

In 1993, Children's Services saw 100 children in 77 families, 160 children in 91 families in 1994, and 85 children in 61 families between April and August of 1995. Intense work with children, their families, and involved agencies operates primarily on a crisis intervention model. Family therapy explores the meaning and effects of trauma on the family. Meanwhile, after a six-session assessment, the traumatized child begins once or twice-weekly psychodynamic psychotherapy for a minimum of one year.

Treatment for complex PTSD in adults begins with an assessment session followed by a treatment session. The focus of treatment is changing the disturbed thinking processes that occur following traumatic events.

Theory

The primary theoretical orientation of the clinic is cognitive–behavioral theory with a major focus on modifications of cognitions/schema. Clinical work is more exposure-based with primary emphasis on cognitive restructuring. This approach recognizes that dealing with problems centered around the meaning of the traumatic event is fundamental. Reframing, giving testimony to reacquire meaning, and building understanding are important techniques. Research studies of treatment approaches, including exposure therapy based on deconditioning survivors of torture, presently are being conducted. The

Traumatic Stress Clinic is in partnership with the UCL Medical School to conduct this research.

Community Involvement and Training

Clinic staff network with other agencies; for example, staff go into the schools after an incident has occurred. Staff also offers training to other agencies, including members of the bereavement service. They do not conduct mediation. Some staff have offered expert witness services as part of forensic work. Trainings range from introductory courses on trauma to advanced clinical workshops. Some short courses run monthly. One major area of training is for counselors working with bereaved and traumatized children and families.

Debriefing and Critical Incident Stress Management

The center offers urgent treatment for recently traumatized people who have significant psychological difficulties, but it no longer uses the debriefing approach (Turner, November 20, 2000, personal communication). The earliest responsibilities of a debriefer were threefold: education (about stress, acute traumatic stress, and posttraumatic stress), reassurance, and screening. A two- to four-session model for group debriefing included an extensive amount of exposure to the traumatic event, offerd early intervention, and triaged those who might need more help. This debriefing process was salutogenic for most participants. Thus, debriefing was offered as an early intervention designed to normalize the response to a traumatic event that had occurred within the previous 2 months. After the initial 1- to 4-hour debriefing, survivors participated in six to eight sessions of treatment based on a cognitive–behavioral approach.

STRESSCARE, TAVISTOCK, ENGLAND

Stresscare is a British charity founded to offer support and treatment to sufferers of severe trauma. It is set up as an informational, educational, debriefing, counseling, training, and treatment organization of several geographically widespread facilities. The program, presently in formation, is expected to set up a pilot center in Plymouth by the year 2000 and in London and other major cities thereafter.

The model on which Stresscare is being built is a continuum of care model that is comprehensive. Decreases in defense spending and closure of operating military centers led to Stresscare's conceptualization, and after a 4-year period of development, its creation. This nonprofit charity eventually aims to have eight centers with outreach facilities forming a network across the United

Kingdom. As an oasis of calm, tranquillity, and a place of hope, any Stresscare center will be well-organized, safe, and professionally run by competent, trauma-trained staff. The common features of all centers will be competency, professionalism, accessibility, confidentiality, effectiveness, and receptivity.

Mission

It is no good to give money to rebuild bodies of those made poor and sick by trauma if a center also does not give the professional help to heal damaged minds and families through information, education, debriefing, counseling, and training. The aim of Stresscare is to offer support, counseling, and therapy.

Clientele

Treatment will be offered to anyone suffering from the trauma of an unusual and stressful event including military and emergency services; civil, marine, and air disaster survivors; sexual abuse and war atrocity survivors; and refugees and hostages. The program also recognizes the need to heal the family. The primary clientele groups, however, would be civilian and younger sufferers, with particular emphasis on sectors of the community who currently have not been sufficiently recognized. They particularly include younger members of the emergency services and other vulnerable occupations. Particular attention will be placed on prevention and information, alongside treatment and cure.

Staffing

Staffing of Stresscare will include psychologists, psychiatrists, social workers, art therapists, employment and training counselors, sexual abuse and trauma counselors, lay caregivers, and volunteers. Staff will have long-term contracts and be licensed/certified by the Association of Traumatic Stress Specialists as well as be members of applicable professional British institutes and associations. Medical care will be provided indirectly through referral. Supervision will be provided through a counseling institute, and the National Health Service and social services will maintain quality control and carry out evaluations. A group debriefing for staff will be held at least once monthly. Trustees of Stresscare are recognized experts in the field of trauma.

Funding

Stresscare is a nonprofit organization funded through lottery, millennium and European funding, and matching and government grants, as well as commercial and private donations.

Community Services

Stresscare operates with National Health, social services, and community trusts. Stresscare staff and board members will offer consultation to anyone in the trauma/disaster field who requests assistance. Stresscare will offer training and supervision in trauma and posttraumatic therapy to community professionals, lay caregivers, and emergency services/law enforcement organizations.

Theory

The theory base of Stresscare is eclectic; staff will utilize many different types of theory bases in their work.

Services

Through enlargement and enhancement, Stresscare aims to provide a civilian alternative to the existent services of Combat Stress, Royal British Legion, and other charities involved mainly with military trauma sufferers. Stresscare staff will provide individual and group counseling, psychotherapy, advocacy, political action, and lobbying in order to move traumatization into recovery. Referrals will come from other professionals (psychiatrists, psychologists, doctors, social workers, and designated channels for referral from other agencies), among others. Clients will be seen initially with an aim to set a specific end point of treatment, with 6-month and 1-year aftercare reviews with built-in support programs. All serious cases will be considered, with the nature and extent of trauma and PTSD diagnosed through clinical interviews. When appropriate, referrals to other agencies would be made, thereby creating a networking agency to link with other service providers in the various related fields of practice. Another eventual goal is to set up drop-in and help-line facilities.

UPPSALA ACADEMIC HOSPITAL TRAUMA PROGRAM, UPPSALA, SWEDEN

Dr. Tom Lundin and his staff implemented the development of the Traumatic Stress Unit as an outpatient clinic attached to the Department of Psychiatry at Uppsala Academic Hospital in Uppsala, Sweden in January 1998. The first 6 months essentially dealt with organizational issues, changes, and development; the actual program began in July 1998. The specialized unit is one of several subspecialty units attached to general psychiatry services (others include sleep disorders, eating disorders, and affective disorders programs). It is part of a University Hospital and therefore fees are low.

Mission

The mission of the program has several components. The first is to develop/collect a body of knowledge in the field of traumatic stress. The second mission is to give services to traumatized persons who are already diagnosed or have treatment-related problems related to complex PTSD. A third mission is to teach and supervise those staff working in the program and in the hospital as a whole as well as provide consultation.

Staffing

The staffing of the program consists of teams of 20 well-trained individuals who are nurses, psychiatrists, psychologists, and social workers. The program does not use volunteers. The staffing model the program is based on a model developed and implemented by Dr. Lundin in Stockholm, Sweden; this program had a staff of 15.

Clientele

The model program worked with refugees from war zones and torture survivors, as well as survivors of differing types of traumatic events including rape, accidents, and the Estonia disaster. Clients may come from all over Sweden and have been referred from their home clinics.

Theory

The program is based on an eclectic model of trauma. The best treatment includes biology and psychology together within a biopsychosocial theory base. It recognizes that traumatized people come to some kind of existential questioning about what has happened to them and therefore also involves some aspect of spiritual theory. The theory includes principles related to focused work, work with emotions, education, and debriefing. The model of debriefing used is a cognitive model developed by Erikson. Newer theoretical models and interventions such as EMDR also are incorporated. One area of theoretical concern is theory related to peritraumatic reactions. This includes examination of the situation around the trauma: before the traumatic event, during the event, and right after the event.

Assessment

Dr. Lundin and colleagues developed their own instrument, a self-rating scale called the Peritraumatic Reaction Profile Scale (PRP Scale). This instrument includes questions about dissociation, cognition, and life and death. They also assess with the Impact of Event Scale (IEC), the Structured Clinical

Interview for DSM-IV (SCID), and a personal interview. Of interest in assessment is the increasing number of dissociative disorders being seen. Diagnostic work is essential and must be carefully done, particularly when looking for biological markers in differing types of traumatic stress syndromes. Assessment also aims to provide a clear diagnosis of comorbid disorders. Assessments are done on an outpatient basis. If an individual comes from another part of Sweden for treatment, that person stays in a hotel. The average number of sessions for assessment is three (range two to five).

Treatment

Treatment is individually based and includes counseling, pharmacological intervention, and newer treatment strategies such as EMDR. There is no group treatment done at the present time. Treatment ranges from provision of traditional support, to short-term treatment in a dynamic, cognitive approach, to longer-term therapy. Art therapy will be implemented in the future. An important part of treatment and research is a careful consideration of the effectiveness of the entire range of serotonin-specific reuptake inhibitor drugs. The average length of sessions for EMDR can be three to four sessions. Psychopharmacology prescription can involve two to three sessions. Traditional psychodynamic, short term treatment generally lasts between 8 and 20 sessions. In general, persons with simple PTSD are treated at their home clinics. In many instances, the role of the clinic is to make recommendations for treatment and return individuals to their homes. The clinic staff also does not treat cases of acute stress. Hospitalization of clientele is rare; the only individuals hospitalized are those who are psychotic or actively suicidal.

Training

The program offers training to various groups in the community including emergency personnel. The intent is to develop training materials. Staff members receive regular training and consultation. Team conferences occur weekly for 1 hour as do case consultations. Staff members participate in a half day training conference yearly. The program also participates in the Uppsala Psychotherapy Conference Trauma Days, a yearly 2-day event. The clinic also has a mission to participate in community development and some kind of activity for professionals outside the organization and for the public. A final training activity is a week-long postgraduate training course.

SUMMARY

What leads to the creation of a trauma center? In many instances, it is the vision of one individual or a group of individuals. Dr. Tom Lundin illustrates this observation. He has brought his ideas and practices with him as he has moved from one city in Sweden to another. Designing trauma instruments, working with survivors of a large-scale disaster (the sinking of the ferry *Estonia*), and dealing with other trauma survivors are only part of his programmatic interventions. Many of the centers described in this chapter not only treat trauma victims, they also conduct research, offer educational trainings, and write for publication. Their efforts illustrate the ideal role of the trauma center: multilevel practice and intervention.

7

Centers Specializing in Trauma and the Workplace

Several of the centers interviewed for this volume deal specifically with workplace trauma. They are located in various countries throughout the world, ranging from the United States to Australia to Germany. These centers often provide crisis intervention services to organizations and companies, help businesses develop crisis plans, and work with management as well as staff.

CRISIS MANAGEMENT INTERNATIONAL, INC., ATLANTA, GEORGIA

Crisis Management International (CMI) consult with corporations regarding the human side of crisis/disaster and provides traumatic stress intervention, crisis readiness programs, PTSD litigation assistance, and injury-related workers compensation services. Prior to creating CMI, president and CEO Bruce Blythe co-owned the nation's first employee assistance program (EAP) business. Crises strained the resources of the EAP staff and they were not trained to work on-site with traumatic incidents. In 1988, Blythe and his partner sold the EAP business to AETNA and began Crisis Management International.

According to Blythe, CMI's corporate mission is to provide "high end, quality services" and "have the best network of crisis and traumatic event professionals in the world." What differentiates CMI's corporate crisis capabilities from other organizations is:

1. The caliber of people employed through their stringent selection process
2. Standardized, formalized training for consultants in crisis management and threats of violence
3. Capacity for very large, as well as smaller, corporate interventions

4. Unmatched availability of consultants in all 50 states and worldwide with both rapid response and the ability to stay on site
5. CMI's comprehensive "structured management response" utilized in thousands of corporate settings

Mission

CMI supports and advocates a workplace culture that conscientiously affirms the psychological safety and well-being of its employees. The goal is to promote prevention-based solutions to workplace risks, hazards, and crises that threaten work productivity and employee morale. To that end, CMI identifies measures, applies strategies, and provides intervention support to nurture the highest level of preparation for the "human side" of risk and crisis management.

Staff

CMI has a CEO (Bruce Blythe) as well as full-time employees (five clinicians, two office managers, a marketing director, and a chief operating officer) and hires consultants in 50 states and several other countries to work in the threat of violence and crisis intervention areas. The network of consultants consists of licensed mental health professionals and former FBI agents. Contractors are recruited at conferences, such as International Society for Traumatic Stress Studies (ISTSS) and Association of Traumatic Stress Specialists (ATSS), and many are certified through ATSS. Availability of providers all over the world with rapid response and ability to remain on site is unmatched and differentiates this organization from others. Approximately 350 individuals are available to respond to threats of violence and crisis situations. Licensed mental health professionals who respond to crisis situations are trained by CMI. Corporate staff provide quality control and work with consultants as a team in an open atmosphere.

Crisis management associates are part of an international network of licensed mental health professionals trained to respond to crises in the corporate world. Corporations have fee for service contracts with CMI to provide training materials, forms, support for crisis readiness training, and associates when personal responses are needed. CMI maintains an umbrella of 5 million dollars in professional liability insurance. However, each licensed crisis management associate must maintain personal professional liability coverage.

Services

Services provided by CMI include crisis and violence prevention planning, threatening behavior defusing, postcrisis trauma intervening, bomb threat response planning, scientific content analysis (SCAN) (linguistic deception detecting), crisis policy and procedure developing, aggression management training, and traumatic response readjusting. CMI consultants do not do direct, long-term treatment per se. Their approach is crisis-oriented and may last up to 6 weeks, as with Hurricane Andrew. Immediate response can be given 24 hours a day 7 days a week. The focus of trauma intervention and service provision is early intervention and may include successful resolution of a crisis with minimal disruption in the workplace, as well as individual assessment and referral to community responses. This rapid response crisis intervention is cost-effective and results in less time lost for employees, lower treatment costs, lower cost for medical treatment and rehabilitation, and less expenses for litigation. CMI assesses the need for services initially and during the course of intervention; in addition, CMI assists in planning appropriate intervention follow-up services. CMI staff monitor all services rendered under its contracts and uses extensive intake, assessment, referral, and follow-up forms and procedures.

CMI utilizes SCAN, which is an analytical/linguistic study of a person's words to detect deception or isolate language that is sensitive and shaped. SCAN relies on interviewing and the use of transcripts of recorded discourse. For example, recalling of information by someone is generally given/presented in the past tense. Deceptive information or information about sensitive issues are often given in the present tense. SCAN can help with assessments of dangerousness and can lead to recommendations for management action.

A major aspect of postcrisis services provided to clientele is group and individual debriefing. Revenue comes from consultations for corporations, government agencies, and other employers. The CMI "Postcrisis Response Manual" is a structured management response plan to address traumatic stress and outrage responses of employees affected by a corporate disaster. The manual answers questions such as: What do I do immediately? What do I do in the next few hours? What about tomorrow? How do I respond? The manual orchestrates time-sensitive delivery of a structured response after a workplace tragedy. Day one interventions may include psychological first aid, next of kid notification, crisis communication, de-escalation meetings, and family intervention. Day two interventions may include management briefings, group debriefings, and individual assessment. Day three interventions may include follow-up for at-risk individuals and back-to-work issues.

CMI may be called on to do a violence preparedness audit: "a structured procedure that analyzes and evaluates workplace violence risks in order to develop comprehensive controls and countermeasures." The audit has been developed through violence prevention and defusing experience with hundreds of organizations and analyzes risks, reviews existing controls, recommends new controls and procedures, recommends specific policies and procedures, presents an implementation schedule, and periodically reviews ongoing preparedness.

In situations with threats of violence, primary prevention sets up systems to prevent conflicts from erupting; secondary prevention occurs if a person is making threats and the contract employee of CMI helps to stop the situation from growing and/or escalating. Tertiary prevention occurs when someone has acted out a threat of violence and crisis interventions occur to lessen the impact through critical incident stress management (CISM) and CMI's structured management response.

The "Threat Response Team Procedural Manual" contains step-by-step procedures and options to assess and defuse threatening behavior. A structured format for documenting management actions is included in the manual. The bomb preparedness audit is a comprehensive analysis to identify preventive controls and management response plans for bomb threats or actual bombing. The audit addresses a physical security plan, a bomb threat response plan, and a bomb incident plan. Hostility management training presents skills and techniques that answer the question of how to handle an individual triggered into imminent aggression. This training presents "to-the-point" usable methods and strategies to reduce and defuse aggression and imminent violence without provoking attack, including verbal persuasion skills, spacing principles, and nonverbal techniques. Included in the training are brief lectures/presentations, role-play demonstrations, simulations, and imagery methods. Key concepts covered include, among others, managing and de-escalating anger, communicating with enraged individuals, the power of questions, provocation avoidance, persuasion techniques, indications of imminent attack, importance of physical stance and balance, and safe escape techniques.

CMI consultants may be called in after inadequate intervention has been done by other agencies or EAPs. CMI tends to take a more comprehensive look at situations; for example, 32 clinicians were used at one time by CMI in Oklahoma City to perform crisis-oriented activities (e.g., debriefings) centered around the bombing. The longest post-air crash on-site stay for consultants has been 6 weeks. As airline representatives disengage from a site, so do consultants hired by CMI.

Theory

One theory on which CMI operates is structured management response. Bruce Blythe has developed CMI's model of trauma response, which uses the Mitchell model (Everly & Mitchell, 1997) of debriefing to some degree; however, on the other hand, it has gleaned appropriate parts, tailoring the model to fit corporate settings. A systemic approach to corporate crises includes a structured management response to help individuals and corporate staff. The educational theory base helps management to "do the right thing" and uses ventilation and normalizing with individuals. CMI works with systems, not just victims, on a long-term basis. CMI already has contracted with two major insurers and is listed in corporate crisis and workplace violence response policies (underwritten). CMI works closely with most of the major insurance companies in the country in crisis response, violence prevention, workers' compensation intervention, and managed disability services.

Training

CMI has developed training materials for both crisis management interventions (postdisaster response) and threats of violence intervention. Training is provided to persons and organizations. Training for professionals who will respond to threats of violence and crises is structured and standardized. On request, CMI provides educational training and consultative services to selected organizations to set up crisis readiness programs. Other training programs provided by CMI include policy and protocol for assessing and handling dangerous person situations. CMI also helps organization design crisis management plans. CMI communications have developed videos for visual support for crisis intervention. CMI provides training in corporate crisis response and threat of violence consultation for mental health professionals.

CLAIMS MANAGEMENT INTERNATIONAL, ATLANTA, GEORGIA

Claims Management International examines psychological injury claims and does file review and analysis of those claims. Pamphlets about managed disability and workers' compensation are included in the appendices.

Research

CMI has hired a psychological research firm to develop a questionnaire to give at follow-up interviews. Research of the impact of work with survivors of Hurricane Andrew and the Oklahoma City bombing has been completed previously. At present, CMI hires a firm to do the actual research presentation of results. It conducts research as part of an intervention and at 6 weeks postintervention. Debriefed and nondebriefed persons are compared to see whether there are significant differences in recovery. In one study of government employees in Oklahoma City, respondents were tested 3.5 months after the bombing, prior to intervention, and then 22 days postintervention. Symptoms that decreased postintervention, among others, were thinking about why the bombing occurred (a decrease from 79% to 56%) and poor appetite (a decrease from 45% to 19%). Statistically significant symptom improvement occurred in 28 categories, for example, problems sleeping, depression, intrusive thoughts, and thoughts of death. Interventions for the employees included group debriefings, individual assessment and assistance, and follow-up.

OCCUPATIONAL SERVICES OF AUSTRALIA, EISTERNWICK, AUSTRALIA

The occurrence of traumatic events in the workplace is always a possibility. Occupational Services of Australia aims to help workplace staff reduce levels of stress and cope with marital/family conflicts, problems at work, finances, substance abuse, and other areas of difficulty. Occupational Services intervenes through an employee assistance program and promotes early intervention. Occupational Services is the largest private provider of EAPs in Victoria, Australia, providing programs to over 90 public and private organizations. It is the Victorian representative member of the Network of Employee Assistance Providers of Australasia. EAPs provide proactive intervention before employee problems adversely affect productivity. Occupational Services also assists organizations on all levels to enhance employee and organizational well-being and performance. Services include individual intervention, trauma response (debriefing and defusing), group intervention, training, consultancy and organizational intervention.

The organization was created out of a sense of turmoil after two psychologists were downsized by a governmental organization. Eight psychologists pulled this organization together because of need. The EAP components were founded first and the "trauma part" developed more recently. Fees charged to organizations fund this commercial organization. These fees are contracted annually and depend on usage. The organization gets no direct governmental support and is a private, for-profit, organization.

Staff

Eight full-time mental health practitioners are based in Melbourne, as are six part-time employees. Not all these employees are clinical psychologists. Two of the four psychologists primarily do training for organizations. Staff members are forging links with clergy to build a referral basis and organizational support. There is an appointed external psychotherapist who functions as an adviser/supervisor to the organization and who does training in critical incident stress management and debriefing. Every 3 months the staff participates in a 2-day workshop that includes marketing strategies, lecture, motivational exercises, and fun. The organization uses no volunteers in service provision.

Training and Community Intervention

Staff members of the organization train others in critical incident stress management. One training program is an intensive 5-day program. The training provided is based on the organization's own model of debriefing. A major objective is to train internal staff in organizations, not just get peer support from them. Director Les Posen has worked a great deal with victims of crime and has had some forensic work experience.

Clientele

The primary clientele groups of Occupational Services of Australia are organizations and the employees of those organizations.

Theory

The theory base on which the actual trauma work is based is primarily cognitive–behavioral with some psychodynamic influence. Mr. Posen has trained in EMDR and uses it in a very circumspect manner.

Services

Organizations contract with Occupational Services to provide EAP services, EAP services plus trauma debriefing, trauma debriefing alone, or critical incident stress management planning. The staff members of the organization recognize that trauma care intervention should begin as soon as possible after an event. Critical incident defusing and debriefing services are provided, if possible, within 4 hours after a critical incident. The debriefing occurs either on-site or off-site depending on the severity of the circumstances.

"Trauma at work" assistance consists of training/education of staff and actual trauma counseling in the form of critical incident stress defusing and debriefing. Defusing is the initial ventilation of emotional and reaction to a critical incident after emergency procedures are complete. Staff usually conducts a defusing within 4–6 hours after an event. Debriefing, a longer problem-solving session, generally occurs within 1 week of an incident if its need is indicated at the time of the defusing. Occupational Services has the potential to provide longer debriefings, off-site EAP counseling follow-up for affected employees and family members, and standard recontact with employees to check on their progress.

EAP counselors maintain a list of private practitioners for persons who need longer-term counseling and therapy. These psychologists are in private health provision; psychiatrists are part of the national medicine system. There is a need to track referrals, services, and maintain good records. Confidentiality of these materials is highly regarded. The organization also has "in-house" assessment instruments staff members utilize. Counselors may work at a larger company, for example, 1 day a week. Others work off-site. Services are provided in a flexible manner. Some organizations have on-site groups.

SIAM: GESELLSCHAFT FÜR SICHERHEITSTECHNIK UND ARBEITSMEDIZIN mbH (SOCIETY FOR OCCUPATIONAL SECURITY AND MEDICINE, LTD.), MANNHEIM, GERMANY

SIAM is dedicated to the prevention of work accidents and occupationally related diseases as well as the integration of psychologically (as well as physically) injured and/or handicapped employees through psychic reinforcement after occupational trauma. The primary focus is prevention of traumatic reactions in and care of employees involved in bank robberies, as well as firefighters, rescue workers, and chemical industry employees, as well as other occupationally damaged (Arbeitsunfälle) individuals. The organization was created because of the needs of laborers in general and bank robbery victims in particular. SIAM has provided educational materials for these victims. SIAM is an independent commercial organization for profit that is part of occupational medicine. SIAM does mailings and seeks referrals under the auspices of occupational medicine. SIAM provides acute help through defusing, debriefing, and counseling with trauma victims. SIAM also phones families of victims and plans strategies to avoid secondary traumas. Staff of SIAM believe that healing occurs in the context of a personal relationship between patient and the doctor–therapist. The services are offered as medical help because of the stigma attached to receiving mental health treatment.

Staff

Personnel of SIAM are physicians, psychologists, paramedics, firefighters, and members of rescue organizations. Some SIAM members are ambulance drivers. The teams are composed of one to six members, depending on the event. Team members are trained in the critical incident stress management model of defusing and debriefing and arrive at the scene "in ambulance style." Staff have no strict work schedules and limit the time of their engagement at the scene. New members generally are recruited by older members who tutor them. The entire team has been trained and is supervised by an American trainer in Europe. The head of a team is a trained physician; however, team members also change roles and the team changes composition to avoid compassion fatigue and stereotyping. Teams are encouraged to take sufficient rest breaks and have confidential talks to limit fatigue Members also can limit the extent of engagement since there is not a strict work schedule.

Theory

The model of trauma used depends on the character of the event and is generally cognitive–behavior or psychodynamic. Debriefing–defusing is based on the Mitchell model (Everly & Mitchell, 1997). The effectiveness of intervention is evaluated through observation of the duration of treatment and how persons return to their professions. The emphasis is less on the theoretical base and more on a "good restart" in life.

Intervention/Prevention

Team members meet with bank staff personnel who then go to the robbed branch immediately after the event. The meeting helps to educate bank staff about trauma and traumatic impacts. The team offers contracts to banks and endangered institutions to train their employees how to deal with dangerous situations through role-plays in their branches and also how to conduct debriefings and screen those in need for further help and support. SIAM responds to acute need. It presents a unique combination of medical knowledge, critical intervention knowledge, and personal experience of staff in critical situations.

SIAM offers some group and individual counseling, both prior to and after an event. Staff members can provide medications if necessary but prefer to avoid the use of drugs. SIAM maintains contacts with victims and with therapists and help-seeking victims. Persons who conducted debriefings maintain day and night phone contacts with their clientele. SIAM also trains customers and nonpresent staff members as to how to avoid secondary trauma. SIAM also conducts follow-up debriefings.

Thus clients include banks, firebrigades, rescue organizations, and the occupationally damaged (Arbeitsunfälle), as well as their family members. Victims pace all procedures and set time limits and end points. SIAM maintains client confidentiality from the workplace institution as well as other organizations (e.g., police). Communication with organizations occurs only with clients' knowledge and agreement.

SIAM responds in time of acute need and therapists provide for chronic need of clients. It is less important to arrive at a "right" diagnosis than to meet the victim's needs flexibly and to see to his or her welfare. Treating institutions give feedback to SIAM and SIAM staff leave the exact diagnosis to them.

Illustrative Case

A bank robbery takes place. The bank staff calls the SIAM team and the team meets at the bank's branch. Staff members sit next to victims who know them from previous trainings and stand with them during police interviews and possible confrontations with suspects. Staff members talk to the victims, and explain acute reactions and how to deal with them. Next, depending on the event, there are individual talks or defusing groups. Staff members give victims their phone numbers so they can call those members who accompanied them directly, day or night. If possible, SIAM staff members call on victims' family members and give them explanations and provide help. Staff members also provide care to the heads of the bank and try to help them with any feelings of uncertainty toward the victim. The team then schedules appointments for second and third debriefings.

Training

SIAM offers training to organizations as a preventive intervention based on the wishes of employers and needs of staff. SIAM has developed training criteria. Trainers have knowledge of psychological situations and the possible damages caused by a traumatic event. SIAM rarely offers consultation because single contacts with victims do not provide real help.

SUMMARY

Where do traumatic events occur? They occur in many locations, including the workplace. However, few centers are dedicated to trauma in the workplace. What conclusions can be drawn from this chapter? It is important to work with corporations and organizations to make sure that they have "just in case" response plans in effect. Most organizations will never have the need for a crisis response plan. But what if that organization is a public school? No trauma organization was available to spearhead the interventions after the Littleton, Colorado shootings in the spring of 1999. Only through the dedication and efforts of trauma specialists such as Carol Hacker and colleagues did the "work" of intervention get done and done well.

Many school systems are beginning to develop crisis response plans as a reaction to the rash of school shootings. Falls Church City (VA) public schools began their efforts prior to these tragic events. As school social worker, Dr. Mary Beth Williams has helped to create that plan. Judy Becker, Coordinator of Student Services, and Dr. Williams have worked to develop organizational charts, response protocols, and handouts for staff members and parents. The hope is that these plans will never be used: no teachers will die from accidental circumstances or sudden illness; no students will commit suicide, die in accidents, or be murdered; no major disaster will strike the school system. They recognized that, in all probability, something would happen to implement the plan. In June, 2000, it did. One Monday evening, an 11-year-old rode her bike speedily down a hill, slipped on wet leaves, hit the side of a van, and died. This event had widespead system impact and led to multiple debriefings and interventions. Then, the following Thursday evening, a senior committed suicide, again bringing the crsis team to action. These crises, though not of the scope of the Littleton shooting, had impact across schools and the community. Because the workplace was prepared with a crisis plan, the long-term impacts were lessened. Perhaps the message of this chapter is to include workplaces in the realm of consideration as necessary settings for crisis intervention. Traumatic events do occur anywhere and no workplace is immune.

8

Hospital-Based Trauma Centers

Many of the trauma centers throughout the world are affiliated with private or public hospitals. These centers offer a range of programs and services including short-term hospital stays to day treatment programs to longer inpatient treatment. A key concept for all hospital programs is the use of the therapeutic milieu as a tool in healing.

THE BENJAMIN RUSH CENTER, SYRACUSE, NEW YORK

The Benjamin Rush Center is a private, for-profit psychiatric hospital and is the first private psychiatric hospital in upstate New York to offer a complete trauma recovery program for men and women suffering from the "debilitating effects of severe psychological trauma." The program began in 1993 and is designed to offer services to men and women ages 18 and older in a safe environment. The program offers a comprehensive range of specialized groups and individual therapy along with expressive therapy. It also includes a dissociative identity disorder (DID) track designed to help patients restore their ability to function. The DID track is designed to help persons with severe dysfunctional problems and distress due to prolonged episodes of psychological trauma. The program includes a variety of individual and group counseling elements ranging from trauma education to specialized expressive therapy to family conflict resolution. All programs are presented in a safe environment designed to help victims end their cycle of pain. The program also offers a personal development program to help clients choose an individualized treatment program from the various components of the centralized program. Recently, the dialectical behavior therapy track, based on Marsha Linehan's work (1993), was also developed. Many patients with trauma histories meet criteria for borderline personality disorder and benefit from these skill training groups on mindfulness, distress tolerance, and emotion regulation. All patients are screened by clinical staff to see if they would benefit from this dialectical behavior therapy programming.

Dr. Karen Wolford was the clinical supervisor of the Trauma Recovery Program, which began in 1993. In 1997, Dr. Christine Allen became the clinical supervisor to the program and Dr. Wolford now serves as the on-call supervisor. The hospital itself began in 1929 and has a staff of over 300 for its 107 beds. The hospital is designed with safety in mind and has a therapeutic environment with gardens, open areas, and courtyards. It is the only such facility within a 10-county area. As of 2000, director of psychology Jack Wohlers, PhD, oversees the psychotherapy groups and trauma education groups developed to discuss symptom management of psychological trauma. He is available at 800-647-6479 for information about trauma education.

Mission

The mission of the Trauma Recovery Program is to provide a safe, therapeutic, structured environment for people to address psychological trauma caused by overwhelming life experiences. The goal of the hospital is to help each patient regain health and the ability to function in normal daily activities, giving them the tools they need to enjoy a better life by teaching them healthier ways to resolve future problems. The focus is on the "person" rather than just the "illness."

Clientele

Traumatic experiences endured by clients are not limited to sexual abuse. The program supposedly serves persons age 18 and up. Over a 3-year period, there were approximately 400 admissions and the length of stay generally was 2–3 weeks. Treatment is paid by private and public insurances, including Medicaid and Medicare. Referrals come from many sources. In addition, the hospital advertises its programs. Clients, however, actually range in age from 5 to over 65 and come from an area of 13 counties in upstate New York with additional referrals from counties outside the region. Most clients in the Trauma Recovery Program are adults or older adolescents. Officially, the children's trauma program began in spring 1996. The hospital also has extensive managed care contracts.

Assessment

Clients are given no trauma-specific testing. However, a trauma event screening instrument or Subjective Units of Distress Scale (SUDS) may be administered by unit staff. Further psychological testing is available on physician's order. In addition, the counselors on the unit, in conjunction with the treatment team, assess the appropriateness of each patient's participation in the trauma track based on the nature of the traumatic events, presence of posttraumatic or dissociative symptoms, and the patient's overall mental status and willingness to participate in programming that deals with their trauma history.

Staffing

The primary approach to treatment is the team approach. At the time of questionnaire completion, the staff participating in the Trauma Recovery Program includes a female psychologist, two counselors, and two expressive therapists, as well as a male social worker. In addition, a variety of hospital staff also were available to the program (RNs, LPNs, psychiatrists, and the program director who has a masters in nursing). Nursing students and interns may observe in the program. The program is supervised by a PhD psychologist.

Twice monthly formal supervision with the staff in the program occurs with ongoing informal supervision as needed. The hospital has experienced a period of restructuring in recent years but the Trauma Recovery Program has remained a viable track within a larger service.

Theory

The treatment model utilized by the program is Judith Herman's model of treatment (Herman, 1992b). The treatment methodology is primarily cognitive–behavioral.

Program/Services

The center offers a comprehensive range of specialized groups and individualized therapy, along with extensive therapy designed to deal with key issues in the client's life. This track is designed for adults 18 years of age or older. The center also had a partial hospital program. The program is designed to confront issues of stigma, shame, anger, isolation, and rejection. Clients are connected with others who share similar histories in an attempt to help them gain a sense of control in daily living. The partial hospital program closed after 1 year due to lack of reimbursement.

When children have been diagnosed with DID or other similar diagnoses, it is often difficult to design the "right" kind of program to fit that child's needs in the normal school setting. Among the goals of helping the child are to encourage participation in psychoeducational group sessions, to cooperate with a behavioral focus, and to work together with the outpatient therapist(s).

Within the Trauma Recovery Program are specialized programs and centralized programs. Specialized programs for survivors *only* include trauma recovery psychotherapy (individual and group), trauma recovery education, and expressive therapy to work through thoughts and feelings through the use of music, movement, drama, drawing, and sculpting. Centralized programs include Adult Children of Alcoholics (ACOA) groups and groups dealing with spirituality, anger, anxiety, assertiveness, loss, conflict, depression, healthy sexuality, parenting, decision making and problem solving, relating, self-esteem, chemical dependency and relapse prevention, and spirituality. Trauma recovery education helps clients learn to recognize and contain their symptoms and behavior. Expressive therapies help them work through undisclosed or unconscious thoughts and feelings. Persons who come to the hospital have the option of participating in a personal development program, the foundation of which is communication, as well as parenting skills and relationship skills. Other groups are healthy sexuality and sexual diversity groups.

Training

Staff offers training to professionals in a variety of workshops and aim to educate the community through the media (television, radio, newspapers). Specialty areas of training include trauma assessment and inpatient treatment of trauma. The organization has developed proprietary training materials and a curriculum. Staff also has developed a brief screening instrument for PTSD.

THE CENTER: POSTTRAUMATIC DISORDERS PROGRAM, THE PSYCHIATRIC INSTITUTE OF WASHINGTON, WASHINGTON, DC

The center offers treatment for adults exhibiting acute symptoms related to posttraumatic and dissociative disorders resulting from significant childhood trauma. The program is designed to provide rapid stabilization and essential training in self-management skills through a variety of treatment modalities. The center maintains separate inpatient and partial hospitalization programs. Located in a private, locally owned hospital, the center provides a continuum of care to its clients.

Mission and Goals

The treatment philosophy of the center focuses on personal empowerment through education.

The goals of the center's program are to:

1. Assess individual needs and determine focused goals
2. Stabilize and resolve crises
3. Identify and modify maladaptive coping skills
4. Educate patients in effective self-management techniques
5. Encourage increased levels of functioning
6. Prepare patients for rapid return to outpatient treatment

An additional goal is to provide education and serve as a forum for discussion and collaboration among local therapists, community agencies, and the center's treatment team.

Theory

The center uses a stage-oriented model of treatment for working with posttraumatic and dissociative disorders. This model emphasizes ego strengthening and skill building, facilitates maintenance of functioning throughout treatment, and helps clients make the best use of health care resources. Stages of treatment include (1) pretreatment assessment; (2) early stage of safety and stabilization; (3) middle stage of trauma resolution; and (4) late stage of self and relational development. Therapeutic work overlaps through all the stages and is done within a stabilization framework of pacing and timing.

Early stage safety is the most important stage of treatment in terms of providing personal stabilization and a foundation for additional therapeutic work. Most of the work done inpatient at the center is in this stage and is directly related to the client's capacity to function. Clients master skills relating to healthy boundaries, safety planning, contracting around termination and disclosure/confrontation, self-nurturing and self-soothing to modulate affect, modulation and management of spontaneous reactions and flashbacks as well as dissociative episodes, and understanding of the human response to trauma.

The middle stage of work begins only after stabilization skills are internalized and used as needed. During this stage, the client revisits and reworks the trauma(s) and processes and integrates traumatic material and affect. During this stage as well the client usually experiences pain and profound grief and needs the earlier-learned skills to provide the framework for the work. Additional support is usually necessary for the client during this stage.

Late stage treatment deals with issues of identity, relationships, intimacy, sexuality, and current life choices. Clients frequently develop a new sense of self apart from the trauma and deal with existential crises. They try to find meaning from the integrated trauma. This stage involves the exploration of new options for the future and is action-oriented.

Staff

The program's directors are Joan A. Turkus, MD (medical director); Christine A. Courtois, PhD (clinical director); and Mary Ann Dutton, PhD (director of research, program, and staff development). On staff are a variety of psychiatrists, psychologists, nurses, social workers, expressive therapists, and counselors to provide multidisciplinary treatment.

Assessment

Pretreatment assessment is comprehensive and includes attention to diagnosis within the posttraumatic/dissociative spectrum, as well as other diagnoses, current symptomatology, safety issues, and comorbidity (including substance abuse, medical illness, eating disorders, affective disorders). All five axes of the DSM-IV are completed. Assessment includes evaluation of current stressors and available resources before a treatment plan is developed.

Clinical Services

The treatment model of the center is a continuum of care with four core components: inpatient hospitalization, partial hospitalization, intensive outpatient programming, and outpatient groups. The presenting needs of the patient determine the level of services. The latter three levels of care are provided in the day center program. Treatment programs for clients are individualized, based on mutually determined goals. Treatment strategies are developed and reviewed on an ongoing basis. Treatment is based on a stage-oriented model. Treatment team members work in conjunction with clients' outpatient providers to support ongoing treatment. Attention is given to providing treatment in a responsive, flexible, cost-effective manner.

The inpatient program of the center offers highly structured daily treatment utilizing a cognitive–behavioral and affect-based approach. The program is grounded in a safe and supportive environment and offers 24-hour nursing care, psychiatric treatment, social work services, expressive therapies, and group therapies. The program includes multidisciplinary therapeutic groups.

The partial hospitalization program are offered through the day center. This highly structured treatment program is open Monday–Friday between 9 AM and 3:30 PM. It helps participants learn self-management techniques for daily living and facilitates progress in outpatient therapy. Clients participate in sequenced therapy and educational groups focusing on the development of coping skills. The program is flexible and patients and their outpatient therapists design the treatment schedule whenever possible. These services can be used as a stepdown from inpatient treatment. The day center can be used as a preventive intervention to forestall acute hospitalization.

The core treatment components of partial hospitalization and intensive outpatient programs are group therapy exploring the impact of trauma on past and present, and skill building for ongoing stabilization, expressive therapy using personal creativity to enhance therapeutic work, knowledge and skills groups as topic-oriented psychoeducational groups, self-management groups using containment skills and self-supportive techniques, and case management (one to one) to clarify patient goals and treatment plans and to coordinate with outpatient providers.

Some clients participate in the evening/weekend program. Clients in this program have moved beyond initial treatment and can maintain a level of stability that allows them to function in the outpatient environment. Groups serve as an adjunct to individual outpatient therapy and are designed to help participants improve general functioning and interpersonal relationships and address trauma themes. Participants are actively employed or are students or volunteer workers, are in outpatient treatment with a therapist willing to communicate with staff, are able to meet behavioral and attendance expectations of the group, and are without active self-harming behaviors. Groups offered include traditional group therapy, expressive therapy, and thematic process groups organized in a 10-week cycle around educational topics, coping skills development, and problem-solving activities.

Training and Community Involvement

The center develops training series for area providers that has continuing education credit. These sessions may be held bimonthly through the hospital grand rounds series and include guest speakers and discussion groups. Topics include domestic violence, family issues in the treatment of trauma survivors, psychopharmacology and posttraumatic disorders, healing skills for trauma survivors, and expressive therapies, among others.

SHEPPARD PRATT TRAUMA DISORDERS SERVICES, BALTIMORE, MARYLAND

Sheppard Pratt Health System was founded in 1853. The Sheppard and Enoch Pratt Hospital is a private, 322-bed, not-for-profit psychiatric hospital with a comprehensive continuum of care for treatment of people with trauma disorders. The Inpatient Trauma Disorders Unit is for persons 18 years or older who are dangerous to self or others, newly diagnosed and unstable, significantly impaired with PTSD or a dissociative disorder, and/or requiring inpatient diagnostic consultation. The 20-bed unit has private rooms. Patients live in a managed milieu to teach grounding and containment skills. They receive intensive individual, group, and family therapy, cognitive–behavioral therapy, vocational, occupational, and expressive therapy, and assessment and treatment of comorbid disorders. The highly structured program focuses on symptom containment and rapid transition to outpatient treatment.

Outpatient clinical services are provided for persons who can function outside the hospital setting. Services from clinical social workers, psychologists, psychiatrists, and advanced practice nurses include individual psychotherapy; group, couples, and family therapy; diagnosis and treatment consultation; psychopharmacological evaluation and management; agency consultation; and clinical supervision. Daily group therapy facilitates stabilization and includes cognitive–behavioral, process-oriented psychotherapy, occupational therapy, and art containment groups.

The trauma disorders day hospital provides a safe, structured environment for patients transitioning into the community after hospitalization or those who need additional support without inpatient care. This multidisciplinary program is a skill-building approach with team and patient collaboration. The treatment plans are modified by team and patient as the patient progresses toward self reliance. The day hospital operates Monday to Friday, 9 AM to 3:30 PM.

The intensive outpatient program provides daily late-afternoon therapy groups including cognitive–behavioral, process-oriented, occupational, and containment art therapy. It operates Monday–Friday from 4 to 5:30 PM. The Center for Trauma Assessment offers structured diagnostic interviews and psychological assessment for diagnosis and evaluation. It also offers reliability protocols for accurate diagnosis. Numerous research projects on phenomenology, diagnostic assessment, and clinical outcome for trauma disorder patients are conducted by the hospital in collaboration with researchers from the National Institutes of Mental Health, the University of Southern California, and other institutions of higher learning. Director of the Trauma Disorders Service Line is Richard J. Lowenstein.

Sheppard Pratt also offers child and adolescent services for trauma-based disorders or suspected trauma disorders. The hospital offers individual outpatient therapy, specialized psychological assessment, diagnostic and therapeutic consultation, agency consultation, and liaison with other child and adolescent services including the adolescent day hospital and the Forbush School.

The Baltimore, Maryland Study Group of the International Society for the Study of Dissociation (ISSD) provides monthly educational and support groups for professionals working with trauma-based and dissociative disorders. The meetings are held on the first Monday of the month. An additional educational forum for providers interested in children and adolescents with trauma-based disorders is the childhood trauma disorders grand rounds.

SANCTUARY @ FRIENDS HOSPITAL, PHILADELPHIA, PENNSYLVANIA

Sanctuary is an acute care, short-term, trauma-based inpatient therapeutic milieu utilizing a multimodal team treatment approach. The program establishes a balance between three fundamental patient needs: to be safe, to be nurtured, and to have clear boundaries and limits. This voluntary inpatient unit admits people of different ages, backgrounds, genders, and presenting problems. As a therapeutic community, Sanctuary offers patients an opportunity to learn about the effects of trauma and to rehearse new ways of dealing with interpersonal situations that are not based on reenacting the abusive past.

Sanctuary is managed by the Alliance for Creative Development (ACD), which is the multidisciplinary outpatient group practice and management company formed in 1980 specializing in the treatment of general adult and adolescent mental health problems. ACD currently contracts with Friends Hospital to provide the management and clinical team who operate Sanctuary, while the hospital provides the nursing staff and support services. Sanctuary originated when a core group of ACD clinicians recognized that a majority of their general psychiatric inpatients had a history of surviving serious trauma, usually child abuse, and that this exposure to trauma had played a fundamen tal role in the evolution of their psychological and physical problems. It became apparent to these clinicians that trauma survivors required a therapeutic environment that could be more responsive to their needs. This led to the creation of the trauma based model in 1986. ACD is funded by client self-pay, insurance reimbursement, and a private corporation, while Friends Hospital is a not-for-profit entity.

Mission

The mission of the Sanctuary program is to provide a healing environment for survivors of trauma. The program is designed to be a temporary refuge and retreat within which significant life change is encouraged, supported, and directed.

Staffing

The executive director of the Sanctuary program is Sandra L. Bloom, MD; the medical director is Lyndra Bills, MD; the program director is Joseph Foderaro, LSW, and the clinical coordinator is Ruth Ann Ryan. Staff members include board-certified psychiatrists, licensed psychologists, licensed clinical social workers, creative therapists, and nurses. The program uses laypersons, including program graduates, to provide information about needed program improvements. The minimum number of staff needed to run the inpatient program with 24 inpatients is five nursing staff, two psychiatrists, three social work care managers, three primary therapists, two creative therapists, and the program director. Each patient is assigned two contact people from the nursing staff, a social worker, a psychiatrist, and an individual therapist. The program director, medical director, and a nurse clinical specialist provide supervision. Inpatient staff participate in structured clinical management meetings three times a week. Outpatient staff also have regular educational, supportive meetings as well as an open newsletter.

Clientele

Patients are admitted to Sanctuary for the treatment of acute symptoms that have necessitated hospitalization. Suicidal thoughts and behaviors, self-mutilation, severe depressive states, eating disorders, continuing abusive relationships, overwhelming anxiety, and paralyzing phobias are typical reasons for admission. Primary victims served are victims of rape trauma, physical and sexual abuse, domestic violence, motor vehicle accidents, and medical procedures. Secondary victims served are witnesses of violence and/or family members of those involved with violent acts. Only 5% of clients are treated during an event/incident and 10% are treated during early postevent. Approximately 20% of clients receive treatment at the late postevent stage and the large majority (65%) of clients are more chronic and distant from the original traumas.

Assessment

Assessment occurs through a standard clinical interview that includes a multidisciplinary team approach coupled with trauma-based tools such as the Dissociative Experiences Scale (DES), Symptom Checklist-90 (SCL-90), depression and anxiety scales and a trauma self-report measure. Some case assessments include a neuropsychological evaluation, Minnesota Multiphasic Personality Inventory (MMPI) and Rorschach. Diagnosis for PTSD is based on DSM-IV and disorders of extreme stress, not otherwise specified (DESNOS) criteria are also used for an additional diagnosis. Comorbid diagnoses that occur generally include depression, substance abuse, dissociative disorders, anxiety disorders, eating disorders, somatoform disorders, and many medical problems.

Treatment

The context of treatment, the therapeutic milieu, is considered to be of primary influence in the Sanctuary program. Community meetings are held twice daily during the week and once a day on weekends. Psychoeducation, through formal group process and through repeated articulation of community norms, are seen as vital tools of treatment. Sanctuary uses a level system to help maintain community standards of conduct.

Many treatment modalities are used and are tailored for each individual patient. In addition to individual psychotherapy, these include art therapy, movement therapy, trauma art, psychodrama, cognitive–behavioral therapy, family therapy, video dialogue, conflict resolution groups, and stress management groups. Early stages of treatment are focused on reestablishing safety as the patient is helped to gain control of self- and other-destructive and compulsive behaviors that originate in previous traumatic experiences. Once safety is established, patients are helped to assimilate, understand, put into perspective, and integrate fragmented pieces of trauma memories, feelings, and thoughts. Reconstructive work is planned so that patients stop and redirect traumatic reenactments while grieving losses. In the social setting of the milieu the patient is encouraged to reconnect with fragmented parts of the self, the past, and the social group.

Therapy groups are an extensive part of treatment. Short-term treatments are tailored to the individual client. Outpatient options may include more intensive services (more than once per week sessions). Brief therapies, using the SAGE model for triage, are time-limited individual or group treatment. Most long-term treatments are supportive, although some clients with severe trauma and dissociation are seen for insight-oriented therapy.

Theory Base

Members of the Sanctuary treatment team share certain basic, trauma-based assumptions that Dr. Bloom articulated in her book about their work *Creating Sanctuary: Toward the Evolution of Sane Societies* (1997). These include the following:

1. Patients begin life with normal potentials for growth and development, given certain constitutional and genetic predispositions, and then become traumatized. Posttraumatic stress reactions are essentially reactions of normal people to abnormal stress. (Posttraumatic stress disorder)
2. When people are traumatized early in life, the effects of trauma frequently interfere with normal physical, psychological, social, and moral development.
3. Trauma has biological, psychological, social, and moral effects that spread horizontally and vertically, across and down through the generations. (Multigenerational transmission)
4. Many symptoms and syndromes are manifestations of adaptations originally useful as coping skills, which now have become maladaptive or less adaptive than originally intended.
5. Many victims of trauma suffer chronic PTSD and may manifest any combination of the symptoms of PTSD.
6. Victims of trauma can become trapped in time, their inner experience fragmented. They are caught in the repetitive reexperiencing of the trauma, which has been dissociated and remains unintegrated into their overall functioning. (Traumatic reenactment)
7. Dissociation and repression are core defenses against overwhelming affect and are present, to a varying extent, in all survivors of trauma. (Dissociation)
8. Although the human capacity for fantasy elaboration and imaginative creation are well established, memories of traumatic experiences must be assumed to have at least some basis in reality. (Traumatic memory)
9. Stressful events are more seriously traumatic when there is an accompanying helplessness and lack of control. (Helplessness)
10. Traumatic experience and disrupted attachments combine to produce defects in the regulation and modulation of affect, of emotional experience. Human beings require other human beings to respond to their emotions and to help contain feelings that are overwhelming. (Attachment)
11. People who are repeatedly traumatized may develop learned helplessness, a condition that has serious biochemical implications. (Helplessness)
12. Trauma survivors often discover that various addictive behaviors restore

at least a temporary sense of control over intrusive phenomena. (Addictions)

13. Survivors also may become addicted to their own stress responses and as a result compulsively expose themselves to high levels of stress and further traumatization. (Traumatic addiction)
14. Many traumatic survivors develop psychiatric symptomatology and do not connect their symptoms with previous trauma. They become guilt-ridden, depressed, and exhibit low self-esteem and feelings of hopelessness and helplessness
15. Trauma victims often have difficulty managing aggression. Many survivors identify with the aggressor and become victimizers themselves. A vicious cycle of transgenerational victimization often ensues. (Violence, anger, aggression, perpetration)
16. The more severe the stressor, the greater the likelihood of post-traumatic pathology. The same is true the more prolonged the exposure to the stressor, the earlier the age, the more impaired the social support system, and the greater the degree of exposure to or involvement in previous trauma
17. Attachment is a basic human need from cradle to grave. Enhanced attachment to abusing objects is seen in all studied species, including humans
18. Childhood abuse often leads to disrupted attachment behavior, inability to modulate arousal, and aggression toward self and others, impaired cognitive functioning, and impaired capacity to form stable relationships
19. Although it may be a lifelong process, recovery from traumatic experience is possible. Over the course of recovery, survivors may temporarily need safe retreats within which important therapeutic goals can be formulated and treatment can be organized
20. We are all interconnected and interdependent, for good or for ill. Safety must be constantly created and maintained by everyone in the community as a shared responsibility
21. The whole is greater than the sum of the parts

SAGE is a treatment model and philosophy that embodies the Sanctuary model of care and applies those principles to residential, partial hospital, outpatient, and self-help settings. SAGE is an acronym for the four important aspects of recovery that the Sanctuary team believe are the most important if people are to recover from trauma: safety, affect management, grief, and emancipation. People who have been traumatized have lost the sense of safety in their lives. The first step in recovery is to reestablish the feeling of being safe. This is always where treatment begins and recovery cannot progress until safety has been established. We feel emotions in our bodies as well as our minds and when people have experienced overwhelming stress, something goes very wrong with the ability to experience emotions normally as well as to the ability to experience the full range of normal emotions. Affect management deals with the stage of recovery in which people must learn how to manage their emotional arousal in a less destructive way. Grieving refers to the inevitable sense of profound loss, sadness, and despair that accompanies a traumatic experience and that must be experienced and worked through if normal life is to be restored. Emancipation encompasses all that goes into full recovery from trauma: social reconnection, finding meaning, and establishing a survivor mission.

This model is meant to provide a structure and framework for the evaluation and treatment of people who have been traumatized as children and/or adults. SAGE represents aspects of recovery, and, although Safety is always the first step and Emancipation usually the last, in actual life, these aspects tend to intertwine, interconnect, and present on-going challenges at each life stage. Future episodes of danger or grief are likely to reawaken old wounds. Therefore, the goal of recovery is to provide the tools necessary to guarantee that a person will be equipped to deal with future experiences without turning to behavior that is destructive to self or others. The goals of treatment for Sanctuary patients are the goals best articulated by Dr. Mary Harvey (1996): gaining authority over the remembering process, the reintegration of memory and affect, the ability to tolerate affect, symptom mastery, self-esteem and self-cohesion, the ability to create and sustain safe attachments, and the ability and willingness to make meaning out of the past traumatic events.

Research

Sanctuary is conducting research to evaluate and learn from its treatment programs. Research data is presented on the research and resource page of the Sanctuary home page (www.commex.com/sanctuary/sanc.htm). Currently, self-report measures are being used to assess the trauma-based therapeutic milieu approach.

Community Activities

The ACD is a multispecialized group of clinicians who provide outpatient general mental health care at five Pennsylvania locations. The ACD offers a wide range of therapeutic modalities and services to adolescents and adults. The clinical core group of staff at ACD has been together for 18 years.

Shrink-in-a-Box is the framework and standard for trauma-based telepsychiatry. It offers psychiatric consultation to any setting with telecommunications capabilities as well as consultation, teaching and supervision for the patient and caregiver. Shrink-in-a-Box also offers telepsychiatric treatment using video dialogue. Sanctuary Systems Consultants (SSC) is a group of senior Sanctuary/ACD staff who tackle complex individual, group, and system problems. They have provided consultation to several hospitals in the United States, Canada, and Great Britain that have sought to set up similar trauma-based treatment programs.

Staff does psychoeducational training and action-oriented training that gets trainees to participate in activities with staff (e.g., coleading groups). Training topics include how trauma theory applies to other venues, the implications of violence in society, and psychoeducation. Training standards are set by a senior clinical team. Staff offers consultations to individuals, clinicians, systems, teams, and families. They also give talks about violence and trauma within the community at schools and agencies. They have presented educational information to managed care companies and legal system representatives. Two of the group serve as expert witnesses. In addition, staff do negotiation/mediation with institutional systems including businesses and hospitals.

Needs and Contributions of the Organization

The knowledge base of Sanctuary and ACD needs to be increased and updated with current knowledge. As the knowledge base expands, clinical treatment methods also will expand. The program at Sanctuary has provided a nonhierarchical approach to looking at clients that is a unique. Patients are able to tell staff what they want and what they think as they help to design their own treatment. At the same time, staff and trainees have opportunities to get involved, participate, and try out new techniques and modalities with groups. Staff and trainees "switch hats" within those settings. The Sanctuary program hopes to expand the milieu to provide more opportunities to engage with peer and patient advocates.

Sanctuary has made a contribution to treatment in terms of the trauma-based milieu and has helped to standardize a model for treatment. The organization hopes to develop a more standardized treatment approach that is trauma based and could apply to all settings and patients. Clinicians at ACD and Sanctuary excel at the "hands-on" level. A shortage of financial resources in an ever-diminishing health care environment makes further growth difficult and even endangers the survival of this innovative treatment approach.

THE MEADOWS, WICKENBURG, ARIZONA

The Meadows residential treatment program helps patients develop a better sense of who they are and teaches a better way of living. The Meadows helps patients learn to face the world in a mature and appropriate manner. It combines intensive group therapy and other therapeutic approaches, including shame reduction and family of origin work. Treatment is guided by a multidisciplinary team and is guaranteed to be confidential.

In the 1970s, the Meadows originally was a drug and alcohol treatment center owned by a large corporation. It was recently purchased by a group of investors. Director of nursing Pia Mellody began to talk about the underlying traumas that drive addictions around 1979.

During summer 1997, Meadows developed a strategic alliance with an inpatient treatment program for women with anorexia, bulimia, and related disorders called Rosewood. Located near the Meadows, the program uses the therapeutic model developed by Pia Mellody. Staff of Rosewood can access services of the Meadows for family members, as well.

Mission

The Mission of the Meadows is to enter into a partnership with patients, staff, referents, and investors to provide the highest level of care through service, communication, and clinical excellence.

Philosophy and Theory

"Where recovery becomes reality" is the theme of the Meadows. The Meadows recognizes that chemical dependence is a primary disease and no other therapeutic work can be done until its process is arrested. The foundation of treatment services is based on the belief that most people who are suffering from chemical dependency, compulsive, addictive behaviors, eating disorders, psychosexual disorders, depressive disorders, and dependent personality lifestyles generally have been exposed to traumatic events, such as child sexual abuse. The Meadows investigates early childhood issues to determine the extent to which they affect the present addictive process. Childhood trauma often results in the impairment of the individual's social, occupational, and/or life functioning abilities.

The theory base and model of trauma is cognitive–behavioral and experiential as well as post-inductive. The latter theory is based on the work of Pia Mellody. In her book, *Facing Co-Dependence* (1989), she presents ways to deal with codependency issues by teaching patients and their families to build appropriate self-esteem, set functional boundaries, own and expand one's own reality, take care of adult needs and wants, and express and experience reality moderately (being in moderation).

Staff

About two-thirds of the staff members are female. Disciplines included in the staff makeup are medicine, counseling, psychology, nursing, and management. Staff need both professional training and knowledge and experience in 12-step work. All counselors on staff are themselves in recovery. Supervision for staff is provided by the assistant executive director, the director of counseling, director of nursing, and the medical director. Each department has its own quality control indicators. To prevent compassion fatigue, staff members are given time off with pay, accumulate earned time, and participate in outside training. Staff members are offered EAP services, family leave, disability insurance, medical insurance, a 401K plan, and extensive staff training in postinduction therapy, and sexual addiction and sexual abuse treatment.

Clientele

Clients to the Meadows generally have grown up in dysfunctional, less-than-nurturing or abusive environments and often have developed addictions to numb themselves. Although the program has approximately 70 beds, generally only 30–50 clients stay there at any one time.

Assessment

Assessment begins with a telephone call. Upon admission, assessment is done by nursing staff, psychologists, and a psychiatrist. Leisure activities, nutritional and spiritual activities are also investigated. Patients receive a physical and if indicated vocational, educational, speech/language, and hearing assessments. The nursing assessment is done upon admission. The health and physical assessment/evaluation is done within 24 hours. A psychiatric evaluation takes place within 72 hours and the psychological evaluation occurs within 7 days. Among the instruments used are the MMPI-2 and the Beck Depression Inventory.

Treatment

Through treatment, the patient beings to develop his or her own boundaries and ego strengths. The Meadows serves people for approximately 35 days. If more services are needed, patients are referred to an extended care facility. The facility offers inpatient services and a one-week outpatient program called the Survivors Program. In patient treatment utilizes group work, lectures, 12-step meetings, therapeutic activities, and specialty groups. More treatment in areas of sex addiction is being planned. A major goal of treatment is to help people grow up and take responsibility for themselves so they are no longer victims. Service run $750 per day for room and board, $992 for psychiatric acute care/detoxification, and $670 daily for intensive partial services.

The treatment team and nursing department makes triage decisions on how to treat clinically and financially qualified patients. Patients review their treatment plans with case managers and express any concerns in a weekly community meeting. Treatment is guided by the work of Pia Mellody and her postinduction therapy and Patrick Carnes and his treatment of sexual addiction. A variety of treatment modalities are used including individual therapy, lectures, group discussions, experiential techniques, and extended workshops.

Workshops and Training

The Meadows offers workshops to meet the needs of residents, alumni, and the general community. These workshops are designed to supplement the inpatient treatment program. Among these programs are the Survivors Workshop, a week-long workshop that investigates the origins of adult dysfunctional behaviors and issues through educational and experiential processes. In this workshop, participants get in touch with and resolve feelings following traumatic events in the past. The workshop has three phases: informational phase (learning about boundaries), debriefing phase (delving into and recollecting the past), and experiential phase (reexperiencing childhood in a safe and nurturing environment to reclaim power). Other workshops are Survivors II; the family workshop designed to help family members establish supportive and healthy recovering environments; the couples workshop to help couples explore difficulties and join together in recovery; the love addiction workshop that looks at compulsive behaviors of love addicts; the sexual compulsivity workshop designed to promote change in the lives of sexual addicts through experiential activities and specific tools; and the eating wellness workshop designed to help those with eating disordered behaviors.

The Meadows provides advanced training for professionals that teaches them to:

- Identify and address early childhood issues fueling addictions and psychological disorders
- Learn etiology, symptoms, and treatment of addictions and psychological disorders
- Learn practical applications of primary treatment modalities
- Apply family treatment modalities in a practical manner

The mission of the Meadows is to provide training in the use and application of Pia Mellody's postinduction therapy. The Meadows provides education as well as hands-on experience. In September 1996, Dr. Patrick Carnes joined the staff of the Meadows to foster quality scholarship and participate in quality scholarship, research, and training in the field of addiction and recovery.

Most students begin their training by participating in a survivors' workshop. This workshop is part of the inpatient treatment program and also can be an independent program. This workshop focuses on the first 17 years of life and on whether or not the years were nurturing or problematic. The second phase of training is in postinduction therapy. Lectures, discussions, and experience cover the etiology, symptomatology, and treatment of codependence using this method. Phase III of training is a 2-week period that is spent working within the primary group experience as an intern. The second week focuses on the family week experience. Students participate in small group discussions, observe dynamics, and assist in counseling.

THE COLIN A. ROSS INSTITUTE FOR PSYCHOLOGICAL TRAUMA, TIMBERLAWN MENTAL HEALTH SYSTEM, DALLAS, TEXAS; FOREST VIEW MENTAL HEALTH SERVICES, GRAND RAPIDS, MICHIGAN

The Colin A. Ross Institute for Psychological Trauma was founded in 1995 with three purposes in mind. The institute aims to provide clinical services to hospitals treating dissociative disorders and trauma. The program was affiliated with and managed the dissociative disorders program at Charter Behavioral Health's facility in Plano, Texas. However, in August 1997, the program relocated to the Timberlawn Mental Health System in Dallas, Texas, an academic hospital in operation for over 80 years. Added to services given by the inpatient, partial, and outpatient programs is on-campus housing availability for day hospital patients.

The institute continues program research that Dr. Ross has been conducting for over a decade and aims to educate the public about dissociative disorders and childhood trauma. Dr. Ross has noted in various publications and on video that approximately 5% of the general adult psychiatric inpatient population has undiagnosed dissociative identity disorder. The institute is a private corporation that specializes in the management of psychiatric treatment programs; it provides inpatient and partial trauma programs and offers numerous services including the designing, managing, and staffing of trauma treatment programs, professional training programs, educational workshops, a Speakers Bureau, and consultation services. The institute was created to contract with hospitals to run trauma programs in a cost-effective manner while providing high-quality service.

A second trauma program at Forest View Hospital in Grand Rapids, Michigan opened in February 1998. Forest View is a sister hospital to Timberlawn Hospital and is also owned by Universal Health Services, Inc. (UHS). Forest View also provides inpatient and partial hospitalization services for trauma patients within the trauma model focused on the problem of attachment to the perpetrator, the locus of control shift, and other core developmental trauma-related problems.

Mission

The mission of this new clinical treatment program is to offer high-quality, effective treatment to people with trauma-related disorders, to assist in treatment planning with referring therapists, and to engage in clinical research to refine diagnosis and treatment of trauma. The philosophical basis of this mission is that trauma is an etiological hazard in many psychological illnesses.

Clientele

Historically, the clientele of the institute generally have been survivors of sexual abuse. However, the institute also treats survivors of other traumatic events as well as the families of those whom they treat. The most underserved population by the institute are children and adolescents. On average, a patient is 35, female, and may be on disability (50% rate).

Staffing

Dr. Ross is medical director, creator, and owner of the institute. Clinical staff include nurses, social workers, licensed professional counselors, psychologists, physicians, psych-techs (part of the nursing staff with bachelors-level of training), certified recreational therapists, art therapists, and chemical dependency counselors. Lay caregivers and volunteers are not used. The staff use a team approach. The majority of staff are licensed and certified by their specific boards. The institute also has a community liaison/marketing section and an administrative arm.

Theory

The theory base of the Ross Institute is based on cognitive systems and psychodynamic principles. Most staff follow primarily a cognitive–behavioral orientation. Treatment is logical and follows a series of steps and includes many components of grief work. The programs of the institute are based on the trauma model of psychopathology that is medical, psychiatric, scientific, and biopsychosocial in nature. The core assumption of the model is that chronic, severe childhood trauma is a major driver of serious psychopathology, including dissociative identity disorder. Normal adults who are exposed to acute catastrophic trauma also exhibit a dissociative identity disorder symptom profile, but to a milder degree. Treatment is based on a trauma model of psychopathology that views serious, chronic childhood trauma as a major risk factor for many types of mental disorders. The theory base leads to a non-event-specific treatment approach; in other words, treatment does not look at, abreact, or deal with every single trauma event that has occurred. Instead, a more system-oriented approach is used. One theoretical principle that is addressed in treatment is ambivalent attachment to the perpetrator, particularly as a driver of dissociation when children must attach in order to survive yet try to pull away from the pain of the traumatic events. Thus, the only way to stay attached to an abusive person is to dissociate. The new treatment model proposes that attachment conflicts are the core cause of dissociation and the locus of control shift is a core cognitive error in victims of chronic childhood trauma.

The view of the institute toward "false memories" is that patients need to be responsible for their own thoughts, feelings, behavior, and memories. It is not the task of the institute to "validate" memories or conclude that they are not real. Patients are helped to sort out the reality of the past as best as is possible, but memory content is not the primary focus. The healing elements of treatment are in the process and structure, not in the content level. However, the institute has collected much anecdotal and some research data to indicate that repression of memory does occur.

Assessment

Assessment is ongoing, although an initial, thorough assessment is done at the beginning of treatment and patients are assessed twice weekly as to fit of patient and treatment plan. DSM-IV criteria are used for PTSD diagnosis. Comorbid diagnoses seen most frequently include dissociative disorders, depression, anxiety disorders, and substance abuse. The psychosocial assessments are usually done by a social worker; however, each potential patient is assessed by a physician before admission.

Clinical Services

The institute offers a wide range of treatment modalities including cognitive therapies and experiential treatment modalities. Cognitive therapies are designed to help clients correct specific cognitive distortions and cognitive deficits. Expressive modalities help clients develop awareness of self, recover traumatic memories, and work through emotions. Didactic interventions help educate clients about trauma and PTSD.

The Ross Institute also has a day treatment program, which treats trauma-based disorders in a day treatment setting and works in conjunction with the inpatient trauma program. The program includes a process group to deal with feelings, coping, and interpersonal skills; art therapy to express feelings, thoughts, and behaviors through artistic techniques; an education group; an experiential ROPES therapy using psychodrama; anger management groups; video therapy, cognitive therapy, recreation therapy, and individual therapy. The day treatment program provides structure, intensity, and supervision 7 days a week (if necessary) and allows patients to live independently. Stable patients are encouraged to use weekends for rest and skill practice. As Dr. Ross has noted, combining trauma-specific psychotherapy with standard treatments for true comorbidity is synergistic and results in better outcomes than either modality alone.

A psychiatrist leads the clinical team and sees patients five to six times weekly. Therapists also see patients three to four times weekly for individual therapy. Patients participate in approximately five different psychotherapy groups daily. Most treatment is short term. The inpatient program generally averages 17 days and the day hospital program averages about 19 days. Treatment looks closely at psychosocial stressors in patients' lives at the time of admission because people who have historical trauma do not typically come in because of the trauma; they come in because of system dysregulation due to some type of external stressor. Some patients may be seen several times over a 2- to 3- year period in an intermittent brief treatment model.

Community Involvement

Therapists are encouraged to visit the Ross Institute. While visiting, they are able to experience several of the program's group therapy interventions including ROPES, video therapy, and cognitive therapy. They are included in a multidisciplinary treatment team meeting, interact with staff and clients in the milieu, and receive 90 minutes of supervision from Dr. Ross. Visiting therapists also are given state-of-the-art information about trauma and its treatment.

The institute maintains a speakers group to provide quality speakers on psychological trauma and its consequences. The institute also provides consultation to many health care organizations throughout the United States. The institute has a website (www.rossinst.com). The Ross Institute also offers educational workshops, consultation services, and professional training for mental health professionals; also, it can design, manage, and staff trauma treatment programs in other facilities.

Training offered to professionals has specific goals and objectives and offers continuing education credits. Training materials have been developed and a training curriculum is in its formative stages. Educational programs are targeted primarily at mental health professionals. These programs involve the institute in the public domain.

Dr. Ross has developed a training video, "Treating Trauma Disorders Effectively, " which gives a comprehensive overview of clinical interventions with trauma patients and teaches advanced techniques for treating dissociative identity disorder, PTSD, and trauma-related depression, and other conditions through case examples, dramatic reenactments, and narrator discussion by Dr. Ross. The approach in this video promotes therapeutic neutrality and provides examples of the problem of attachment to the perpetrator.

The Future of the Organization

In 5 years, the institute hopes to be multifaceted, with a large research arm, an educational component, and a very large treatment component. The institute also may expand from being hospital based only to include more halfway or residential treatment situations and more day treatment programs that are not medically based. Its services will grow in the areas of research, treatment, and education, in spite of limited health care dollars.

HOMEWOOD HEALTH CENTER'S PROGRAM FOR TRAUMATIC STRESS RECOVERY, GUELPH, ONTARIO, CANADA

Since fall 1993, a specialty unit for adult survivors of childhood trauma has operated as part of the Homewood Health Center, a 312-bed psychiatric hospital in Guelph, Ontario, Canada. This unique intensive, voluntary program is the only one of its kind in Canada and offers an intensive 6-week trauma recovery program, the Program for Traumatic Stress Recovery. Initially, the program served only adult survivors of childhood abuse and trauma; it now serves anyone who is traumatized as well as family members, spouses, and significant others as secondary victims. This for-profit organization is the only one of its kind in the country. A combination of client requests/needs, program management, and potential for financial success led to its development.

Mission

The mission of the program is to offer a safe haven wherein healing can occur through specialized therapy within a community in which survivor helps survivor. The community creates a warm, secure environment for recovery. The mission also is to provide excellent inpatient care and to serve patients to the best of the program's ability in a client-centered manner while focusing on safety and empowerment. The goals of this voluntary intensive program are helping patients to create physical, emotional, and relational safety; to examine patterns of revictimization and traumatic reenactments; to reduce symptoms; to modulate affect; and (at times) to "metabolize" trauma.

Theory

The theoretical basis of the program is the work of Herman (1992b) and van der Kolk (1989). Their models of treatment recognize the impacts of early trauma on childhood development and the development of complex PTSD. One specific component of the trauma model used in the center is "traumatic reenactment" via maladaptive behaviors used to work through past trauma in the present. Traumatic reenactment, a modern reframe of repetition compulsion, serves as a daily frame for the existence of those maladaptive behaviors, viewing them as unsuccessful efforts to work though past unwanted traumas in the present. The program's holistic model of intervention is predominantly eclectic, incorporating medical, cognitive–behavioral, spiritual, contextualistic, and psychodynamic principles. Additional helpful theoretical models for the program are complex PTSD (disorders of extreme stress) and the therapeutic community milieu model as proposed by Bloom (1994). This latter model recognizes that social wounds require social healing.

Staff

Staff of the center is primarily female. Staff includes two program coordinators, two psychiatrists, and a variety of nurses, psychologists, psychology assistants, social workers, art therapists, dance/movement therapists, recreational therapists, occupational therapists, practical nurses, a chaplain, pharmacists, and an accessible family doctor. More of each staff category is needed.

The center does not use lay caregivers or volunteers, but plans to use persons who have completed the program as resources in the future. Supervision within the staff team is done by outside facilitators and peers. The hospital has a wellness program to combat compassion fatigue and the team have half-day workshops, as well. Staff had no specific trauma training when the program began and trauma specialists were brought in to help. The treatment team shares responsibility and accountability for treatment and nurses coordinate patient care.

Clientele

Clientele are generally in their 30s and 40s and are 80% female. They typically self-refer or are referred by a therapist. Most have chronic PTSD (approximately 90%) with comorbid diagnoses of major depression, anxiety disorders, dissociative disorders, mood disorders, obsessive–compulsive disorder, and personality disorders.

Funding

This for-profit facility receives basic funding for treatment from the provincial government. Profit revenues come from an additional accommodation rate for semiprivate and private beds. Third-party payers, usually insurance companies, cover the accommodation rate for the majority of people. The treatment mandate is currently limited to inpatient treatment due to these funding arrangements.

Clinical Services

Although a patient is assigned an individual nurse who provides some individual intervention, counseling is almost exclusively provided in group settings. Groups include a daily psychotherapy group; creative therapy groups of dance, movement, art, and spirituality; and educational and skills development groups that focus on grounding, boundary setting, self-esteem building, and safety planning. Patients also are provided medications and some advocacy services, usually with third-party payers.

The overriding principle of treatment is "safety first" within the community milieu and the general goal of treatment is to help patients create physical, emotional, and relational safety within the here and now. The program does not do organized memory work or provide debriefing services. It is a time-limited, 6-week program. After a 3-month hiatus, patients can return for another 6-week stay. Patients are admitted on a weekly basis. During the first 5 days of participation, they complete an assessment, which includes a mental status exam, relationship history, trauma history, nursing history, and psychological exam [including MMPI, Clinician Administered PTSD Scale-1 (CAPS-1) and -2 (CAPS-2)]. The assessment process lasts one week as program and patients get to know and evaluate each other.

To be admitted into the program, patients need to be group ready, that is, have the ability to function adequately in groups and the community. Each patient attends daily community meetings and weekly "wraps" as part of learning to develop healthy relationships and boundaries. Other requirements for admission include a preassessment review as to suitability, extended sobriety, and absence of extreme levels of dissociation. Many patients do need longer lengths of service than the program provides. In view of this need, the program hopes to expand and add an outpatient component.

The three main elements to the treatment protocol recognize that (1) healing takes place within relationships and, to that end, a community milieu has been established; (2) creation of safety in physical, emotional, spiritual, and relational spheres is paramount; and (3) challenging problematic behaviors that may be linked to past traumatic experiences that interfere with healthy living in the present (e.g., healthy reenactment) is a major goal.

Community Involvement

The program serves as a resource for clients receiving primary treatment from other therapists or clinics. The program is not strictly a local community resource and has participants from an international community base. Staff offers informal consultation to others within the hospital but not to outside agencies. Staff is beginning to be involved in community advocacy/social change. A joint project with the program and outside agencies developing prevention strategies and seamless service for violence against women has just been funded by the government. In addition, the program has started to train therapists from other communities.

Research

Upon admission, over 90% of patients qualify for a PTSD-positive diagnosis. At discharge, 45% do not meet threshold criteria and 87% report improvement in symptoms. In a study of 114 participants (13 males and 101 females) with a PTSD-positive diagnosis on the CAPS-1 who were tested at admission and discharge, 54 (5 males and 49 females) also participated in a 3-month follow-up study. Measures of dissociation, hopelessness, depression, anxiety, anger, and self-esteem as well as the Symptom Checklist-90 (SCL-90) were administered. Participants who met CAPS-1 criteria then took the CAPS-2 to establish current PTSD symptoms. The CAPS-2 and other measures were given upon treatment completion as well as 3 months postdischarge. Of the 96 persons who completed the CAPS-2, 40 (38.4%) no longer met PTSD threshold scores upon completion of the program. Participants also reported a significant decrease in depression, anger, hopelessness, dissociation, and anxiety. However, treatment gains were not maintained at 3 months postdischarge, although most measures maintained statistical significance. The CAPS-2 was not administered at this time; therefore, there are no results on whether PTSD symptoms also continued to be reduced. A 1-year follow-up using Briere's Trauma Symptom Inventory (TSI) is being conducted as well (Briere, 1995). Results suggest that symptom reduction can be achieved through stabilization by a present-centered treatment focus that strengthens skills to respond to current needs. The program has now attracted the research interest of several local universities and collaborative projects focusing on quality of life outcomes have been started.

In an additional study, 134 participants (19 males and 115 females), 20–56 years of age, volunteered for admission versus discharge phase of the study. Sixty-five participants continued at 3 months postdischarge; 69 participated at 1 year postdischarge. These participants completed the CAPS, the Symptom Checklist-90 Revised (SCL-90-R), TSI, and a survey questionnaire providing information about significant life changes, suicidal behaviors, hospital admissions, and available support networks. The objective of this study was to assess whether treatment gains were maintained over time (admission, discharge, 3 months postdischarge, 1 year postdischarge) and whether frequency and intensity of symptoms decreased by participation in the program. For 46.09% of the respondents, symptoms did not meet frequency and intensity for diagnosis of PTSD upon completion of the program (all were PTSD positive at admission). The majority of participants had supportive connections within their home communities. The results suggested that participation in the program effectively reduced the frequency and intensity of PTSD symptoms through stabilization and by taking a present-centered focus.

TICEHURST HOUSE HOSPITAL TRAUMA CENTER, NORTH WADHURST, EAST SUSSEX, UNITED KINGDOM

This 3-year-old program is a brief group-treatment format, with an initial highly structured residential phase followed by one year of support with three standard group reviews at 6 weeks, 6 months, and 12 months. Patients in the program are located in a separate building from the main hospital in order to enhance a rehabilitation atmosphere, to depathologize and normalize treatment. The program at Ticehurst represents experience-led developments to an original similar program run in the Royal Air Force beginning in 1991, following the Gulf War. The program has been published in an article by Busuttil et al. (1995).

Mission

The mission of the program is to restore control and a sense of independence to persons who have experienced a loss of control and loss of independence after traumatic events. All participants currently suffer from PTSD

(DSM-IV criteria). The main strategy of the mission is the cognitive and emotional processing of traumatic memories.

Clientele

Between four to six persons, male and/or female, ranging in age from 18 to 70 plus, participate in the closed program at one time. No children are included in the program. Clients come mainly from the United Kingdom; others have originated from other English-speaking countries. They have experienced traumatic events across the entire range of road traffic accidents, assaults, and attacks. Clients generally are not diagnosed with complex PTSD.

Theory

The Ticehurst House Hospital program uses a systems approach that is biopsychosocial in orientation. PTSD is conceptualized as a survival adaptation based on traumatic memories that have become blocked or inaccessible, usually in individuals with strong psychological defenses (avoidance). Just as early processing of the traumatic memory complex usually results in good outcomes, the expectation is that delayed processing also should lead to considerable recovery or personal development. Debriefing, using the standard format of Mitchell/Dyregrov (Everly & Mitchell, 1997), is used during the initial phase of the residential program in an attempt to revitalize memories of the critical incident. It demystifies what happens after an event, looks at feelings, provides explanations, and uses humor.

Staffing

The clinical director of the program is Dr. Gordon Turnbull. Currently, the program also had three primary debriefers, three doctors who offer support debriefing for the primary debriefers, a part-time relaxation therapist, and two secretarial staff. One of the three primary debriefers is a registered psychiatric nurse; one, a retired police inspector; and another, a trained group analyst from the Tavistock school. The program hopes to have a psychologist and a social worker on staff and will have another consultant psychiatrist shortly.

Clinical Services

The program is a 2-week program. Leaders review previous groups and "catch up" on other duties including writing and research during intervals between groups. Only one group participates at one time.

Since January 1997, Ticehurst House Hospital also has offered treatments for complex PTSD. The unit philosophy embraces the DSM-IV category of PTSD, acknowledges the proposed category of DESNOS, and addresses the results of chronic traumatization by emphasizing the value of a combination of educational and treatment approaches. Individuals suffering from complex PTSD are individually assessed before admission to the highly structured 60- to 90-day residential program. A therapeutic community milieu with focus on rehabilitation, restoration of normality, insight formation, and education is the aspiration of the program. Complex PTSD issues and symptoms are visualized as the result of repetitive injury rather than psychiatric illness. Individual and group follow-up are available; however, the emphasis is on completion of major therapeutic goals within the residential phase of the program. Cognitive–behavioral techniques are used throughout and progress in the residential phase as well as eventual outcome are monitored. This program is unique and is offered only within the United Kingdom at this time.

Phases of Treatment for the Regular Program

Phase 1 provides assessment using a thorough clinical interview. In that interview, candidates to the program are evaluated for their suitability to group work, their motivation to work, and their trauma history. They take several psychological tests including the General Health Questionnaire (GHQ-28), the Impact of Event Scale (IES), the Beck Depression Scale, and the CAPS. They also complete questionnaires about intimacy and relationships, and caffeine, alcohol, and tobacco usage.

Phase 2 introduces the participants to the group. There are two 5-day modules with a weekend off. The first day includes trust exercises to build bonds in the group and emphasizes why group members are there. The format has a strong educational element and teaches the "Ticehurst concept" of PTSD. By the middle of the second week, a group has developed and members seem able to talk in new ways. Each member also has an individual meeting the first afternoon of the program, at the end of the first week, and in the middle of the second week.

Phase 3 is the debriefing phase. During this phase, group members present their personal accounts of their traumas. The two debriefers assigned to the group listen actively and serve as facilitators and catalysts. Each member of the group is given half a day to present his or her history. The sharing of traumas also builds strong bonds between group members.

Phase 4 is called the "lines" phase. Each member presents a chronological map of his or her life and identifies positive and/or negative events that have occurred. Each event is rated as positive or negative on a 1–5 Likert scale. The participant also identifies coping skills used to overcome these events. This exercise identifies significant past life events and the pattern of characteristic coping strategies used. Upon completing "lines," group members share them and receive peer appraisal of coping mechanisms, issues, and patterns. Members trade coping skills with one another and group members do not tolerate ducking issues by one another.

Phase 5 is the "ladders" phase in which members construct a ladder depicting realistic ambitions. The lowest rung represents the lowest point of an individual's life, rung 2 is chosen to be where the individual perceives he or she is now, and rung 3 represents the top ambition of where the individual wants to be. The member puts in other rungs in the middle.

Close relatives are encouraged to visit and receive education. Many have secondary PTSD. Individual therapy may be provided, depending on geographical factors. Those out of area who need individual therapy are linked to appropriate therapists back home. Other therapeutic services include aromatherapy and recreational exercise daily.

Assessment

Members are assessed at 6 weeks, 6 months, and 1 year both in a group meeting and in individual assessments with the same two debriefers who participated in the initial group.

Funding

Ticehurst House Hospital is a private hospital. Persons who participate in the program either are funded through private medical insurance or through interim payments as part of a compensation program or postsettlement packages after legal adjudication. Health authorities through extra contract referrals may buy extra services as part of health packages, as well. The all-inclusive cost of the program is approximately $5500 (3800 pounds). Some clients are referred by their general practitioner. Others are referred by corporations (e.g., the British Broadcasting Corporation) and the military, emergency medical services and law enforcement organizations.

Research

Results of a study of 34 Gulf War veteran subjects at the Royal Air Force Wroughton Post-Traumatic Stress Disorder Rehabilitation Programme that used a similar treatment protocol revealed a high significant global response to treatment. At 1-year posttreatment, 85.3% of the subjects no longer met PTSD-positive (DSM-III-R) criteria in veterans who had been diagnosed through a comprehensive assessment protocol. At 6-weeks follow-up, improvement had occurred in most subjects. The findings strongly endorsed the use of psychological debriefing in the treatment of PTSD even if the debriefing was implemented well after traumatic exposure and was used with individuals who had been traumatized by different stressors. Addressing coping mechanisms within the treatment process also was probably important in relapse prevention.

Training

Staff provides training in nonmodular format to a variety of groups including health professionals, lawyers, law enforcement, and emergency medical services personnel. Training presents the Ticehurst model of PTSD and suggests interventions. The facility has provided training to Broadmoor Prison Hospital service workers, emergency services in Sussex, the Metropolitan Police Service, and the Wiltshire Health Authority, the last by helping to develop a disaster-planning program. Education also is provided to staff.

SUMMARY

Hospital-based trauma programs have been greatly impacted by managed care (particularly in the United States) and limitations imposed by insurance companies. No longer are there weeks-long inpatient stays for traumatized individuals (in the United States); Unless a person is flagrantly suicidal, the goal seems to be to manage symptoms, medicate, and then move the patient out. The primary approach to care is an approach that focuses on quick management of acute symptoms to save money combined with some education and, in some programs, emphasis on empowerment. Financial issues have forced trauma centers to change programs and even philosophies.

Many hospital-based trauma centers do continue to offer a continuum of care that ranges from inpatient treatment, to partial hospitalization, to day treatment, to outpatient follow-up. These programs, because of their "24–7" nature, offer many opportunities for research, differential diagnosis, and long-term follow-up. There is no better setting to study the impact of (as well as the development and implementation of) the therapeutic milieu. Perhaps, as the pendulum of health care provision swings away from an emphasis on provision of brief therapy, the allowable length of stay in hospital-based trauma centers will increase. Hospital-based centers can do much more than stabilize, prescribe, and manage acute symptoms. What better place to process the terrors of the past than in the safety-based contained environment of a hospital-based trauma center? Americans in particular should take note of the Ticehurst House Hospital model and its longer-term emphasis on follow-up and care. It is a model for extended treatment of complex PTSD, as it combines a 2-week intensive inpatient stay with periodic reassessment.

9

Centers for Holocaust Survivors and Their Families

Before there was Vietnam, before there were connections made between trauma and sexual abuse, before any of the *Diagnostic and Statistical Manuals* wrote about trauma and posttraumatic stress, Holocaust survivors and their families were experiencing the long-term aftereffects of their horrendous experiences. Yael Danieli's research (1988, 1998) and work with survivors and their families was the impetus for others and gave the prototype for survivor-related programs. Several of these programs are described in this chapter.

GROUP PROJECT FOR HOLOCAUST SURVIVORS AND THEIR CHILDREN, NEW YORK, NEW YORK

The Group Project for Holocaust Survivors and Their Children was established formally in 1975 by volunteer psychotherapists in the New York City area. It was cofounded by Yael Danieli and Lisette Lamon Fink. Like many other survivors, Ms. Lamon Fink, originally from the Netherlands, died of cancer, prematurely, in 1982. The project was created to counteract the profound sense of isolation and alienation among Holocaust survivors and their children and compensate for their neglect by the mental health professionals who typically participated in the conspiracy of silence that existed between survivors, their children, and society since the end of World War II. It was not intended to be a mental health facility; the name was thus chosen to be without mental health connotation.

The project gives survivors and their children the opportunity to share and reflect on their memories and experiences, past and present, in individual, family, group, and community settings. It capitalizes on group and community therapeutic modalities and provides individuals with a sense of extended family and community. It also provides mutual support to counteract the sense of alienation and isolation among victims/survivors.

193

The Group Project has developed a national and international network with similar initiatives in Los Angeles (California), Paris (France), Germany, Israel, and other locations. It is a living community in that it responds to many of the complex life needs of its membership.

Mission and Goals

The mission of the Group Project is threefold: (1) to help survivors and their children share, articulate, and integrate past and present concerns into their lives in a meaningful way; (2) to train professionals to work with Holocaust survivors and their children, as well as victims/survivors of other traumata; and (3) to make the concerns of survivors known both to the general population and to the mental health community.

The goals of the Group Project are preventive and reparative. They rest on the assumptions that:

1. The integration of Holocaust experiences into the totality of survivors' and their children's lives and awareness of the meaning of post-Holocaust adaptational styles liberates them from the trauma of the Holocaust and facilitates mental health and self-actualization
2. Awareness of transmitted intergenerational processes inhibits transmission of pathology to succeeding generations, since children of survivors consciously and unconsciously have absorbed their parents' Holocaust experiences into their lives

The ultimate goal of treatment of Holocaust survivors and their children is psychological/internal liberation from the trauma of victimization and its effects. The central therapeutic goal of integrating rupture, discontinuity, and disorientation informs the diagnostic and therapeutic choice of constructing a multigenerational family tree. Integration is the central and guiding dynamic principle; that is, integration of the trauma into the life span so that it becomes a meaningful part of the survivor's and the survivor's offspring's identity, hierarchy of values, and orientation of living.

Staffing

A great deal of the administrative work of the Group Project is voluntary. There are numerous volunteer groups within the Group Project. Some do administrative duties; others do home and hospital visiting. At the height of its influence, the project had between 12 and 15 participating clinicians in New York City alone. Each member of the network has seen patients in his or her own offices and charges a fee.

Theory Base

The ultimate goal of treatment is psychological/internal liberation from the trauma of victimization and its effects. Integration is the central and guiding dynamic principle. The task of therapy is to help survivors and their children achieve integration of an experience that has halted the normal flow of life. Integration and recovery, at least at the cognitive level, involve developing a realistic perspective of what happened, by whom, to whom, and the acceptance of the reality that it happened the way it did; what was not under one's control and what could not be and why. The theory (Danieli, 1988, 1998) recognizes that two other tasks are to counteract psychological aloneness and reestablish and maintain a sense of belongingness and familial/social/cultural continuity.

A major tenet of the theory is the intergenerational perspective. This perspective reveals the impact of trauma, its contagion, and repeated patterns within the family. It may help explain certain behavior patterns, symptoms, roles, and values adopted by family members of Holocaust survivors, as well as job choices, sources of vulnerability, and sources of resilience and strength. From this family systems perspective, what happened in one generation affects what happens in the younger generation, though the actual behavior may take a variety of forms. The trauma and its impact may be passed down as the family legacy even to children born after the trauma. Other theoretical concerns are issues related to aging and countertransference.

Clinical Services

The group modality has a unique reparative and preventive value in meeting the needs of survivors and their children. Group and community therapeutic modalities serve to counteract a sense of alienation and isolation and affirm the central role of "we-ness" in their identity as victim/survivors and the need for a collective search for meaningful responses to their experiences. By participating in groups, survivors and offspring who were plagued by mistrust and the feeling that nobody who had not undergone the same experiences could "really understand" them could at last talk about their memories and experiences. The group gives opportunities to express, name, verbalize, and modulate feelings. It is a safe way for members to explore fantasies, to take on roles of murdered relatives or victimizers, to observe and identify victimization-derived behaviors in themselves and others, and to use peer clarification, confrontation, and interpretation for change. It also is a forum to test out new behaviors and receive feedback. The group modality also is helpful to compensate for countertransference reactions. The group functions as an ideal absorptive entity for abreaction and catharsis of emotions, especially negative ones, that are otherwise experienced as uncontainable.

The Group Project provides individual, family, group, and intergenerational community assistance in a variety of noninstitutional settings. Each prospective participant is interviewed to determine the appropriate therapeutic modality. Many choose to combine a variety of modalities. The project has opportunities to participate in a variety of types of therapy as well as self-help groups:

1. *Awareness or rap groups.* These groups are attended separately by survivors, their children, and both generations. They meet weekly with trained leaders for 6–8 weeks. Their goal is to help participants become aware of and to share common experiences. The group may disband at the end of the time period or may continue as a self-help or therapy group.
2. *Self-help or kinship group.* These groups are open-ended and have no leader. Members may not work though complex issues of power versus helplessness because they are leaderless. Instead, the groups support participants in conducting oral history interviews with their families. These aid in learning more about the Holocaust and in discussing and acting on sociocultural and political issues. They also have social and cultural events.
3. *Long-term therapy groups.* These groups usually have seven to nine members who meet weekly for an indefinite period.
4. *Mixed groups.* These groups are attended by both survivors and children of survivors, but not from the same families, who may find it impossible to communicate with members of their own families.
5. *Family groups.* Family members address and work through family issues.
6. *Multiple family groups.* In these groups, more than one survivor family addresses intrafamilial issues. The group meets until satisfactory progress is achieved.
7. *Intergenerational community meetings.* Every 2 months the Project invites all group participants, their families, and newcomers to share mutual past and present concerns. These meetings actively encourage and substantiate the sense of community. At them, volunteers are assigned to visit the ill and comfort those who are troubled. There also is a phone network. The group also mourns and commemorates those who have recently died and congratulates and celebrates members' achievements. The meetings allow participants to take their time to open up, to listen, to learn from others, and to experience personal reactions. The meetings offer a safe opportunity for social learning.

Project members participate in individual therapy. Although the expression of intense negative emotions is more threatening in individual than in group therapy, individual therapy gives a safer place to express, explore, and work though parts of themselves that are secretive, embarrassing, or shameful before those parts are shared in the group. Persons who need individual therapy are referred through the Group Project.

Training and Community Service

The Group Project actively takes part in the functions of other related organizations. It provides training/supervision seminars for professionals who work with all victimized populations. The project also educates the community at large through speaking engagements and media presentations.

The project has kept an ongoing data bank including written and oral recordings of almost all its activities. This data bank has been the source of many publications. There are thousands of hours of taped treatment sessions and training seminars that await transcription in order to complete a systematic program of research.

Dr. Danieli is a founder and past president of International Society for Traumatic Stress Studies (ISTSS). She has served as a consultant and has helped to set up similar projects around the world. She teaches, lectures, and supervises therapists in person or by phone. Dr. Danieli also conducts a biweekly countertransference and trauma seminar (every second Saturday).

CAFÉ 84: A DAY PROGRAM FOR JEWISH SURVIVORS, STOCKHOLM, SWEDEN

In 1945, approximately 10,000 Romanian, Hungarian, and Polish Jews came to Sweden from the concentration camps of Europe for convalescence. At first, they settled in Malmo; approximately 4000 remained to start a new life. By 1984, it became obvious that these survivors needed more than the normal social services to help them deal with the past. In 1984, Jewish leaders, through the intervention of the Jewish Community Council of Stockholm, conceptualized Café 84, a special day care center for survivors. The café was designed to facilitate socialization, to meet psychological needs through small group experiences, and to create intimacy to enhance working through mourning. Psychologist Hedi Fried, herself a survivor of Auschwitz, was hired to head the organization. Funding for the program was primarily through the Jewish Community Council with some assistance from the Swedish government.

The program began for a small group of survivors with serious symptoms and opened with a traditional Friday night Kabalath Shabbat candle-lighting ceremony. Within a few months, the program included approximately 30 regular attendees on Fridays and 5 to 10 on other weekdays. Eventually, over 40 persons attended on Fridays and others came more irregularly.

Common past experiences bind the members together to create a bond of acceptance and understanding. Activities include films, study groups on Jewish history, Friday celebrations, and informal discussions. Formal group treatment is not the method of choice. Instead, groups provide a warm, supportive atmosphere and the leader is a trusted "transference object" who helps members work through traumatic experiences and work through symptoms resulting from repressed memories. In 1988, there were over 100 active members.

Café 84 presents a unique approach to addressing delayed symptoms of concentration camp survivors. It has involved a large number of survivors from the Stockholm area in regular group activities in an informal group setting. It has used groups led by a survivor psychologist using nonconfrontational techniques and serves as a model for other similar programs.

As the potential population from which members come has aged, the program has changed to meet the needs of older persons. By the mid-1990s, the program had about 200 active participants with 20–40 attending one of the regular daily meetings. The greatest numbers attend on Friday evenings for Shabbat services.

The approach by Café 84 is noninvasive. The atmosphere is similar to an Eastern European coffeehouse with food and coffee, love, caring, and support. Over the years, members have become more comfortable discussing their own experiences during World War II. The program has had visits from dignitaries, movie stars, visiting rabbis, and Elie Wiesel, Nobel peace prize winner. Members have learned to nourish one another and themselves and have developed friendships and courtships. Members have found each other and created a place of warmth and belonging.

THE NATIONAL CENTER FOR PSYCHOSOCIAL SUPPORT OF SURVIVORS OF THE HOLOCAUST AND THE SECOND GENERATION: AMCHA, VARIOUS LOCATIONS IN ISRAEL

AMCHA is a Yiddish word derived from Hebrew. As a codeword, it helped survivors identify fellow Jews in war-ravaged Europe. AMCHA also is the name of a nonprofit, voluntary organization founded in 1987 by Holocaust survivors for survivors in Israel. These survivors believed that it was time for Israeli society to deal with the Holocaust survivor population and their psychosocial needs in a specialized, differential way. AMCHA provides nonmaterial psychosocial support through its four branches in the four main cities of Israel (Jerusalem, Ramat Gan, Haifa, and Beersheva). AMCHA opened a Tel Aviv outlet in 1995 to handle increased volume of appeals. As an illustration of the level of services given by AMCHA in 1995, in the Jerusalem branch during that year individual therapy hours totaled 5423; group hours, 853 hours; documentation of survivors' stories, 160 hours; and home visits by 72 volunteers, 3024 hours. In addition, 140 survivors participated in the moadon-social club. A total of 31,700 treatment hours were provided in 1995, and the estimate for 1996 was 35,700 treatment hours.

Israel has many Holocaust survivors at high risk for mental health problems. In 1994, 45% of Israeli residents over 65 years of age were survivors of the Holocaust. There may be 500,000–700,000 second-generation family members and close to 300,000 direct survivors of the Holocaust in Israel.

AMCHA does preventive work and offers community mental health services. General mental health services in Israel have deficiencies in relation to problems of survivors. As public awareness changes and public demand for services has grown, so has AMCHA. Services are provided through Israel's Ministry of Health.

Dr. Danny Brom is the research coordinator of AMCHA. Brom defines trauma as an event accompanied by extreme helplessness which severely disrupts "normal" life (expectations) and is negative to the person. A traumatic event also is the response to the event, ranging from short term coping and integration into the personal life history to full-fledged PTSD and dissociative disorders.

Mission and Goals

AMCHA provides a framework for mutual support that helps Holocaust survivors and their families with memory processing, with working through grief, and with treating psychosocial problems. The goals of AMCHA are:

1. To increase awareness among professionals, therapists, and other persons having contact with the Holocaust survivor population in various settings
2. To bring to people's attention that the Holocaust survivor population is aging
3. To help people recognize that the aging process is a trigger that arouses repressed memories and creates agitation in the client's inner world
4. To break the conspiracy of silence that has characterized the state and people of Israel
5. To replace silence with the needs and desires of survivors to listen and be heard

The mission of AMCHA is simple: AMCHA listens; AMCHA understands; and AMCHA helps.

Funding

Since 1988, AMCHA has offered Israeli Holocaust survivors and their families subsidized services that are not inexhaustible. Twenty-five percent of the budget of AMCHA comes from client fees and 15% from governmental subsidies. Other sources of funding (up to 85%) come from donations and endowments from abroad, especially Holland, Germany, and Austria. AMCHA had a financial crisis in 1994 when demand exceeded revenue. At that time, the board of directors severely cut back organization's activities and accepted no new clients except in emergency situations.

Clientele

Clients are either Holocaust survivors or second-generation family members. The presenting problems of these clients are not necessarily related to the Holocaust. Services are prioritized to survivors who are now elderly and have many psychosocial needs and who often are very lonely. Since its inception, AMCHA has dealt with thousands of cases. For example, in 1995, AMCHA received over 1100 new requests for assistance from survivors and their families. Many of the later reaction patterns of survivors are excellent social integration, psychological restrictions and symptoms, late decompensation and breakdown, late grief work, and spiritual transcendence. Some problems relate to psychological inflexibility, anhedonia (inability to feel or experience pleasure), lifelong symptoms of trauma, and/or problems with intimacy. Many survivor clients have "hardened" through stubbornness, anhedonia, and other adaptive behaviors. Nonclinical survivors tend to have a greater degree of cognitive restriction, less emotional responsiveness, worse emotional coping strategies, more emotional distress, more psychiatric symptoms, and better instrumental coping skills. Stress and pressure, for example, threats of terrorism, national existential threats, and/or death threats, wreak havoc on aging survivors.

Approximately 65,000 Israeli residents were under 15 years of age when they were survivors of the Holocaust. Now, 50 years later, they are eager to process memories and deal with survivor's guilt, work through recurring fears of abandonment and sadness, and deal with late grief and mourning. They often want to search for their origins as they deal with these identity crises and often they show depression, identity disorder, psychosomatic illness, and decompensation as late consequences of the Holocaust.

AMCHA has at least 13 client target groups. Each demands a specific strategy and level of expertise. Survivor client groups include nonclinical elderly, elderly with psychogeriatric crisis and posttraumatic stress, middle-aged "child" survivors, Russian immigrants with massive trauma histories, and very orthodox religious survivors. The second-generation clients include old second-generation clients (early post war second generation), younger second-generation clients (generally born in Israel), recently immigrated individuals, and heavily traumatized clinically needy second-generation clients. Other clients include spouses of Holocaust survivors and second-generation clients, third-generation clients, members of helping professions, and trainees specializing in PTSD treatment.

Theory

The general theory of treatment followed by staff at AMCHA is psychodynamic. Staff generally do not see PTSD; instead, they see complex trauma and disorders of extreme stress. AMCHA professes a developmental perspective of trauma. Interest in how trauma gets integrated into life with clients who are receiving very late intervention is paramount.

Staffing

The staff members of AMCHA are primarily part-time professional employees numbering over 120 psychologists and social workers. Psychiatric consultants are also available. Many of the staff members are second generation themselves. Universities (School of Social Work, Tel Aviv; Psychology and Social Work Schools of Bar Ilan University, Hebrew University of Jerusalem) place fieldwork students with AMCHA. AMCHA also has a large corps of volunteers. For example, in Jerusalem, 73 volunteers perform many roles and functions. Supervision for staff is provided by senior staff and there are also supervision groups. Staff members feel very committed to the cause.

Assessment

When survivors and second-generation clients come in, they have a diagnostic intake interview that looks at what it is they are seeking. Clients are screened and staff members try to get to know them in order to place them in appropriate services.

Services

Treatment within AMCHA is based on the following principles:

1. Treatment is based on clients' needs.
2. Treatment may open a "Pandora's Box" of repressed experiences, memories, and tears that need to be worked through firmly and carefully.
3. Treatment attempts to set inner chaos in order.
4. Treatment involves principles of integration and individuation.
5. Treatment increases an awareness of the "self" as part and parcel of the family and as a part of society (Weiss & Durat, 1994).

AMCHA provides a variety of clinical services. Individual, couple, family, and group psychotherapy sessions are provided to clients. The professional staff of social workers and psychologists evaluates and treats individual clients. Over 32,000 therapy hours were provided by AMCHA in 1994. AMCHA estimates the cost of keeping an individual in therapy for a year is approximately $2000. Individual therapy still is generally psychodynamic, somewhat neglecting the trauma issue. Budget constraints generally limit individual therapy to 2-year periods for Holocaust survivors. Second-generation family members are generally seen for longer times.

A group therapy session is an "oasis of healing" and costs approximately $225. In Jerusalem, therapists conduct monthly group meetings for children of survivors. Kleber and Brom (1992) have written about their model of intervention. In these groups, those in attendance quickly opened up to talk about what it was like to grow up with survivor parents. Group participation has not been constant and attendees struggle with a need to know more about the experiences of their parents and how to get them to tell more without causing them great pain. These open-group monthly meetings required no prior commitment so that individuals could regulate attendance according to their own needs.

AMCHA also provides support groups. Support groups are based on the needs of client populations. Formats include therapy groups and discussion groups for survivors and child survivors, discussion groups and psychodrama sessions for second-generation clients and spouses. Some sessions are open to the public; others are not.

All AMCHA branches have *maodon* (social clubs). The homelike atmosphere of these clubs encourages a drop-in program in addition to regularly scheduled activities such as educational classes, nutrition management, lectures, and workshops on Holocaust-related topics. Many older survivors have a strong need to participate in social meetings wherein the Holocaust is not necessarily a central theme. The atmosphere of the social club is enabling and supportive. In this environment, it is legitimate to be a survivor. The club is both a formal and informal meeting place without therapeutic obligations. It provides an answer to loneliness and isolation and an unanswered need to relate to others. The club acts as a bridge between theory and practice and may bring potential clients closer to actual treatment. Locating the club in the AMCHA center legitimizes a visit to the club and is in itself a treatment element. Clients can come casually dressed and not have to hide their tattooed arms or be ashamed of their pasts. Meetings are held twice a week and become a source of stability and security.

There also is a program of documentation to record testimonies and personal stories of survivors to provide legacies for future generations. The cost of a complete documentation is $400. Specially trained professionals guide clients through the process of documentation before and after the Holocaust as well as during the Holocaust itself as they record on audio- or videotape. Persons who accompany the interviewee are prepared as witnesses to the testimonies to pay complete attention to the stories being told. The files are not open to the public. Video- and audiotaping have brought up many issues in families and survivors as survivors use the process to organize varied heavy memories that have been flooding through their minds in order to make those memories more bearable as the survivor deals with retirement, aging, and separation from children through impending death.

AMCHA maintains the Yom Hashoah telephone hot line as a lifeline for survivors and their families who experience pain on the National Day of Remembrance. In 1995, the 50th anniversary of the liberation of Europe, over 600 survivors called the open phone lines. The majority were elderly survivors who told their own stories. In 1996, during a 24-hour period, nearly 1000 callers told their stories on the special hotlines.

AMCHA has an extensive network of volunteers who provide listening and caring to many survivors, their families, and second-generation clients. Volunteers take on roles of teachers, administrators, matchmakers, and confidants. Many volunteers visit elderly, homebound survivors weekly or teach classes in drawing, ceramics, writing, and other subjects. The volunteer program began in 1988 and has grown tremendously. For many survivors, the volunteer is the individual's only contact with the outside world; the volunteer helps with grocery shopping, transportation to doctor's appointments, and with red tape involved in social service contacts. Volunteers receive a special outing or festive meal each year in thanks for their giving of themselves.

Debriefing

AMCHA staff has provided expertise to those working with trauma victims in war-torn countries. AMCHA counselors were dispatched after rescue efforts for terrorist victims were completed. They worked with paramedics, ambulance drivers, teen volunteers, and others who experienced stress by their experiences. Dr. Brom is searching for a model of debriefing that includes follow up. Debriefing also includes a preventive component.

Research

The research programs of AMCHA deal with personality, diagnosis, epidemiology, and service delivery. Research activities are concentrated in two major areas. The first study is of clients who have completed therapy at AMCHA within a year of the study. The aim of this study is to improve the course and quality of therapy; researching success of therapy documents the needs of the survivor populations as well. The second study compares "child" survivors with a control group of nonsurvivors to learn about current psychological and social status of the child survivors. Another research project aims to track the progress of Russian immigrants who are Holocaust survivors.

Training and Community Services

AMCHA is a center for specialized training. It provides inservice training for staff on trauma-related topics. Staff members have study days to pursue training and education. AMCHA has not developed formal training materials. Two AMCHA therapists traveled to war-ravaged Croatia to work with UNICEF's psychosocial assistance program. AMCHA publishes *The AMCHA Link*. AMCHA provides programming for the community on Yom Hashoah and other significant dates and works to increase the communal awareness of problems of Holocaust survivors. Training, conferences, and courses are sponsored and staffed by AMCHA in cooperation with Tel Aviv and Bar Ilan Universities. Director of AMCHA John Lemberger was invited to participate in an official conference on genocide in the capital of Rwanda in order to help develop a policy to treat persons who survived the Tutsi ethnic slaughter by rival Hutus in 1995.

The issue of repatriation of funds from Germany to Israeli citizens has led to some work with forensic issues. Clients may ask for help from AMCHA as they seek funds. Friends of AMCHA organizations have been developed around the world. AMCHA also hosted the first International Institute for Professionals Working with Holocaust Survivors and the Second Generation (July 1994). The book, *A Global Perspective in Working with Holocaust Survivors and the Second Generation*, edited by Director John Lemberger (1996), is a compilation of papers from this conference. Topics addressed are psychosocial effects of the Holocaust on survivors, problems of survivor guilt, familial and collective identity, and the merits of various models of assistance and psychotherapeutic interventions.

THE CENTER FOR THE STUDY OF GENOCIDE, VIOLENCE AND TRAUMA, NEW HAVEN, CONNECTICUT

This center is described in Chapter 6 because it is still in conceptualization.

SUMMARY

As these thoughts were written, thousands of Kosovoar Albanian refugees were beginning to return to their homes, if any homes remained undestroyed. NATO troops were beginning to uncover the magnitude of atrocities that had been perpetrated against these people and my thoughts return to the Holocaust. The horrors of war extend across decades and generations in the primary victims of Kosovo and in the primary and secondary victims of the Nazi persecutions (the second and even third generations).

On a more personal note, the life of the first author of this volume was shaped and channeled by Holocaust survivors George and Esther Kemeny. Who would have ever thought that carrying a 4-year-old girl on his back as he walked along the banks of the Ohio River and talked about the horrors of the Holocaust would "pave the way" for my entry into the trauma field as practitioner, author, researcher! Esther Kemeny alone remains as my connection with that childhood past. She has given her testimony for the Survivors' Project in San Francisco and now wants to "tell her story." As her surrogate daughter, it will be my honor and duty to help with that telling. Only through personal narratives of those who remain, only through work with today's youth who need to hear the stories (as my dear friend and colleague Hedi Fried told her story to the middle-school students of George Mason Middle School in Falls Church, Virginia), will the survivors be memorialized and remembered. As Dr. Yael Danieli has said, the epitaph of those who died in the Holocaust must be made visible and real, more real than the smoke in the sky that was all that remained after they were sacrificed.

10
Centers Designed
to Work with Refugees

Many of the centers have been created with the specific purpose of working with refugees and survivors of war-torn countries. In the past few years, the war in Bosnia–Herzegovina has been very prominent in the news and in its impact. This war has led to the dislocation of hundreds of thousands of individuals and the creation of many centers and programs. The most comprehensive of these programs are those in Slovenia, the Rehabilitation Center for Torture Victims in Copenhagen and its "clones," and the programs growing out of the Department of Social Work in Zagreb. These programs offer much information to persons who are seeking to create comprehensive trauma centers as well as suggestions for future center development.

THE SLOVENE FOUNDATION, LJUBLJANA, SLOVENIA

In 1992, Slovenia had about 70,000 refugees from Bosnia and Herzegovina living within its borders. Many of these refugees came from rural regions. Some were illiterate, with low educational levels and a peasant background. About half of the fathers in these families had worked away from their homes and the women and children remained on small farms or in privately owned homes. Many of these homes were destroyed during the conflict. The majority of the women did not work outside the home; 36% of them had at least three children.

By 1993, 35,000 refugees remained in Slovenia; by 1994, 29,000, over half of them children and youth. These war-traumatized children needed help to organize their lives, particularly through a supportive school experience and a structured, predictable environment. In spite of the traumas they experienced, the majority of these children have not suffered direct devastation nor are they disturbed. Many have developed good coping skills. This is good news in light of estimates that at least 900,000 children from the former Yugoslavia have been psychologically traumatized by the war. At least 150,000 of these children have been exposed to terror. As of September 1992, 1,417 children had been killed and 29,169 had been wounded.

A History of the Camps in Slovenia

After the refugees arrived in Slovenia, the majority were accommodated in 28 collective shelters; the remainder stayed in private accommodations, mostly with family members living in Slovenia. The shelters were run by the Slovenian state and did not have self-government; in the initial phase they were led in many instances by persons who were unemployed public workers with no appropriate education or training The leaders received low salaries to "run" the centers; with some exceptions, the centers had no social workers. In one center, two social workers worked occasionally. A few weeks after the arrival of the refugees, mental health teams were organized under the auspices of the Counseling Center for Children, Adolescents, and Parents. These activities were financed by UNHCR and foreign donors from the very beginning. The teams developed outreach activities and visited collective shelters all over Slovenia on a weekly or monthly basis. They provided some psychosocial help to families. Primarily, their activities were focused on providing help to children and adolescents. Only a small number received psychological help as clients of the Counseling Center in Ljubljana. In 1994, these psychological programs for refugees were transformed into the Slovene Foundation. Ultimately, under the umbrella of this nongovernmental organization, the Center for Psychosocial Help to Refugees was created.

The Velike Bloke Center at Cerknica held 450 refugees in the first year; in 1995, 251. This center was an old military barracks. In time, inhabitants planted vegetable and flower gardens; the center had a disco for the teens and a kindergarten for 40 children run by 3 refugee women. Food was brought to the center twice daily from a central kitchen in Cerknica and the 251 people stood in line to get food they did not like. Director Natasa Jerman, concerned by this situation, decided to build a functioning kitchen in which inhabitants could do their own cooking. She also constructed warm water showers. However, in spite of these improvements, each day began and ended like the others, controlled by fate, without a purpose or goal for the majority of the inhabitants. A poem by Raza Mehmedovic, summarized some of the feelings of the center's inhabitants:

> There is the row of men, irritable.
> Noise. Lumped together.
> Early in the morning is the first sign
> Of their non-existence.
> Like a parasite,
> You wait, going towards
> What was cooked somewhere and reaches you.
> You stand in a row, bundles between you.
> The second, the fifth, and so on

> Heartweary, you go on your way,
> Back to your room,
> That you share with 30 others, who are just like you.
> Rows of beds, like the military,
> The hard sheets are gray with no bit of beauty.

(Poems have been translated from German by M. B. Williams from a paper called "Dangube: Weggestellte Menschen-abgestellte Zeit: Die bosnischen Flüchtlinge in slowenischen Lagern" by Maja Wicki and furnished to the author by Dr. Mikus-Kos during a trip to Slovenia and the centers.) Meanwhile, the refugee center in Hrastnik had 170 inhabitants; Roska in Ljubyana, 656; two refugee centers in Maribor held 859. The center in Hrastnik was created from the narrow wooden barracks built for Bosnian miners and construction workers who were migrant workers to Slovenia before World War II. In this camp, Swiss volunteers built a kitchen and eating room where three refugees could cook meals appropriate to the majority of Muslim inhabitants.

Maja Jagnjac, 14 years old, describes the conditions in the camps and her reactions:

> Again, a day that goes by with me being a refugee.
> Again, foreign faces of foreign people.
> I don't want to be here.
> For months I have had the same thoughts.
> What existed earlier, remains all that is remembered.
> Why the war?
> Why the tears, the suffering?
> Why not laughing and luck?
> For too long I am going around on the strange earth,
> For too long, I am warmed
> By a foreign sun.
> I don't want all of this.
> What I want is,
> To go through the streets of my city.
> To hear the church bells and the call to prayers in the evening.
> I want simply to return home.

People in the towns around the camps try to ignore the presence of the refugees. The natives have their houses and gardens, their apartments, their cars, their summer houses in the mountains. Most of them are not interested in the lives of the refugees; they do not want their lives disturbed. Only if someone needs a few construction workers or during harvest someone needs to have apples or pears picked quickly does that person remember that the refugees are cheap labor. Afterward, particularly in the winter months, the refugees are forgotten. No one wants to give them a voice or an opportunity to be self-determined. Aida Supuk, 15, describes what it feels like to be in this situation.

> To be homeless is difficult,
> To be a refugee is also difficult,
> Days and nights and hours are difficult,

It is hard to wait, that somewhere something will be given to you,
It is hard, to be sad day after day,
It is not easy, to be sick,
It is not easy, to hold back the sadness,
It is difficult, to hear the black news,
It is still harder, to experience that your family is hungry,
You are sick, when fate is so dark.
You become sicker, when your people are murdered.
It is hard, when the shoes of hope sink,
It is hard, when you are not in your home, not in your country.
It is not easy, if you lose all hope,
It is hard, if your enemy steals away luck for you,
It is hard, if no one understands you in a foreign land,
It is hard, if you are able to trust no one,
It is not easy, to see other lucky faces,
It is not easy to be a refugee.

The Slovene Foundation

The Slovene Foundation (Slovenska Fondcija), established in November 1992 and registered at the Ministry of Internal Affairs, is a national philanthropic, nonprofit, nonpolitical, nongovernmental association of individuals, associations, and groups. Dr. Anica Mikus Kos, a consultant child psychiatrist and director of the World Health Organization (WHO) Collaborative Center for Child and Adolescent Mental Health, is president of the foundation. The foundation has collaborated with numerous organizations including Johns Hopkins University and volunteer organizations.

Mission

The mission of the Slovene Foundation is to develop philanthropy and voluntary work in the social field; to promote values of voluntary work in the social field; to raise public awareness; to activate the society for solidarity actions; and to educate young people for responsible citizenship. An additional mission is to provide psychosocial help to refugees from Bosnia and Herzegovina living in Slovenia.

Funding

The Slovene Foundation is financed through membership fees and donations.

Staffing

The staff patterns of the Slovene Foundation include the general assembly consisting of all members, which meets once yearly and passes major resolutions and is the supreme organization; board of managers, which is the executive organ; council, an advisory group consisting of Slovene public figures; supervisory board supervising the financial operation of the foundation prepares the annual report; and tribunal of honor, which treats misconduct of the members.

Services

The activities of the Slovene Foundation include development of programs of voluntary work; education and training for volunteers and coordinators/managers of voluntary organizations; development of a network of voluntary organizations; publications on voluntary work; fund raising for voluntary organizations and disbursement of funds on a competition basis; linkage with international voluntary organizations; creation of a data base on voluntary organizations and activities in Slovenia.

The Center for Psychosocial Help to Refugees

The Center for Psychosocial Help to Refugees was founded in April 1994 under the umbrella of the Slovene Foundation. While the program does outreach work with the entire refugee population in Slovenia, staff members give priority to children and teens. The center focuses on community development, psychological and psychiatric help, and education and training. The purposes of the center are to provide mental health for refugees, especially for children, adolescents, and parents; to provide community mental health work and preventive activities; to train educational, medical, and social workers as well as teachers and other psychosocial helpers from Slovenia, Bosnia, and Herzegovina; to develop mutual help and self-help models; to cooperate with and build links with humanitarian and refugee organizations from within and outside of Slovenia; to analyze mental health-related circumstances and problems important for healthy psychosocial development of children and adolescents; to publish representative materials describing the center's activities and professional findings; and to organize activities of foreign mental health professionals to transfer experiences, models of help, and knowledge to refugees (see Fig. 10.1). Other priorities include provision of learning assistance to children, care for unaccompanied children, organization of summer holiday programs for children, advocacy of children's rights, provision of excursion programs for children, work with parents, provision of financial help to adolescents for schooling, and advocacy of children's rights.

Among the beliefs of the center are that the essential life conditions of refugees must be met through provision of housing, food, health care, employment, and respect; the most valuable form of support is enhancing coping capacities and empowering refugees for autonomous life; and the most important protective factor for children is giving them the opportunity to attend school and obtain vocational training. Prevention of school failure and drop-

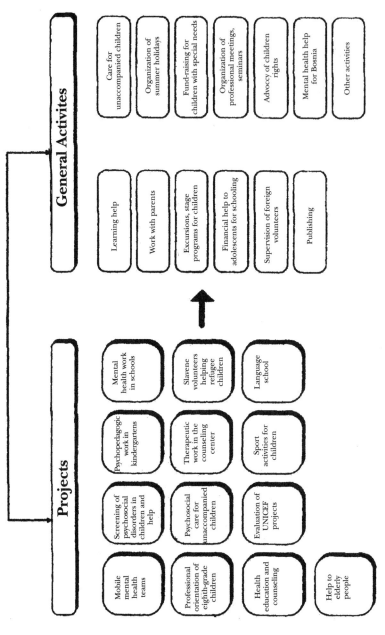

Figure 10.1. Slovene Center for Psychosocial Help projects and general activities.

ping out is very important as well. Mental health activities should be integrated into primary health care, health education, kindergartens, primary schools, sports activities, and other activities. Helpers should work *with* refugees, not *for* refugees. Mental health and psychosocial programs are most efficient when they engage refugees and helpers from host countries together. Psychosocial and mental health programs for refugees should use existing domestic regular services as often as possible while linking these services in continuous collaboration.

Funding

The Center for Psychosocial Help to Refugees is financed primarily by UNHCR, which provides 50% of the funding in return for performance of psychosocial services for UNHCR. Other sources of funding include WHO, the French government, Foundation de France, Fluchtlings Hilfe Direkt (Germany), Save the Children, and others.

Staffing

The center employs a full-time secretary, two part-time office workers, as well as many volunteers who are Slovenes, foreign volunteers, and refugees from Bosnia and Herzegovina. A certain number of refugees are working in the psychosocial projects. They are financially rewarded for that work.

Clientele

The clientele are refugees from all over Slovenia, especially children and adolescents.

Services Provided

Services provided by the Center for Psychosocial Help to Refugees include supporting education of refugee children at all levels, developing outreach population-oriented modes of global psychosocial help to refugees, providing psychotherapeutic help for refugees, and implementing health education programs as models to reach the most deprived and least educated refugees. Other services provided include the activities of mobile mental health teams that reach out and offer help to traumatized people living in the collective shelters and pay regular visits to schools for refugee children. The teams do needs assessment, support and initiate activities designed to protect the mental health of children in the schools, discover those who are in most need and organize professional help for them, offer immediate help in crisis situations, support activities that protect the mental health of vulnerable population groups, monitor the psychosocial situations in collective shelters and in primary schools, and inform the responsible service providers and institutions about their findings. One other service is the provision of care to unaccompanied children. Persons who are working in this area monitor the situations of unaccompanied children and provide psychosocial support and some material help.

Mental health teams have helped to establish kindergartens designed to normalize preschool life through programs that help with stimulation of development, that prepare children for school, that stabilize children emotionally, and that help to protect the children's mental health. The teams identify children with trauma disorders and developmental disabilities in order to make appropriate referrals.

The center provides mental health activities in schools, as well as education to and training of teachers of refugees. This education and training is important if they are to recognize emotional and learning problems among their pupils. They learn how to provide instruction to and for traumatized children in a way that is supportive to those children. The center also provides mental health counseling for the children and women. Bosnian children were able to be included in regular Slovene elementary schools beginning in Autumn 1995. The center organized a support network to help the children integrate into this educational environment while being supportive to Slovene teachers. Language schools teach French and English to refugee children. Holidays in foreign countries are organized for students by these programs. The children then have the opportunity to spend 3 to 4 weeks abroad to practice the language skills learned in the classrooms.

Volunteers provide many helping activities. They befriend refugee children, provide learning assistance, and organize leisure time activities. Mental health workers supervise the volunteers' helping activities. The program also improves relationships, modifies distorted perceptions and misconceptions about members of the other nationalities through mixed groups of youth (Bosnian and Slovenian), reduces prejudice, and increases cultural tolerance.

The center provides help to the elderly who are alone in collective centers. The center stimulates young Bosnian persons to care for the elderly, to help them in their daily activities, to bring them lunch, and help with laundry. The project provides practical psychosocial help to elderly refugees, increases communication with and among the elderly, and encourages the elderly to get active.

The Consulting Center for Children, Adolescents and Parents, Ljubljana: WHO Collaborating Center for Child Mental Health: Unit for Trauma Treatment

The Consulting Center is a nonprofit governmental institution founded in 1955 that combines clinical work with preventative activities and training. The Consulting Center is the most important outpatient mental health service for children and youth in Slovenia. The center is a government-supported, nonprofit organization and is directly responsible to health and education authorities. It was appointed as a WHO Collaborating Center for Child Mental Health in 1995.

The trauma center was created as a department of the institution. The trigger for its creation was the arrival of traumatized refugee children who appeared at the institute as clients. Previously, the center primarily had treated children and adolescents who had been exposed to family violence, the suicide of a family member, and traffic accidents. Thus the needs of victims and their families, the needs of the broader community, and the need for knowledge about trauma led to the creation of the trauma center in 1993. The work of the center is described in Figure 10.2.

Mission

The mission of the trauma center is to provide direct preventive and therapeutic help to children and adolescents exposed to traumatic events, as well as to help their family members and other caregivers. Another mission is to spread knowledge about trauma to settings that impact the everyday life of children, for example, kindergartens, schools, health services, and law enforcement agencies.

Only a minority of children and adolescents with trauma symptoms are users of mental health services; therefore, knowledge about trauma should be spread among caretakers in a broad fashion. Efforts to prevent further adversities and to introduce protective factors and processes into the children's lives are important aspects of the work of the center. The guiding therapeutic principle is to enhance the client's own resources and coping capacities.

Funding

Funds for the Consulting Center come from two major sources: 50% of funds are given annually by the health system and 50% come from the education system. Resources are strictly limited.

Staffing

The center has 27 full-time employees including seven clinical child psychologists, three psychologists, three child psychiatrists, two social workers, three teachers, one speech/language therapist, and one director. Nonprofessional staff include four secretaries, one courier, one cleaning woman, and one accountant. There are also seven part-time employees including one psychiatrists, one child neurologist, two psychologists, and three special education teachers. All full-time employees are female except for the courier. There are three coordinators for clinical work, educational activities, and research. The

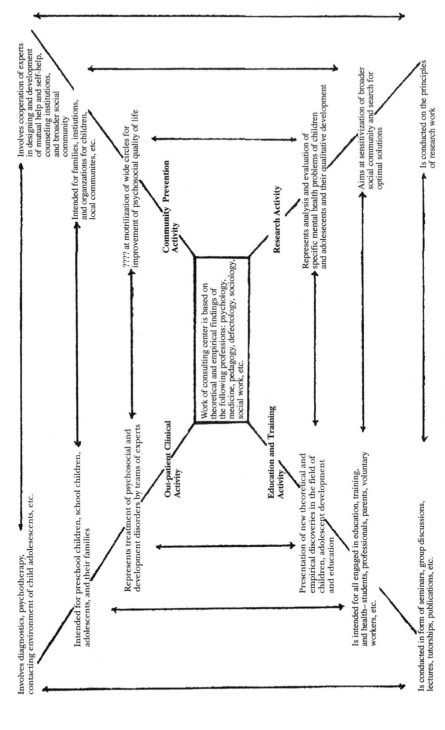

Figure 10.2. Work of the Consulting Center.

center also utilizes many volunteers in a variety of capacities, for example, approximately 100 high school and university students help children and adolescents as peer helpers/friends. The students make a 1-year commitment (academic year) but many commit to help for 2–3 years. About half of these staff members work with traumatized children.

The staff members are supervised by senior psychologists and psychiatrists. There are regular team conferences, professional staff meetings, and daily meetings. These activities and an occasional "anti-burn out program" help to prevent burnout and compassion fatigue. The director supervises and evaluates staff. Seminars are designed to provide staff with theoretical information and therapeutic approaches and interventions for working with traumatized children and adolescents are provided to staff.

Between 1992 and 1994, mobile mental health teams for refugees worked under the umbrella of the center. Teams included eight Bosnian doctors, two psychologists, and one social worker. The team members gathered research in a sample of 286 8th grade students from 30 elementary schools. These students completed a variety of instruments including the Impact of Event Scale (IES) and a Childhood War Trauma Questionnaire. Of these 286 children and teens, 18% had experienced a direct threat to their lives, 32% had been exposed to shelling and shooting, and only 12% had not been exposed to a war event.

Clientele

The populations served by the trauma center are primary victims, secondary (family) victims, and tertiary (caregiver) victims. Primary victims are children and youth from the entire country of Slovenia. Priority is given to clients who have the most serious problems as identified during the first contact. Clients complete questionnaires on a yearly basis about satisfaction with and opinions about services provided. Many of the clients are refugee children and adolescents. The center treats about 300 refugee children and about 2000 Slovene clients yearly, as well as their parents, teachers, and other caregivers. The clients are referred by primary health care services, schools, and kindergartens. A majority come on their own incentive. The Slovene Foundation's Center of Psychosocial Help to Refugees also refers refugees to the center.

Theory

Both the counseling and the trauma center integrate cognitive–behavioral, contextual, psychodynamic, systemic, family, and other theory bases and approaches in treatment. Theoretical principles stem from a holistic biopsychosocial paradigm that integrates knowledge from these three areas. The outstanding characteristic of treatment is a holistic approach that pays immediate attention to the helping and healing resources that are available in the child's environment. Natural resources may be more reliable and stable than direct professional help. Mental health professionals have a role in activating and organizing the various supportive and protective processes utilized. The work of treatment recognizes culturally appropriate approaches and also includes outreach interventions to improve the child's everyday life situation.

Assessment

Assessment of a patient uses clinical psychiatric and psychological interviews, and measures, scales, evaluations of psychosocial functioning, and data provided by caretakers about personal life situations. The initial assessment takes two to four sessions and is conducted by senior psychiatrists or clinical psychologists. The center has developed questionnaires, used existing instruments (e.g., the IES), and adapted others for this task. A PTSD-positive diagnosis uses criteria from ICD-10 and DSM-IV. The conclusions reached from the assessment are used to plan for treatment, to gain a commitment to engage in treatment, and (less often) to determine disability claims and assist with forensic evaluations.

Services

Treatment interventions include individual counseling, group counseling, psychotherapy, relaxation exercises, social work interventions, remedial teaching, advocacy, system intervention/political action, and provision of medication. The trauma center also provides debriefing services/methods combined with other techniques to offer support to a child in his/her everyday life condition as another part of the integrated treatment approach. The outcomes of debriefing are evaluated clinically through measurement of reduction of symptoms, observation of changes in coping capacity, and improvements in psychosocial functioning. Forensic work is done primarily with children exposed to family violence (sexual abuse, physical abuse of the child, physical abuse of the parent, homicide of the mother), traffic victims, and accident victims.

Trauma center staff members between 1992 and 1994 participated in

1. Mobile mental health teams that reached out to traumatized persons at collective shelters and schools. Team members did needs assessments, offered support and organized group activities in schools to protect the mental health of children.
2. Care for unaccompanied children. The center did assessments, set up interventions for and with children (e.g., helping a child enter school or kindergarten), set up volunteer friends programs, and involved the children in activities and outlets.
3. Kindergarten programs normalized the preschool life of refugee children. The programs helped children prepare for school, stimulated

their development, stabilized their emotions, and identified children with disorders in order to refer them for services.

4. Mental health activities in schools educated teachers of refugees how to recognize emotional and learning problems, how to provide instruction to traumatized children, and how to refer children for mental health counseling. The center also provided psychological support for teachers.
5. Adolescents (8th graders and teens) were helped to enter secondary schools and vocational training programs.
6. Therapeutic intervention to children, adolescents, and their parents who were referred was provided.
7. Volunteer programs.

Services are provided to persons with ongoing needs over long periods of time; at the same time, new clients are accepted. There is no end point in length of time services can be provided.

Training and Consultation

The center offers training to professionals (psychologists, health workers, teachers, social workers) and laypersons (volunteers, helpers). The majority of training occurs in workshops designed to teach practical skills as well as theory. Training standards are set by the Ministries of Health and Education, by professional organizations of Slovenia, and by the Consulting Center's regulations. The center offers training in trauma and PTSD in children and adolescents, psychological trauma in child health care settings, dealing with trauma in the school setting, providing psychological first aid to traumatized children, enhancing coping capacities of traumatized children, providing trauma treatment through specific techniques (e.g., desensitization, relaxation), traumatic loss and bereavement in children and adolescents, conflict resolution techniques, and preventing staff burnout.

The staff of the trauma center provides prevention activities to primary and secondary schools and medical settings and educates the public about trauma through media, public forums, and conferences. The center staff also has expertise with violence-related and accident-related traumatic incidents. The trauma center is highly involved in community action, advocacy, and social change.

THE AMANI TRUST, HARARE, ZIMBABWE

The AMANI Trust, established in 1993, is a Zimbabwean registered nongovernmental organization (NGO) that provides rehabilitation services to human rights violations' survivors, particularly persons who have experienced torture and repressive and institutional violence. The trust operates in Harare and the Northeast region of Zimbabwe (Mt. Darwin District since 1995 and Centenary District since 1997). The Northeast region has a population of approximately 240,000 persons and has considerable poverty. It operates on a nonprofit basis and provides services free of charge, depending on voluntary funding for its survival.

The community-based program has assisted health personnel and torture survivors to deal with problems and organized violence using an empowerment approach. This approach works well, has strong support from the health service, and may provide a useful new model for management of torture survivors. The basic model for developing a district psychiatric service has three phases:

1. Basic training of health workers; identification, assessment and counseling of survivors.
2. Advanced training in counseling skills, district team building, home visiting, and networking.
3. Consolidation of the district team and community work.

The AMANI Trust incorporates a holistic approach to the assessment and management of survivors of torture and psychosocial trauma. The approach to rehabilitation is based on principles of community-based delivery of services, individual assessment and counseling, home visiting and family therapy, development of community support networks, training of community health workers, development of district psychiatric services, and ongoing research and monitoring of programs.

Mission

The mission of the trust is to rehabilitate torture survivors so that they can return to the community to lead full, productive lives. The missions also are to provide services for the rehabilitation of victims of human rights violations, particularly torture, repressive violence, and institutionalized violence; to participate in the creation of a human rights climate by instituting programs of training and education, especially within health and allied professions; to offer ongoing training in the detection and treatment of the sequelae of torture and psychosocial trauma; to liaison with other national and international bodies who share AMANI's objectives; to undertake research into the effects of torture and human rights violations; and to provide information and documentation on the effects of torture and psychosocial trauma.

Funding

A variety of donors and organizations have supported the AMANI Trust. Among them are the Swedish Red Cross, the United Nations Voluntary Fund for Victims of Torture, the Swiss Embassy, the International Rehabilitation Council for Victims of Torture, and the Danish International Development Agency, among others.

Clientele

The AMANI trust serves two categories of victims. Primary victims have had direct experience of organized violence and physical torture. Some have experienced deprivation, sensory overstimulation, and psychological torture. Others have witnessed violent death, extreme violence or torture. Secondary victims are those indirectly affected by organized violence and torture, such as spouses and families of torture survivors, families of the disappeared, communities experiencing high levels of violence, and health and other workers who care for torture survivors. The majority of clients are males. Few of these males have more than primary school education and 74% are unemployed or in unskilled employment. Most do subsistence farming and experience general social adversity. They are more socially isolated and earn little.

In the Mt. Darwin District, between 1995 and 1996, 386 torture survivors and their families were in the AMANI Trust caseload. The trust trained 55 nurses from the two hospitals, 22 nurses from the rural health clinics, and 8 rehabilitation technicians. Fourteen nurses participated in the advanced counseling course. In the Centenary District in 1997, 12 nurses from St. Albert's Mission Hospital and 7 nurses from rural health clinics were trained. In 1996, the trust identified 7 families for family therapy; in 1997, 15 families. In 1996, 112 new survivors of violence were assessed and 94 were on the waiting list.

Assessment

The assessment procedure developed by the AMANI Trust seems to be valid and reliable and has shown that there may be characteristics of Zimbabwean survivors that differ from other survivor populations. In fact, the measure of PTSD shows no relationship with measures of torture, which is a curious finding.

Services

The AMANI Trust has an integrated series of programs in the Mashonaland Project, which combine to form a self-sustaining district psychiatric service that is capable of supporting torture survivors. Each phase lasts roughly 1 year, depending on numbers to be trained and the size of the district, and uses a two-tiered approach to strengthen existing medical services and strengthen the community. Phase 1 includes basic training of health workers and identification, assessment and counseling of survivors. Phase 2 includes advanced training in counseling skills and district team building. Phase 3 includes consolidation of the district team, community work, and consolidating of food security. The hospital program offers a variety of clinical and consultative services to survivors, including assessment, treatment, and referral; single therapeutic interviews and therapeutic interventions; provision of consultation to hospitals; liaison work with other organizations; and assistance with compensation claims.

The Rehabilitation Technician's Project provides a training program for the rehabilitation technician in the assessment and management of trauma victims, including victims of torture and organized violence. These technicians are trained to assist physiotherapists and occupational therapists in the assessment and management of trauma. The project is a collaboration between the AMANI Trust, the Department of Rehabilitation of Mashonaland Central Province, the Department of Rehabilitation of the University of Zimbabwe, the Rehabilitation Center for Torture Victims (Copenhagen, Denmark), and the Rehabilitation Technicians' Training School. The project has been funded by the Swiss government and has several stages: (1) assessment of 38 survivors for basic research data; (2) development and piloting of an assessment instrument; (3) training of rehabilitation technicians; (4) reassessment of effects of training; (5) assessment of outcomes of treatments provided by technicians; and (6) production of a manual.

In the Mt. Darwin District, 182 persons with psychological disorders were identified at the Mt. Darwin District Hospital and the Karanda Mission Hospital, as well as another 57 disorders of organized violence. Minimal problem-solving intervention was beneficial for these patients with psychological disorders. These groups had very high rates of witnessing of violence, torture, and executions, as well as high rates of disappearances by other family members. After the pilot study, a community-based program was introduced in March 1995. The AMANI Trust also has initiated a forum to establish a district psychiatric policy, organizing trained staff into an organized system. The first step is the formulation of a management and referral algorithm for the Mashonaland District.

The rehabilitation algorithm has five stages: (1) identification (screening or referral); (2) assessment (Self-Reporting Questionnaire-20, Structured Assessment Form, medical history, Clinician Administered PTSD Scale, history of violence); (3) individual treatment (single therapeutic interview, physical therapy); (4) family visiting (home assessment, family therapy); and (5) community program (income-generating skills; permaculture).

The community program aims to create community support networks. It includes family visits (all survivors are visited in their own homes), provision of family therapy in the home, and creation of community development initiatives. The family therapy approach used has been developed by AMANI for the Zimbabwe situation and revolves around a family-witnessing model. AMANI staff conducts community meetings in each area to discuss torture-related issues; these issues primarily revolve around poverty and ways to overcome it.

The trust has begun a program aimed to alleviate poverty. This program focuses on maintenance of food security through a permaculture, income generation through cash crops and small projects, and deforestation and family wood lots. This project also aims to assist individuals and families with legal and social difficulties, particularly if the survivors are seeking assistance (and compensation). The AMANI Trust liaisons with other NGOs in this effort, including the Legal Resource Foundation.

The AMANI Trust launched a small pilot project to assess the efficacy of a time-limited counseling intervention, the single therapeutic intervention. The work used a sample of 20 patients who are being followed in a small clinical trial with 6-month and 12-month follow-ups. The AMANI Trust also conducts research, which is described below. In addition, the trust is assisting the Mt. Darwin District in its development of a district psychiatric plan, which includes survivors of torture.

Training

The AMANI Trust provides training to hospital nurses in an 8-week program that includes detection of disorders, assessment of disorders, problem formulation, counseling, problem solving, forensic assessment, effects of violence, and care for caregivers. The trust also trains health personnel from rural clinics and hospital in the identification, assessment, and basic management of psychiatric disorders in general and torture survivors in particular. The training was provided in a 5-day workshop. The Danish Agency for International Development Cooperation (DANIDA) funded an advanced counseling program for a core group of hospital nurses and funded the development of a referral system. The Rehabilitation Technician's Training Project is described above, under services.

The AMANI Trust also has been involved in various human rights activities. The trust participated in a human rights training course for the Zimbabwe prison service; the workshop led to establishment of a working group of which the AMANI Trust is a member. It also has been monitoring the government's implementation of the UN Convention, has requested that the Zimbabwean government sign and ratify the UN Convention on Torture and Other Cruel, Inhuman or Degrading Treatment or Punishment, and is producing a document to initiate a human rights forum.

The AMANI Trust maintains a web page, www.oneworld.org/. The trust has published several manuals, among them *Chiweshe Nurse Counsellor Programme: Resource Manual* (rev ed, 1997), which provides primary care nurses who work in primary care clinics with skills to manage psychological disorders or anxiety, depression, and alcohol abuse. The manual presents a 5-day workshop to develop problem-solving therapy. *Assessment of the Consequences of Torture and Organized Violence: A Manual for Field Workers* (rev. ed., 1997) outlines a procedure to assess and manage consequences of torture and organized violence in primary care and community care for the field worker with some previous experience (nurses, social workers, trained community workers). It is supplementary to the Chiweshe program. *A Trauma Counselling Handbook* (1998) is a manual for primary care and community workers dealing with sequelae of trauma, primarily trauma of torture and organized violence. The manual includes sections on debriefing, the single therapeutic interview, and family witnessing. The final book is *A Handbook for Nurse Counsellors* (1998), which also is an adjunct to the Chiweshe program and is second-level training for primary care nurses. It aims to provide more advanced counseling skills of identification, assessment, and management, individual counseling, family counseling, group work, and peer counseling.

Research

The trust has undertaken a series of small studies to examine the effects of violence of the 1970s on its survivors. The first is the district epidemiological study, which was a point prevalence study and a pathway study. The results of the former indicated that Mt. Darwin District has a 34% rate of ordinary psychological disorders and an 8% rate for disorders due to torture and/or organized violence. The pathway study of referral networks indicated that patients with conspicuous disorders are younger, have more serious disorders, and take little time (or effort) to obtain formal psychiatric help when they have contact with health facilities. Previous training of hospital staff increased the detection of disorders at the hospital level.

The single therapeutic interview study is a small pilot study of a specific approach to counseling torture survivors. The preliminary results show improvements in all patients, as measured by the Self-Reporting Questionnaire and self-ratings. The family therapy algorithm is a small pilot study that assesses the efficacy of a brief family therapy approach. This approach revolves around a family meeting designed for participants to discuss the effects of torture on survivors and their families. It also aims to increase family support for the survivor. Preliminary results indicate that the approach is leading to some changes in the families' functioning.

THE BELLEVUE PROGRAM FOR SURVIVORS OF TORTURE, NEW YORK, NEW YORK

In March 1995, psychologist Jack Saul, PhD, and physician Allen Keller, the current contact person for the agency, decided to set up a clinic at Bellevue Hospital in New York City to treat torture survivors. Bellevue is a teaching hospital affiliated with New York University and is the United States' oldest public hospital. The Bellevue Program for Survivors of Torture, now directed by Keller, has seen over 200 victims of torture or severe political violence from

50 countries as well as their families. Staff are from the hospital and clients have access to all hospital services. The program offers an integrated treatment approach for the psychological and medical needs of survivors.

Individuals are referred to the program from a variety of services including several human rights organizations such as Lawyers Committees for Human Rights and Physicians for Human Rights, local immigrant communities and advocates, and by individuals. By 1997, the center had established itself as the premier torture survivors' treatment and resource center in New York City. The clinical program is based at the Primary Care Medical Clinic.

Mission

The aim of the program is to reempower survivors and help them rebuild their lives using a culturally sensitive approach that uses clients' cultural and religious resources The focus of the program is to help survivors rebuild their lives while reducing symptoms, assisting with social difficulties, and networking with community organizations.

Staff

The staff of Bellevue's Program for Survivors of Torture meets weekly to discuss its work, the needs of the program, and administrative issues. During these meetings, staff members share ideas, review client progress, and formulate integrated treatment plans. The meetings also provide a forum to share reactions to trauma stories, to receive emotional support from colleagues, and to avoid compassion fatigue/burnout. Health professionals who currently are participating in the program include primary care physicians, psychologists, psychiatrists, gynecologists, rehabilitative physicians, occupational and physical therapists, and social workers. Staff donates "in kind" staff time, office space, and administrative support so that no client will be billed for services, medications, or diagnostic procedures. The current psychological treatment team includes a psychiatrist, 4 senior clinical psychologists, 4 staff psychologists, and 11 psychology interns. Other staff members include program director Allen S. Keller, MD, social workers, and program consultant Dr. Sophia Banu.

The colleague support service helps to prevent secondary traumatization of staff who care for center patients. Support service personnel contact staff members after initial visits and afterward as needed. This early intervention model promotes and maintains psychological health of staff.

Clientele

During 1997, the program provided services to 92 clients from 30 different countries. Sixty-four of the clients were new and 28 clients received follow-up care. Clients made approximately 900 clinical visits in 1997. Since the inception of the program, 136 clients from 36 different countries have received services, including survivors of torture and their families and victims of political violence. Clients have suffered numerous forms of torture and abuse including beatings, burns, electric shocks, cuts from sharp objects, asphyxiation, rape, sexual assault, mock execution, deprivation of food/water, exposure to heat/cold, imprisonment under inhuman conditions, witnessing of torture/murder of others, and forced labor. Physical manifestations of the traumatic experiences include broken bones, joint and muscle pain, headaches, dizziness, neurological damage, burns, hearing loss, and loss of sensation. Other sequelae include memory disturbance, problems with concentration, lack of energy, sexual dysfunction, emotional irritability, loss of trust in the world, insomnia, flashbacks, phobias, difficulty expressing/feeling emotions, depression, anxiety, and PTSD.

Theory

The crucial event in therapy for trauma victims is getting the individual to feel safe, connected, and in control. The next step is to get the survivor to feel connected to society, and finally to integrate the experience of trauma into the scope of the patient's life. Survivors of torture have resources and assets that have enabled them to survive; the aim of the program therefore is to enhance reempowerment. The process of recovery from trauma progresses in stages from the sense of unpredictable danger to reliable safety, from dissociated trauma to acknowledged memory, and from stigmatized isolation to restored social connection.

Services

Psychological services use a culturally sensitive approach to treatment in intensive individual, group, and family psychotherapy. Treatment focuses on symptom reduction, assistance with social difficulties, and networking with community organizations. The program provides both culturally homogeneous and mixed therapy groups when appropriate. Clinicians are encouraged to use a wide range of methods, including art, with survivors, allowing them to communicate that about which they cannot talk. Other treatments that are helpful include cognitive–behavioral therapies, narrative/solution focused therapy, testimony as a therapeutic process, body-oriented therapies, psychodynamic therapists, hypnosis, eye movement desensitization reprocessing, and ethnopsychological approaches.

Clients have access to comprehensive medical care; mental health services including individual, group, and family therapy; rehabilitative services including physical and occupational therapy; gynecological care; and social services providing assistance with housing, education, and employment. Clients are evaluated medically by one of five primary care physicians who provides and coordinates ongoing medical care. Care for chronic conditions as well as preventive care are included. A female gynecologist provides care and individuals have access to all specialty and subspecialty clinics at Bellevue. The goals of rehabilitative medicine are to reduce pain, restore physical function, and restore a sense of control over the body.

Survivors often require intensive social services and support, particularly if they experience culture shock upon relocating. Social work staff offers a consistent supportive presence as they conduct detailed initial intake assessments of social needs and services. Interventions include assistance to help clients meet basic needs of housing, food, and clothing as well as assistance in obtaining medical insurance. Social work staff advocates for clients with outside agencies and help clients deal with the bureaucracies around them. Social work staff acts as liaison between client and administrative staff of the hospital and with other agencies. They offer a community outreach program to visit survivors outside the clinic setting. In this program, they assist clients to adjust to basic activities of daily living.

Training

In the past, the program served as a training and resource center for other organizations assisting refugees and immigrants. The staff of the center has taught Immigration and Naturalization Service agents how to judge whether refugees are truly the victims of torture and deserve protection and asylum. The 2-week course was taught in conjunction with the Center for Victims of Torture in Minneapolis, MN. The training included mock interviews with actors playing the roles of torture survivors drawn from real cases. Specialists gave investigators on-the-spot critiques and suggestions. The program sensitized asylum officers and also dealt with the stress experienced by those officers as they listen to refugees' histories of trauma and torture.

Program staff also are available to present at conferences, grand rounds, and other educational venues. They also are involved in a number of advocacy activities and provide medical affidavits and testimony for clients applying for political asylum. They work at the state and federal level to effect change on issues and legislation impacting torture survivors. Program staff participated in a fact-finding mission sponsored by Physicians for Human Rights to Dharamsala, India, and interviewed Tibetan refugees. The program also has developed a collaborative relationship with Victim Services and has helped that organization to develop a community-based program in Jackson Heights, Queens, New York, called Solace. This latter program provides case management and social services to refugee torture survivors. The Bellevue program provides training to the staff of Victim Services as well as case consultation and medical and mental health services to its clients.

The program conducts an orientation for new staff including psychology interns and externs. All project staff participate in a continuing education

program to learn about innovative treatment approaches and new developments in the field. Guest speakers make presentations to staff. In 1997, 23
psychology interns, 1 social work intern, 3 primary care residents, 2 psychiatry
residents, and 10 medical students received mentorship and training.

Research

The program is collecting information on the effects of torture and
trauma and on approaches to treatment. The program is setting up a research
project to investigate the long-term effects of torture on the survivor and family
and to identify resources upon which survivors draw to aid recovery. Standardized measures of PTSD, a trauma history, and other measures are being
incorporated in this study. The program also has developed a screening questionnaire to identify survivors of torture among immigrant patients. Psychology interns are encouraged to conduct doctoral research projects.

DIRECT CONSULTANCIES: HEALING COMMUNITY TRAUMA AND MASS VIOLENCE COUNSELING, CONSULTATION, AND TRAINING, SAN FRANCISCO, CALIFORNIA

The original organization, created by Holbrook Teter, was named the
Coalition to Aid Refugee Survivors of Torture and War Trauma and was
designed to meet the mental health needs of victims of torture and refugees
from Central America. The coalition began working in San Francisco and the
Bay Area in 1985 to meet the mental health and social needs of refugees fleeing
state terrorism. The work of the coalition was shared with groups in Central
America, people living near contaminated areas of Chernobyl, war-torn communities in the Caucasus and former Yugoslavia, families and individuals
imprisoned in the United States, Cambodian refugees, and others. The members of the organization include agencies and individuals who work in mental
health and social service fields as well as the refugees themselves. The present
organization also works with many other services and agencies, both public
and private. It has little to no funding but receives some help from grants from
health departments and foundations. Goals of the organization are to develop
mental health promotion in the refugee community and networking in local,
national, and worldwide arenas.

Philosophy

There is a need to revisit the trauma experienced by torture survivors in
order to defuse its toxic qualities and to help survivors move on to appropriate
social (or personal) action. State terrorism aims to destroy communities by
rendering opposition to the state inoperative or impossible. The goal of the

state is to crush opposition and prevent change through the use of terror tactics, including torture.

Staffing

There is no paid staff for the organization per se, only volunteers. Some individuals are paid by collaborating organizations. The persons who work with the group are not professionals per se. Staff are very loyal to one another but find funding organizations to be very unloyal.

Theory

Traumatic reactions are normal reactions; breaking the silence, education, and finding a community are all healing interventions. Work with torture survivors aims to lower their emotional distress, which in turn leads to less distorted thinking, feeling, and action. The organization has developed a model for community treatment of trauma as persons learn from each other as well as consult the current PTSD literature.

The role of education is a primary concept underlying the work of the organization. Therapy is "deconstruction": cultural and personal deconstruction (from the past). Therapy deals with perception. Another concept is promotion of human rights: taking action against abuse of human rights for all persons of all races and social orientations. The work takes place in a social and political context in a global arena; spiritual qualities and values are inherent in it. It includes democratic psychiatry. Community treatment deals with perception of "reality" and "reaction." Symptoms of PTSD are able to be seen at community and society levels. A loss of trust, feelings of helplessness, and alienation also may be visible at community levels.

Services

The organization deals with current, acute, and chronic trauma. Services themselves are defined by the needs of the community. Assessments are done for medical referrals or court purposes and services are available to all. Services include education and sharing. Public education is a basic feature of community treatment. In some instances, torture survivors are aided with their applications for political asylum. A new trend for service provision is working with lawyers on prison issues.

Treatment at the community level can counteract demoralization from oppression. Open community discussion of emotional reactions to trauma is an attack on silence, a goal of state terrorism. Assignment of responsibility to death squads, secret police, armies, and governments is part of breaking of silence. Individuals are encouraged to give public testimony about what has happened to them. Other treatment-oriented activities include community planning, collective action, training of community leaders, service provision of jobs, food and shelter, and grassroots organizing to accomplish social change, demonstrations, and cultural presentations.

Publications

A handbook initially published on March 15, 1992, *Promoting Mental Health for Those Living in Contaminated Areas* (Teter, 1992), was written for survivors of the Chernobyl disaster. It addresses practical steps and specific techniques to deal with the psychological problems brought on by that disaster. It provides definitions of environmental disaster, stress, and PTSD. The manual recognizes that, while an environmental disaster is a one-time event, it also is ongoing, pervasive, and has invisible effects of anxiety, fear, uncertainty, and feelings of contamination.

The No Means Press has created a handbook to address the mental health effects of depression and state terrorism. The handbook offers guidelines for prevention, healing within the community, help for individuals, and promotion of human rights. It also can be used as a text for community training and planning (Teter, 1996).

INSTITUTE FOR PSYCHOTRAUMA SWITZERLAND, VISP, SWITZERLAND

The Institute for Psychotrauma Switzerland (IPTS), founded in 1993, is an organization of professionals (as an informal network) located throughout Switzerland who work with primary, secondary, and tertiary victims of any kind of trauma. A traumatic event, according to child psychiatrist and director Dr. Gisela Perren-Klingler (1996), is one through which one or several people are massively endangered in their physical and/or mental integrity. Feelings of helplessness (feeling of being at the mercy of someone else/others), a breakdown in one's own existence, loss of security, and extreme negative stress are central to the experience of trauma. Societies as well as individuals are afflicted with traumatic events and entire populations suffer the impacts of repetitive, chronic trauma. In 1993, when Switzerland enacted the law "Help to Victims of Violence," there was no established organization to provide that legislated help and included no training to helpers. The need for that training and for a network of trained practitioners to operationalize the law led to the institute's creation.

Many of the clients of IPTS also are asylum seekers who have not a refugee status in Switzerland. The organization is decentralized, expansible, and adaptable to new cultural, linguistic, and target population needs. It also could be adapted to Third World countries. All the practitioners also treat nontrauma patients, in order to prevent burnout. The institute consists of a central phone number (free of charge) which is linked to director Dr. Gisela Perren-Klingler's office phone 5½ days a week. During the phone interview, Dr. Perren-Klingler asks the caller about the nature of the trauma, language spoken, region where the caller lives, and other pertinent information. She also considers issues of gender, culture, race, and class when making a referral to a "specialist" who seems the best suitable.

Mission

The mission of IPTS is to provide as specific as possible service (sexually and culturally specific) and as up-to-date treatment as possible.

Funding

Funding is a problem for the center. Practitioners in private practice pay a fee of 100 francs for each patient referred by Dr. Perren-Klingler. However, in some instances, the therapists do not pay that fee. Many of the treatment sessions are paid by "Krankenkassen" (health insurance). Those who have no insurance can negotiate the cost of treatment. The organization also is funded by personal investment.

Staff

Approximately 50 physicians are in the network, primarily in private practice or government service and paid by insurance. They include general practitioners, internists, psychiatrists and child psychiatrists as well as approximately 30 psychologists, 10 social workers, and 15 nurses who work in institutions. Some of the more inexperienced staff show evidence of secondary trauma. All members of the network have had at least 20 days of training in trauma as well as training to combat secondary trauma; when necessary, staff call Dr. Perren-Klingler for consultation. Dr. Perren-Klingler, as referral source for clients, tries to give more difficult cases to those who are more experienced. Since no member of the network performs only trauma work, burnout is not a major issue of concern.

Clientele

Clients range from torture victims to torture perpetrators, from Swiss citizens to foreigners who are experiencing a range of traumatic reactions on a continuum that extends from an acute stress reaction to chronic PTSD. Many of the clients are refugees with an average of 4 years of asylum seekers' status. In order to integrate into Swiss society, even temporarily, return home in a state of dignity, or go into (illegal) hiding, these individuals need interventions. In 1995, the institute had 180 phone calls and Dr. Perren-Klingler referred approximately 30–40% of the callers. The callers ranged from asylum seekers, torture survivors, traffic accident victims, to survivors of family violence, with acute or chronic PTSD or other psychological difficulties.

Assessment

Assessment is left to the clinician who gets a referred patient. The first assessment is made by Perren-Klingler by phone, as to need of intervention, client's motivation, and possible diagnosis.

Clinical Services

The type of treatment that is needed is negotiated by Dr. Perren-Klingler with the client on the phone. The work may include individual and/or group counseling, psychotherapy, system intervention, provision of medication, critical incident stress debriefing (CISD), as well as supportive interventions, depending on the various levels of presentation of the clients. The CISD model used is based on the six-step Mitchell model (Everly & Mitchell, 1997), with the addition of a seventh step that helps the client to construct or invent a closing ritual.

Refugees often do not appreciate the need for psychological/psychiatric treatment for symptoms of PTSD and feel that treatment makes them crazy. Therefore it is important to have therapists/doctors who speak the language treat them. Many of the clients experience reactions ranging from acute stress reaction along the continuum to chronic PTSD.

Reorganization of communities is another aspect of practice through mobilization of traditional resources and coping skills, keeping in mind the culture of the refugees' communities. The cultural concept of "treatment" can hinder traumatic healing. Practitioners work with both the culturally nonspecific reactions of helplessness, the pathogenic nature of silence and shattered assumptions of trust as well as culturally specific reactions. Help primarily consists of giving support and protection and providing security.

"Healing" interventions and methods include breaking the silence in various ways, listening, reframing, doing outreach, providing education, conducting support groups, using community resources through referral, helping with practical problems of daily life, sharing of information, role-playing, sharing humor, using social action, and others (Perren-Klingler, 1996).

Theory

Trauma affects people on a social–societal level. Questions of meaning also have a spiritual/religious component that needs to be addressed. This meaning is easier to deal with on a metaphorical/ritually bound level than on a strict cognitive level. This means giving trauma a "picture" through metaphor and ritual, not just through history. The theory base of the practitioners is cognitive–behavioral, contextualistic, and eclectic with a client-focused, resource-oriented approach. The theory base of debriefing is Perren-Klingler's adaptation of the Mitchell model (Everly & Mitchell, 1997).

A very important theoretical concept is the societal–cultural context and understanding of trauma. Metraux and Fleury (1996) recognized that a community prevention model of trauma is participatory and encourages development of self-help networks, community solidarity, and self-determination. De Andrade (1996), wrote "how trauma is defined determines the model which theorists and researchers use to gather information about its existence" (p. 212). The structure model of trauma that looks at the psychocultural conceptualization is rooted in consideration of the social context of that trauma rather than just the individual psychopathology. The model recognizes that individuals are traumatized within their cultural contexts by violence, social polarization, institutional abuse, detention, and abandonment. The consequences of this type of trauma include disruption of the self and self-psychological functions and mistrust toward others.

Trauma is immense and more evident. The biggest challenge to the trauma field is primary prevention of violence. It is important to use First World professionals to work with human rights violations and do political intervention. However, the First World is not carrying out its social–political responsibility. The trauma treatment community needs more solidarity and more integration in its approach to these violations to stay credible in its therapeutic interventions postevent.

Training

Dr. Perren-Klingler has trained a bicultural group of Balkan/ex-Yugoslavian and Swiss practitioners to deal with trauma in preventive ways, for example, recognizing symptoms and signs of trauma and doing group debriefings with refugee peers. In 1997, she trained Swiss teachers in the French-speaking part of Switzerland in a similar way as well as a bicultural group in Geneva. The trained individuals are what Dr. Perren-Klingler calls "multiplicators"; they work with their compatriots, start groups to train others, and go back to Bosnia with the knowledge that has been learned. One trained individual has begun to debrief nurses; another is now working with Kurds and others in Southern Germany. The refugees who have been trained are German or French speaking, and they have been trained in techniques of debriefing, resource enhancement, and psychosocial activation. Training deals with knowledge, skills, and self-evaluation. Specialty areas for training include short-term intervention, systemic intervention, and assessment of torture and its consequences. The course takes place over an 8-month period. Dr. Perren-Klingler also trains the psychology professional who wants to have more skills in psychotherapy with survivors of trauma.

In late 1997, the Institute Psychotrauma Schweiz founded the Organisation de Victimologie et Psychotraumatologie Europenne (OVPE), with France
and Belgium and soon expanded OVPE to include Germany, Italy, Holland,
and possibly Great Britain, and soon Spain, Portugal, and Greece. The OVPE
has received some funding from the European Community with the goal of
building a complete European network from Greece, Turkey, and Spain to
Ireland and Iceland. The hope is to expand the network to Eastern Europe and
perhaps North Africa, while putting in place minimum training standards for
trauma treatment and CISD (at a European level).

THE SOCIETY FOR PSYCHOLOGICAL ASSISTANCE, UNIVERSITY OF ZAGREB SCHOOL OF SOCIAL WORK, ZAGREB, CROATIA

The Society for Psychological Assistance (SPA) is a registered, nonprofit,
nongovernmental health organization that is open to psychologists, social
workers, psychiatrists, and special educators with clinical, research, teaching,
and applied backgrounds. The SPA has a seven-member executive board and a
five-member supervision board to ensure that the interests of the community
at large are represented in the activities of the SPA. The general assembly
meets annually to develop a work plan for the following year.

The SPA has ongoing partnerships with international organizations such
as UNICEF, the Kempler Institute of Scandinavia, Save the Children (Norway
and Sweden), the Slovene Foundation, and the Norwegian Council for Mental
Health. The SPA has long-standing connections with a variety of international
centers including Johns Hopkins University, the EMDR Institute in Pacific
Grove, California, and the Psychosocial Center for Refugees at the University
of Oslo.

At the community level, the SPA works closely with local authorities,
schools, and social work centers as well as over 25 NGOs from Croatia and
Bosnia-Herzegovina. The SPA advocates for a humanistic approach to helping
populations, groups, families, and individuals in distress and crisis. The organization needs funds to continue its work.

The SPA will continue to respond to the variety of needs of those who need
psychosocial support. The overriding principle is empowerment of clients and
their respective communities. Special care is devoted to serving the most
vulnerable groups—children, adolescents, the elderly, and separated families.
Focus will be on development of preventive programs in the postwar period of
social transition, focusing on prevention of violence in families, children, and
adolescents at risk, women, and the elderly.

The SPA will remain committed to the highest standards of delivery of
training, services, and supervision. These efforts are targeted to foster systemic
change, increase the quality of human services, and help build a civil society.
The SPA plans to establish a series of children, adolescent, and family centers
in the localities of greatest need. The SPA has an excellent track record of

successful collaboration with local NGOs and major international organizations. It had full programming responsibility for projects funded from a variety of sources including USAID, totaling $3,650,000 over the last 5 years. In the near future, the SPA will focus on meeting the needs arising from three parallel transition processes: (1) from war to peace, which is hindered by deep psychological scars, fears, and hate; (2) from centralized to market economy, which engenders anxieties and uncertainty; and (3) transition from nondemocratic to democratic system, which brings challenges for the nongovernmental sector and civil society.

The SPA will continue to pursue the policy of integrating practical experiences in providing psychosocial interventions, critical evaluation, and refinement, and providing a range of training curricula. It will continue to be open to local and international partnership initiatives, willing to share experiences and to work together both nationally and internationally. Its ambition is to remain a leading regional mental health NGO. The information is regularly updated on the SPA's worldwide web pages (http://www.dpp.hr).

As part of long-term sustainability strategy, the SPA needs guidance in accessing the resources that are likely to support its programming activities and operational costs. This includes help in identifying the most likely funding sources and facilitating contacts with them. The SPA also looks forward to expert professional input in particular areas of work, including assistance in development of the crises intervention teams and learning from other organizations of their experiences in working with female victims of abuse, as well as providing training for SPA staff and associates in these issues.

Mission and Goals

The mission of the SPA is to help alleviate the suffering of traumatic stress survivors and to provide psychological and psychosocial assistance to individuals, families, groups, and communities in distress. Goals of the SPA include:

1. The provision of direct psychosocial assistance to survivors of traumatic stress with special focus on underserved populations
2. The provision of psychological support, counseling, and therapy to individuals and families in distress, grief, and crisis
3. The training of professional and nonprofessional mental health care providers; serving as a field center for training university graduate students
4. The development of clinical and community-based needs assessment techniques, protocols, and instruments
5. The development of methods to monitor programs and evaluate impacts
6. The provision of professional support and consultation to organizations and brochures and leaflets to the community at large
7. Assistance to increase community awareness and understanding of stress, trauma, and recovery

Staffing

Current SPA membership is 41 mental health professionals. They are admitted to the organization solely on the merit of their human and professional quality, expertise, and commitment to serve people in need. Full-time staff include five professionals: general secretary, curriculum advisor, project coordinator, psychologist, and social worker. Administrative staff include a full-time administrative assistant and a part-time secretary. The largest number of employed staff was 17 during the major 3-year-old training project. Other professionals are hired part time, including computer and data specialists, consultants, therapists, and trainers. The number of these depends on the workload and availability of projects funded by outside sources and donors. The SPA is able to recruit up to 31 professionals from within its membership at any one time to provide training and treatment services. This framework makes it not only a leading regional mental health nongovernmental community-oriented (trauma) organization, but also a very flexible one, able to respond to a variety of needs. The SPA has an office in downtown Zagreb that includes a training facility, counseling center, and a specialized reference library.

Clientele

The SPA has provided direct and continuous psychosocial assistance services for 5 years to over 3000 persons in collective refugee centers. Seven hundred clients have been served directly by community crisis interventions and individual and group counseling and therapy. A total of 1635 participants from 90 communities completed training courses. These trainees serve about 200,000 clients. Over 700 mental health providers attended professional public lectures sponsored by the SPA. Senior SPA staff taught 220 students at Universities of Zagreb and Sarajevo.

Service Provision

The SPA offered comprehensive psychosocial services between 1991 and 1997 to two collective refugee centers in Zagreb (CSC) and Karlovac (Gaza) housing 3000 refugees and displaced persons. Special care was given to children, adolescents, the elderly, and separated families. Interventions included individual and family counseling, support groups, income-generating activities, structuring of leisure activities, school assistance, creative activities, and trauma treatment.

The SPA started implementation of community-based psychosocial assistance programs to resettlement communities of Slunj and Hrvatska Kostajnica beginning in April 1996. Teams traveled twice weekly to the communities to provide individual and group services to over 200 persons (2200 interventions monthly). Part of the intervention included a weekly radio talk show.

As soon as it became possible to reach the beneficiaries in the former Kraina region and Eastern Slavonia (former UNTAES zone), the SPA started to provide training and support to the local care providers. In spite of many hardships, SPA members and associates offered assistance there because that is where it was most needed. During 1997, they worked with as may as 180 care providers in the area. Part of this work was funded by the United Nations. They also helped establish a counseling center in the community of Bilje, staffed with former trainees.

During the previous 3 years, the SPA worked in Bosnia-Herzegovina, in Sarajevo, both sides of Mostar, Gorazde, Tuzla, Zenica, Bihac, Jablanica, and Sanski Most, to name but a few places that the SPA has worked since 1994, often under direct threat of safety. To the care providers in Eastern and Central Europe, the SPA has offered a program addressing management of stress in relief work with women and children.

SPA developed a predeparture trauma recovery (PDTR) curriculum module and program for persons approved for resettlement in the United States in collaboration with the International Catholic Migration Commission (ICMC). This program has met the needs of 474 Bosnian refugees; 15% of them also received individual counseling.

The SPA operates a counseling center in Zagreb for persons experiencing reactions to stress, trauma, loss, and related psychosocial difficulties. Services provided include individual and family counseling, group work, social coping skill training, and other coping skill training. Services from this NGO community-based mental health service are offered at no cost. Based on these experiences, the SPA plans to develop a network of child, adolescent, and family community centers throughout the country. Establishment of the first two, in communities of Velika Gorica and the almost destroyed city of Vukovar, are under way. These centers will provide a range of services for preschoolers to adolescents and their families when those needs are not met by other human service agencies.

Training

Recognition of the mental health needs of mental health workers in Croatia has been an extremely slow process. Before the Bosnian war, recognition of the hazards of mental health work and supervision as a source of support for mental health workers were nonexistent. When the war occurred suddenly, the needs of victims superseded those of the workers. The Society for Psychological Assistance recognized the needs of mental health care providers and developed a training program to meet their needs. This program began in Spring 1994, initially funded by an International Rescue Committee Umbrella Grant and then by various organizations.

The mental health training program that was created included a 3-day workshop followed by two one-day supervision sessions. The workshop curriculum was based on Lazarus and Folkman's (1984) model of stress and led participants through five steps of (1) recognition of and development of awareness of signs and sources of burnout and vicarious trauma; (2) identification and cognitive reappraisal of professional stressors; (3) increase in awareness of alternative coping strategies; (4) development of practical and achievable individual self-help plans; and (5) encouragement of the construction of supportive mechanisms for care providers. A manual accompanied the course. The SPA established eight program objectives:

1. To gain knowledge about the effects of helpers' stress and indirect traumatization on mental health and to understand the process of burning out
2. To identify signs and sources of stress and ways of coping
3. To become aware of personal professional responsibility to protect mental health
4. To use communication skills to reduce professional stress
5. To appreciate the importance of supervision
6. To learn and practice specific coping strategies
7. To design and implement individual self-help plans to cope with professional stress
8. To facilitate network building and support building among participants

Between March 1994 and October 1996, the SPA provided 16 workshops for 463 care providers who worked primarily with refugees and displaced persons, torture victims, and disabled clients. The majority of the care providers were female (83.6%) and by profession the majority were teachers, social workers, and psychologists (23.6%, 20.2%, and 10%, respectively). Many of the helpers were from Bosnia and Herzegovina. The mental health training model has been extended to helpers who work with victims of war in governmental organizations and helpers who work with populations not directly affected by war. Information gained from the program has been integrated into two new courses at the University of Zagreb.

The SPA hosted a two day interactive meeting for persons working in collective refugee centers to share their experiences in January 1995. The SPA offered a five-day workshop for 40 non-professionals who worked with children in collective centers as well. SPA then published a manual of theoretical information, ready made programs, methods to assess needs and resources of children and questionnaires to assess outcomes.

A 2.5 million dollar grant from USAID and Catholic Relief Services funded the above programs as well as training courses developed for Trauma Awareness and Referral, Leadership and Program Building Training, Basic Trauma and Recovery Training, and Advanced Trauma and Recovery Training. These workshops used participatory small group workshops and specific topic lectures and ranged from 24–360 hours/course. This was part of the three-year old Post-trauma Recovery Training Project that has been the major training effort in the whole region.

The SPA has published numerous leaflets, written numerous manuals and books (Ajduković, 1997; Pregrad, 1997; Ajduković & Ajduković, 1996), and publishes a quarterly newsletter. It operates a professional library focusing on trauma and stress psychology, counseling and group work, and grief and family therapy. The library has over 1200 titles and subscriptions to three Croatian and eight international journals.

The SPA Professional Lecture Series was established in May 1995 by leading international experts in the field of stress, trauma, family issues, violence, and grief. The series has led to networking, information sharing, and idea sharing among mental health professionals who attend.

One of the most important events in recent years was the 3-day international conference, "Trauma Recovery Training: Lessons Learned," held in July 1997. The conference focused on a critical review of the lessons learned through a wealth of trauma recovery training opportunities available during the past several years in Croatia and Bosnia-Herzegovina. A number of mental health professionals from 17 countries met to summarize what they learned about training care providers to better serve the traumatized population. The presentations reviewed past experiences, elaborated on current issues in the field of individual and community trauma recovery, and set the stage for future directions. A heightened awareness of the role of social context and its meaning in understanding trauma and PTSD and appropriateness of the psychosocial model in trauma treatment emerged from the meeting.

The SPA is developing a psychological crisis response team and network at the national level. The project is supported by UNICEF in collaboration with the Ministry of Labour and Social Welfare. The psychological crisis response team works with preschool facilities, schools, centers for social work, children's health clinics, Red Cross branches, and emergency services.

Research

The SPA has demonstrated commitment to continuous evaluation and refinement of its service and training programs. It has developed an evaluation model that has been used to assess the effects of comprehensive training projects at a variety of levels. The feature of this multidimensional model is that it integrated (1) three types of evaluation of needs, program efficiency, and program effectiveness; (2) three evaluation levels: direct beneficiaries, clients' benefits as ultimate beneficiaries, and community impact; and (3) three time points: before training (pretest), after completing the program (posttest), and 6–24 months later (posttest and follow-up). The SPA has developed and implemented specific protocols and instruments for assessing each aspect of service provided. The evaluation used a 14-item Helper Role Scale (HRS), a 21-item Helper Time Effectiveness Scale (HTES), and an 18-item Helper Burnout Scale (HBS). Participants were evaluated at the beginning of a seminar, at the second follow-up supervision 3 months later, and 1 year after training was completed. Participants also provided evaluations through informal feedback and written anonymous evaluations. Postintervention comparisons of mean scores on the three instruments at the first supervision session indicated that the training program was probably effective, with a reduction in stress symptoms, although nothing had changed in participants' work environments. Questionnaires were returned by 122 of 283 participants 1-year postworkshop and change has persisted.

The SPA serves as a consultant for evaluation of the trauma-related and psychosocial assistance projects. An illustration of this is the external evaluation performed using the experimental design of the project "School-based Health and Peace Initiative." The project was a collaborative effort of UNICEF, CARE Canada, McMaster University, and the Croatian Ministry of Education and Sport. It was implemented in Western and Eastern Slovenian elementary schools with a high proportion of children traumatized by the war.

As a complementary activity to evaluation and research, a 3-day workshop on evaluation of the psychosocial and humanitarian projects was developed and held for participants from nine local NGOs from Croatia and Bosnia-Herzegovina. A workbook to accompany this training program was developed. This workshop was the first of the kind developed by a local organization with the profound insight into both the evaluation methodology and culturally specific issues in evaluation of community-oriented trauma assistance projects. The SPA also has translated and adapted numerous psychological instruments and has constructed 20 new assessment instruments to document the impact and effectiveness of its services and activities.

CENTER FOR PREVENTION AND RESOLUTION OF VIOLENCE, ("QA TUTSAWINAVU"), TUCSON, ARIZONA

The Hopi word *tsawana* means "a state of mind that is terror." The Center for the Prevention and Resolution of Violence strives toward a state of mind that is unintimidated by fear from any source, the state of "Qa Tutsawinavu." The center was established in 1992 to work with violence that has occurred and the legacy of that violence. The center is a multicultural treatment, training, and research program that works with at-risk communities to prevent and diminish violence and reconstruct and revitalize lives traumatized by violence. It provides treatment for survivors of severe physical, sexual, and emotional trauma and focuses on psychological, physical, and spiritual aspects of the individual.

The center is a project of the Hopi Foundation, a group begun by the Hopi Indians in Northern Arizona to combine indigenous values with Western technology. The Hopi Foundation began in the 1980s on the reservation; at first it worked domestically and then expanded services to help people from Ecuador, because as the oldest inhabitants of the United States they had the responsibility to help other indigenous peoples in other places. After completing a needs assessment, Dr. Barbara Chester, founding clinical director, shared with the board of the foundation that the biggest need area was in Tucson. She previously had helped to establish the first US center for the treatment of political torture and had experience designing programs. Some of the work of the center is actually done at the centralized clinic; other work is decentralized. The organization is its employees and it is almost entirely a volunteer organization. Management also is line staff and everyone has an integral, nonhierarchical role in service delivery.

In the future, the organization hopefully will be more of a full-time operation with a clinic that is open more than one night a week. It would have a larger space more under the control of its clientele than the medical school that houses it and would be more a community space for those who come for services. The organization is one of the few in the world working with issues of indigenous human rights and indigenous populations that are being displaced.

Mission

The Center for the Prevention and Resolution of Violence (CPRV) is a treatment, training, and research program working with at-risk communities to prevent and diminish violence and to reconstruct lives traumatized by violence. The basic contribution of the program is to give voice to indigenous peoples who are being displaced. The aim of CPRV is to design programs to help fragmented communities and individuals regain a sense of "wholeness." These programs are designed to be replicable models to prevent the occurrence of further violence within high-risk communities. The program also provides services to undocumented refugees who are filing for political asylum. It aims to serve survivors of unsafe settings at a distance from their traumas. The philosophy of the center is that healing has to be approached with an appreciation for the culture of the people who are being healed, people whose strong cultural strengths and skills have allowed them to survive.

Staff

Most services are preformed by volunteers. A refugee coordinator guides the refugees from the time they are in Central America to the time they arrive in Tucson. The coordinator handles logistics of scheduling at the clinic and prioritizes medical and psychological emergencies or persons awaiting evaluation for asylum. The violence prevention program has two advisory committees: one of adults indigenous to Central America and a youth council.

The actual clinic is staffed primarily by medical students as part of the Commitment to Underserved People program and by volunteer professionals. Staff of the psychological services include one psychologist, two clinical social workers, three counselors (2 male, 1 female), a female licensed physiotherapist, and a female massage therapist. Most staff are Caucasian. This multidisciplinary group covers the mind–body continuum.

A mental health coordinator (behavioral health coordinator) does the mental health evaluations; a physician does medical evaluations. The mental health coordinator determines triage of services and confers with the physician about the need for medications and alternative treatments. A traditional Nicaraguan healer also is available to the program. The violence prevention program utilizes trauma survivors and survivor–professionals in service provision. Many were community organizers in their countries of origin and use their skills with the program or serve on the advisory board.

A management team maintains quality control. The team includes the mental health coordinator, the medical director, two medical students, a physiotherapist, and the director of the refugee clinic. The medical director reviews all files weekly and the team then arranges for follow-up.

Funding

The work of CPRV is supported by private foundations, individual donations, and thousands of hours of in-kind contributions by dedicated volunteers. Clinic services are donated by the local medical school as are space, equipment, and some laboratory testing; people in crisis receive prioritized services. Any available funding from private foundations (Charles Stewart Mott Foundation mainly) at the present time is used primarily for the Violence Prevention Program to fund the coordinator position (the person who does the logistics for refugees) and several consultants. The remainder of the program is run by volunteers and laypersons.

Clientele

The center deals primarily with persons from the border area of Mexico. The primary clientele are indigenous people being forced out of their homes in El Salvador and Guatemala. The secondary populations served are the families of those people. Some clients have been victims of torture, witnesses of massacres, and victims of other types of violence. The tertiary clientele of the program is the community of these indigenous peoples.

Service Provision

CPRV has established a violence prevention program to help unify disenfranchised Central American Indians residing in the United States through extensive focus groups designed to identify needs and target objectives specific to their communities. A group for relatives of disappeared persons and a group for women who have been survivors of rape and/or domestic violence are being planned.

The center participated in a pilot project with the Vietnamese Former Political Prisoners Association of Tucson Refugee Education Project. The project provided an integrated holistic health model to political prisoners and their family members. The project may become an ongoing program.

The center works to increase public awareness about and implement changes in government policies that violate basic human rights including the indigenous peoples of Central America. One object of this action is to bring pressure to bear on governments to end torture, oppression, and warfare against those indigenous peoples. The center evaluates people for documentation for political asylum and facilitates the asylum process. A large part of the work done by the center is advocacy, including getting children into schools and services that do not want them and helping them to obtain legal status. The program has a violence prevention program for children under 18 who come as unaccompanied minors or with families. Programs designed to help these children include dropout prevention and provision of English as a second language services.

The center has completed a pilot study of Southern Cheyenne women who are survivors of sexual assault. It participates in a study investigating cumulative trauma, PTSD, traditional culture, and sexual assault in communities with low and high rates of alcoholism. In October 1995, the center cosponsored a conference entitled "Intimate Violence in a Cross-Cultural Context" in conjunction with the Southern Arizona Mental Health Center and other agencies. Center staff trained individuals in the area of intimate violence.

The center provides direct medical services to about 300 people a year through the weekly clinic. Additional services including mental health, physiotherapy, and violence prevention serve approximately 500 persons yearly. Approximately 60–70% of persons seen have a PTSD-positive diagnosis. Comorbid diagnoses include depression, panic disorder, and generalized anxiety disorder. Treatment is both short and long term; many persons have a long-term relationship with the clinic and come back when specific problems arise over time. This is a family practice model that is frequently crisis based, particularly around the time of an asylum hearing or when bad news comes from home.

Theory

The work of the center is based on a philosophy of "whatever works." Since the majority of persons seen by the program are traumatized and come from different cultures and have different worldviews, staff and volunteers try to incorporate culturally sensitive treatment techniques. Posttraumatic therapy, cognitive–behavioral therapy, the testimony method, narrative therapy, eye movement desensitization reprocessing, and other techniques are used when they are thought to be appropriate.

A second theoretical principle that guides the work of the center is based on the Hopi philosophy of "Qa Tutsawinavu." Trauma, war, and violence exist in the world and cause fear; however, the goal of the organization is to create a state of mind that is not influenced or impacted by fear. This philosophy helps people come to positions of inner strength in dealing with their adversities in a proactive way. This is not a rehabilitation model but more a way of looking at the world.

Training and Education

Center staff provides training to other professionals. Goals of training are identification of PTSD in refugee populations, cross-cultural sensitivity, post-traumatic therapy as a treatment choice, and appropriate referral. When referral resources are not available, trainees are taught to normalize traumatic reactions and to give information to clients. The program has developed training materials, curricula, protocols, and handouts that the center would be willing to share.

This description is dedicated to Barbara Chester, pioneer and founder of the organization, who died in 1997. She is greatly missed.

GOVERNMENT OF THE REPUBLIC OF CROATIA OFFICE FOR VICTIMS OF WAR, ZAGREB, CROATIA

The Croatian Psycho-Social Program (CPSP) was created in January 1995 to combat the consequences and treat psychosocial problems resulting from the war in Croatia (1991–1995). The program is based on ideas of WHO (Agger, 1995), and the community-based rehabilitation programs of UNESCO, as well as national experience.

The Croatian psychosocial hexagon is the model for optimal coordination of the three main parts of the program: experts, administration, and victims on governmental and county levels. The program organized 18 county operative headquarters through interdisciplinary counseling centers to open psycho-social programs that treated 3000 victims between January 1995 and June 1996. The emphasis is on maximizing treatment to victims and families of victims in their real surroundings through an integrated approach that delivers services at the "ground level."

Mission

The mission is to build an integral psychosocial program for victims of war and their families and to provide help to victims of war in the family through the work of experts, state administrators, and organizations of war victims.

Funding

A number of economic, social, and financial limitations have led to maximization of available resources.

Staffing

Basic psychological help is provided by an interdisciplinary counseling team of social workers, lawyers, psychologists, and medical workers who utilize stationary and mobile counseling, media, direct group discussion, and telephone hotlines. Three hundred eighty-four educated experts treated individuals and groups in interdisciplinary teams. Staff were obligated to meet weekly for a team synthesis. The teams included health workers (152, or 39%), psychologists (82, or 21%), social workers (41, or 16%), lawyers (32, or 8%), special teachers (26, or 7%), and various others (38, or 10%).

Clientele

Between 1991 and 1995, there were over 50,000 direct victims of the war in Croatia, including 10,668 killed and 37,180 wounded and 2775 missing. Among these victims were 268 children killed and 971 children wounded, as well as 180,000 displaced persons. The surviving persons experienced prolonged, multiple stressors. At the time of the war, the population of Croatia was 4.7 million.

Services

Psychosocial help is provided to victims of war at a variety of levels. One hundred percent of those seen receive help for basic life and emotional needs; 60–80%, unspecified psychological help; 20–50%, basic psychological help; and 5–10% intensive psychiatric help. Only a few receive programmatic help. The goals of the program include work with victims and their families; medical, social, and psychological education, employment, and spiritual help; team work with experts; mobile approaches to ground work in real surroundings; creation of coordinated network (the Croatian Humanitarian Network) with governmental structure, consisting of experts and NGOs; counseling including individual and group/family work with stationary and mobile teams; and an informational and counseling hotline.

Research

Research findings include a 12% PTSD rate in disabled victims and a 14–31% PTSD rate in nondisabled war veterans. Children of victims have increased stress reactions and depression. Families of missing persons cope predominantly with a fatalistic approach to life. Much of this interview is based on Ajduković, Ajduković, and Ljubotina (1997).

THE REHABILITATION CENTER FOR TORTURE VICTIMS, COPENHAGEN, DENMARK

The Rehabilitation Center for Torture Victims (RCT) serves primary victims who are torture survivors, secondary victims who are families of the survivors, and tertiary caregivers in the organization. In addition, the organization educates professionals both in Denmark and abroad, develops new methods to improve treatment and treatment outcome, conducts research, assists in the establishing of similar rehabilitation centers worldwide through setting up the infostructure, and helps to raise funds from governmental (e.g., European Union) and nongovernmental sources. The organization has a physical security system with the ability to activate an alarm in each of the treatment rooms. Staff is trained in evacuation procedures in case of a phone bomb threat or the arrival of a suspicious package.

In 1973, Amnesty International called on international health professionals to prove the occurrence of torture when allegations had been made. Doctors examining torture survivors discovered the severity of psychological consequences of torture and recommended treatment. In 1979, the medical group approached the University Hospital in Copenhagen and asked permission to hospitalize Latin American refugees. Amnesty International established treatment principles, sponsored an international meeting in Copenhagen, and asked the Danish group to create a treatment center. The organization was created in 1982 as an independent, nonprofit organization in a building near to the University Hospital, the first such facility in the world. The second facility was the Canadian Centre for Victims of Torture.

Mission

The RCT works against the use of torture as a means to maintain power through destruction of the identity and health of those less powerful. The journal *Torture* defines the mission of the RCT, an independent, humanitarian, nonpolitical organization. The RCT was established to respond to the continuing needs unique to survivors of torture, rehabilitate victims of torture, contribute to the prevention of torture, instruct Danish health professionals in the examination and treatment of persons subjected to torture, and carry on research into the nature, extent, and consequences of torture.

Staffing

The RCT uses psychologists, psychiatrists, general practitioners, nurses, physical therapists, social workers, and support staff in the clinical department. The head of the RCT is an administrative director; under the director are heads of education, treatment, and project departments. In the project department, staff members are lawyers, anthropologists, cultural socialists, and support services. Librarians run a research library containing information on torture. The organization has limited resources and limited space but could use more staff as demand for services grows. The organization does not use lay caregivers or volunteers. It is not possible for non-Danes to do a practicum at the center. Supervision is provided by a psychiatrist outside the organization for those doing the treatment. Professionals see clients only 50% of the time; the other 50% is devoted to researching, writing, or giving lectures. Staff are highly qualified and trained in their individual professions. All are licensed and certified as health professionals by the government or their professional organizations. A board of directors is composed of members from the Danish Medical Association, Danish Bar Association, and Danish Hospital Association, as well as others.

Clientele

Survivors are referred to the RCT by Danish Health and Social Systems, the Danish Refugee Council, and general practitioners as well as United Nations agencies. Once torture survivors who have sought asylum in Denmark are evaluated, they are referred for ongoing therapy to private practitioners. At the present time, most of the survivors come from the Middle East. In 1982, when the RCT began its work, clients came primarily from Latin America. New survivor groups bring information about and evidence of new methods of torture.

Funding

The RCT is a nonprofit organization offering free of charge services to clients. Funding comes from the Danish government's Ministry of Foreign Affairs, private foundations, the European Foundation, and the UN Voluntary Fund for Torture Victims.

Assessment

Assessment of a survivor is performed at the beginning, middle, and end of treatment. Among the instruments used are the Hamilton Depression Scale, Hamilton Anxiety Scale, Hopkins Checklist-25, Harvard Trauma Questionnaire, and self-created instruments. Staff are reluctant to label clients with a diagnosis in order not to stigmatize them, but they do use DSM-IV criteria for PTSD.

Services

The RCT is the link between survivors of torture and professional services and support networks including doctors, lawyers, social service workers, and volunteers. The RCT provides medical care directly to clients and can refer to a university hospital when hospitalization is needed (e.g., surgery to remove rubber bullets). Two teams of professionals work with clients: one team works with single individuals, and the other with families and family members as well as the torture survivors themselves. The RCT staff has worked with torture survivors from 58 different countries.

Individual, family, and group counseling is provided to individuals and family members. The RCT staff do some advocacy to create awareness among the general public and other professionals about the work of the center. Staff try to avoid any treatment methods that might lead to flashbacks of torture methods (long waiting times, small rooms, water training). Clients are seen after they have escaped, obtained asylum, and generally been on the center's waiting list. Unfortunately, treatment is provided between 2 and 10 years postincident. The minimum length of time in treatment is 6 months; the maximum is up to 18 months.

Theory

Torture survivors were traumatized in a conspiracy of silence and were not allowed to tell what happened to them. In asking for asylum, they were questioned about reasons for applying; however, it is difficult for them to share what they experienced. When they finally come to treatment, the initial task is to establish a situation of mutual trust between client and therapist. A major goal of treatment is to help the client retell what he or she experienced so the experiences can be put "in the right places" as well as help the client learn better coping mechanisms. The minimum length of treatment is 6 months and the maximum length is generally 1½ years. Treatment includes both psychological and physical treatment.

Community Intervention

The RCT organized the International Rehabilitation Council for Torture Victims (IRCT), an informal network of rehabilitation centers worldwide. The IRCT and RCT have relationships with United Nations agencies. The RCT staff publishes articles in professional journals, give interviews to the media about torture, and train health professional organizations' staff.

The RCT staff offer training to professionals in the specialty area of work with torture survivors. They advertise their training seminars to colleagues around the world or instruct colleagues how to apply for training in Denmark. Researchers are allowed to use the RCT's library and conduct research. The RCT staff has developed training materials which they share and have written several books for physical therapists, nurses, and doctors who treat torture victims. The RCT has helped to create a special section of the World Psychiatric

Association that can build awareness of the problems related to torture. The RCT also provides documents for persons involved in forensic work. One publication of RCT/IRCT is *Torture: Quarterly Journal on Rehabilitation of Torture Victims and Prevention of Torture.* The journal looks at torture throughout the world, describes center presentations, publishes declarations for various professional groups, and reviews professional books and programs.

THE REFUGEE PROJECT, SPONSORED BY THE INTERNATIONAL STUDIES PROGRAM AT NEW YORK UNIVERSITY, NEW YORK, NEW YORK

The International Trauma Studies Program at New York University is a university-based center of expertise for local, international, and multidisciplinary collaboration, promoting humanitarian and mental health/human rights work through postgraduate training, research, and consultation, as well as through community-oriented programs. The first postgraduate certificate training program began in October 1998 under the leadership of Dr. Jack Saul. The program offers intensive clinical training for mental health professionals in psychotherapy with individuals, families, and groups, as well as multidisciplinary training in community approaches. Other participants come from the related fields of health, law, human rights, community activism, humanitarian organizations, the arts, journalism, and the media.

The International Trauma Studies Program collaborates with the following projects:

1. Theater Arts Against Political Violence, which is a program that works with survivors of political violence to create performances on human rights issues and the plight of refugees
2. REFUGE: Family and Community Outreach Project facilitates sustainable community-based programs to address the psychosocial needs of survivors of severe human rights violations and their families
3. The NYU Project on Trauma and the Media
4. The Taking Care of the Caretakers Program, which provides psychosocial support services for those working with traumatized populations

The program emphasizes a transcultural view of trauma, preventive approaches, and family and community orientations. It offers advocacy training through active promotion of local, national, and international collaboration across disciplines and service populations. It has a research component with epidemiological studies, service and training needs assessments, and program evaluation. The program also is working closely with the International University Center for Mental Health and Human Rights based in Copenhagen, Denmark.

The Refugee Project

The Refugee Project, sponsored by the International Trauma Studies Program, has developed a variety of approaches to address the mental health needs of refugee survivors of torture and trauma living in New York City. The project bases much of its work with current survivors of political violence on accumulated research and clinical experience with survivors of the Nazi Holocaust and their families.

Many of the survivors of torture and other forms of state-sponsored violence seeking services in New York City are in the process of applying for or have received political asylum and/or refugee status. While waiting months for the applications to be reviewed, they are unable to work legally, receive no public assistance, and are dependent on charitable members of the community for basic support. This vulnerable population is easily exploited in the workplace and often is further victimized by violence on the streets. Estimates are that 10–35% of the refugee communities (which are close to 1½ million) have suffered trauma from political violence. Many have experienced multiple traumas of violence, torture, imprisonment, and/or chronic threat. Until recently, there were no specialized services/programs/centers offering mental health, medical, or social support. Many of these asylum seekers are socially isolated. They are often in a state of continuous stress due to unresolved political and family calamities in the home country, superimposed on the difficulties they have in adapting to their new and often alienating environments.

It is estimated that there are close to 100,000 torture survivors in the New York area and perhaps three times as many who are refugees directly affected by political violence. Torture is most often an assault that has the goal of suppressing and depowering opposition. Thus, it is important to view the process of recovery in the context of collective healing.

The Refugee Project takes the perspective that refugees will rebuild their lives and gradually find ways of healing. The mental health approach of the project is attuned to the hierarchy of needs of the population in need of services, rather than imposing external values and goals. Services are best provided by practitioners from the community who understand the culture, language, and practices of the population(s) served. These approaches are most successful when involving creative integration of scientific knowledge about trauma recovery with the particular sociocultural context of the community. The program provides family support, crisis intervention, home visitation, pharmacological intervention, other medical treatments, as well as new intervention strategies for prevention of difficulties and maintenance of functioning.

Psychotherapy is an alien concept for most refugees. In many instances, mental health professionals (back home) in the countries of origin were associated with stigma of severe mental illness. This fact has led to the development of models for working with survivors that are sensitive to their needs and access their strengths, resources, and coping capacities, however they are defined by the survivor as important to recovery The services that are more appropriate include making contact with family remaining back home, documenting experiences for human rights' organizations, and performing a purification ritual or ceremony to memorialize the dead rather than working on alleviating symptoms of posttraumatic stress. Another important function of the therapist is to help a survivor recover the intuitive and natural resources needed to heal through rebuilding of a meaningful social context.

The creation of small support groups for survivors, consisting of either members of the same country or from different countries, is extremely important. Social supports such as small informal groups of peers promote the process of healing, especially when groups have opportunities for prosocial action and provide a safe place for self-disclosure. It also is very important for many survivors to reconnect with their pretrauma past, particularly with the family from which they were separated.

Testimony and Representation in Art

In the giving of testimony, healing in the private space of psychotherapy gives way to the need for public affirmation, intervention, and recovery of a political or cultural voice. The representation of experiences through public documentation is an important mode of healing. One important means of documentation is the creation of a new venue to bear witness to actors about their experiences and then work collaboratively to create theatrical performances to express them. The shift of view from healing to artistic representation can liberate the survivor by recontextualizing the memories with the support of an engaged group. This type of creativity and others often are central to the process of healing.

Theater Arts Against Political Violence is a theater group that creates performances based on those testimonies. In December 1997, a group of actors and a director worked with staff from the Bellevue/NY Program for Survivors of Torture to train Immigration and Naturalization Service (INS) asylum officers. The actors played torture survivors who were interviewed by INS officers as part of their instruction on compassionate approaches to interviewing. Following the training, the director of the Artaban Theater Company and Dr. Saul started the theater group to raise awareness about the consequences of severe human rights violations and the plight of refugees living in the United States. This theater of witnesses helps to break the conspiracy of silence surrounding torture, political violence, and refugee trauma.

As the project evolved, members of the refugee community were invited to a theater workshop to tell their stories and work collaboratively with the group. A number of refugee communities now participate in the project on an ongoing basis. The processes of theatrical experimentation and performance provide access to a unique combination of communication, witnessing, creative transformation, documentation, storytelling, and education.

SUMMARY

As Jack Saul's innovative work has shown, there always is room for growth and change in the trauma field. No one program has "the answer" or "the perfect organization" to work with refugees. We have learned lessons hopefully from work with Bosnian refugees and African refugees that can be implemented and modified to help the refugees of other conflagrations, including Kosovo. Again, meeting the basic life needs of refugees must be the primary focus of intervention—needs for housing, food, clothing, health care, and meaningful activity. Children need support to obtain an education, to play, and to spend time with peers. Displaced professionals need opportunities to work—as doctors, teachers, and therapists. Hopefully, their efforts can be compensated; but if that is not possible, they must be allowed to volunteer in their chosen fields.

All trauma centers working with refugees participate in the creation of a human rights climate. In addition, knowledge of the culture of the clientele is an essential part of service delivery planning, implementation, and evaluation. Mobilization of traditional, culturally appropriate resources at a social–societal level is essential. As Perren-Klingler notes, trauma must be understood within that societal–cultural context.

Numerous individuals and organizations are working toward linking centers and center directors. Perren-Klingler and others have founded the Organisation de Victimologie et Psychotramatologie Europenne (OVPE). The efforts of the Hamburger Institute for Social Research (Hamburger Institüt für Sozialforschung) under the leadership of Jan Philipp Reemtsma brought together center directors and representatives with the aim of developing an international network for interdisciplinary research that would encourage networking, program planning, resource identification and development, fund raising, and needs assessment. Leadership of the network was tripartite, with Stig Hornshøj-Møller of Denmark, Dr. van Reemtsma, and Klaus Vogel of the Max-Planck-Institute for History. However, the untimely, unexpected death of Hornshøj-Møller brought trauma to that network. The efforts that have been made for networking are only a beginning. It is the hope of the authors of this volume that network directors will join to create a case management program for refugee trauma on an international scale.

11

Trauma Centers for Children

When the authors of this volume were researching trauma centers for children, very few responded. Several of the centers described in this chapter did not reply to requests for information or interviews, or after the description was completed, did not review the material for accuracy. Therefore, the data for those centers from the interviews with Robert Pynoos and William Yule may be somewhat dated. The centers described in this chapter, though, have much to offer as templates for other centers. The most comprehensive of these, CIVITAS, is described below.

CIVITAS CHILD TRAUMA CENTER, HOUSTON, TEXAS

Civitas, a Latin word, translates as "service to community." The Baylor College of Medicine Child Trauma Program is part of the national CIVITAS Initiative established by Jeffrey Jacobs, a Chicago attorney. The goal of the CIVITAS Initiative is to train and bring together professionals from fields that impact the most on the lives of maltreated children. CIVITAS Child Law Center at Loyola University School of Law in Chicago and the University of Michigan School of Social Work CIVITAS Partnership Program were started in 1993.

The CIVITAS Initiative and the Department of Psychiatry and Behavioral Science at Baylor College of Medicine have established the CIVITAS Child Trauma Programs. This program is the first formalized didactic and clinical training program in the United States to teach medical students, psychiatric and pediatric residents, psychiatry fellows, affiliated medical, psychology, social work, physician assistant, and nurse trainees about understanding, evaluating, and treating traumatized children. The CIVITAS Child Trauma Program includes a combination of direct clinical services to underserved children, research investigations, and training in clinical, child welfare, and community settings. The CIVITAS Child Trauma Clinic at Children's Hospital provides assessment and treatment for children of all ages who have experienced neglect, abuse, or other forms of trauma. Referrals come from public and private agencies across the state of Texas.

The CIVITAS Child Trauma Program also has been an active collaborator in the Pediatric Injury Center located in Ben Taub Hospital in Houston, Texas. Ben Taub Hospital is a major trauma center that serves hundreds of severely injured children yearly. The center follows children from immediately after admission through 2 years postinjury; this is a longitudinal, multidisciplinary, proactive model of coordinated care.

The CIVITAS Child Trauma Programs provide direct clinical services to potentially traumatized children, trains dedicated and competent professionals to carry out the services, and trains in the context of research. The innovative programs are multidisciplinary and interinstitutional within cultural, social, legal, psychological, and physical environments. Models developed, piloted, and evaluated by the program are designed to be replicated throughout the United States.

Mission

The major goal of the program is to develop, pilot, and evaluate innovative models for clinical service and clinical training that may be adopted by other sites across the United States. The overarching mission is to understand the impact of good and bad experiences on the development of children and, with this understanding, to change the ways in which we, as a society, care for our children. By decreasing or preventing some of the neglectful and traumatic experiences and by increasing experiences that identify, protect, treat, and enrich high-risk children, we can dramatically influence the direction of millions of lives—and, in important ways, the direction of society.

Funding

The Child Trauma Clinic is supported by foundations and other charitable donations. The majority of families and children who seek treatment have no financial resources and no health insurance.

Staffing

The staff of CIVITAS includes child psychiatrists, pediatricians, psychologists, teachers, social workers, and counselors, as well as clinicians-in-training. Bruce D. Perry, MD, PhD, is the executive director of the program. He is the architect of all CIVITAS Child Trauma Program activities, oversees and participates in clinical activities, participates in and coordinates all research and writing projects, and gives frequent presentations on the topic of child maltreatment. David J. Conrad, LMSW, associate director of the program, also is the program liaison with the Texas Department of Child Protective Services.

The professional diversity of the staff allows for a deeper understanding of the child.

Assessment

The evaluation process at the Child Trauma Clinic is multidimensional and interdisciplinary and generally takes between three and five visits. The child's comfort level increases with each visit and the clinician's understanding of that child becomes more accurate. The child undergoes extensive interviews and standardized psychometric testing. The interdisciplinary team during assessment develops an initial treatment approach based on individual needs of the child and the child's caretakers. Assessment is the key to appropriate treatment planning. The plan often involves multiple recommendations ranging from classroom intervention to support group enrollment to medical treatment to parent training. Children are either referred back to their primary clinician at the completion of the assessment or continue in individual or group therapy with a CIVITAS clinician. Pharmacotherapy usually occurs only in conjunction with psychotherapy.

The CIVITAS Child Trauma Center staff members have developed screening assessments for children entering the Child Protective Services system. Screening data aid in making disposition and service plans; a computerized database manages these data and facilitates periodic reevaluation to guide disposition and service planning. Symptoms of PTSD in children may appear as attention deficit hyperactivity disorder, conduct disorders, anxiety disorders, and affective disorders. A consistent physical finding in these children is autonomic nervous system hyperarousal.

Theory

Perry, Pollard, Blakely, Baker, and Vigilante (1995) have written that the intensity and frequency of trauma determines how the brain internalizes the traumatic event, in a use-dependent fashion. If the threat of trauma is predictable, children find stress more tolerable. When a traumatized child is threatened, more primitive parts of the brain come into play and the child's reaction is more reactive and reflexive. When a child is raised in an environment that has persisting trauma (e.g., domestic violence, physical abuse), that child develops what Perry et al. call "an excessively active and reactive stress response apparatus." The majority of these systems reside in the brain stem and midbrain (e.g., locus coeruleus). This overdevelopment may lead to a predisposition for the child to act in an aggressive, impulsive, behaviorally reactive manner (Perry, Pollard, Blakely, & Vigilante, 1995; Perry, 1993a,b).

Childhood trauma has a profound impact on the emotional, behavioral, cognitive, social, and physical functioning of children. Physical hyperarousal and dissociation are adaptive mental and physical responses to trauma. The developing brain organizes and internalizes new information in a use-dependent fashion. Thus, the more the child is in a state of hyperarousal or dissociation, the more likely the child will have neuropsychiatric symptoms following trauma. If early life trauma results in an abnormal pattern of stress-mediating neurotransmitters and hormones, leading to altered CNS catecholamine systems, then there may be abnormalities related to catecholamine regulation of affect, anxiety, arousal/concentration, impulse control, sleep, startle, and autonomic nervous system regulation.

The brain of a young child is sensitive and more malleable than is the brain of an adult. Children who are victims of traumatic events experience an overactivation of their neural systems. Children's experiences during the first 3 years of life organize the brain and determine how they will function, in large part, for the rest of their lives. Once this window of opportunity passes, many capacities become difficult to modify and develop. Without "exercise," the brain muscle atrophies. Without "love" at critical times, that part of the brain atrophies in a manner that is almost impossible to reverse. The brains of these children develop as if the world is chaotic, unpredictable, violent, frightening, and devoid of nurturance. When the child faces a threat, there is an increased release of norepinephrine and threat-induced hyperarousal occurs, which impacts vigilance, affect, attention, and the startle response (Andrade & Aghajanian, 1984). If the child experiences a trigger reminder of that event or thinks about the event, these parts of the brain may be reactivated and responses may become maladaptive.

When a threat continues, the child may become dissociative and disengage into an "internal" world through daydreaming, fantasy, depersonalization, and derealization. In a dissociative state, the child's blood pressure and heart rate decrease and a different type of response occurs. It appears that younger children who experience immobility, helplessness, and powerlessness are more likely to use dissociative responses in response to a traumatic occurrence. Additionally, females seem to use the response more than males. If a young child dissociates during a traumatic event and then remains in that state through reexposure, the child internalizes a sensitized neurobiology that is related to dissociation; if the child responds by hyperarousal and that response persists, the child may develop persistent hyperarousal symptoms. Thus traumatic events diminish emotional, behavioral, cognitive, and social potentials and capacities. The child responds to a traumatic event based on a variety of factors:

1. Premorbid functioning and history (especially a history of previous stressors)
2. Age—neurobiological response patterns appear to change with age
3. The specific cognitive meaning of the event
4. The specific nature of the trauma
5. The presence of exacerbating (loss of caretaker) or attenuating factors (e.g., early intervention)

Clientele

Between 1994 and 1995, 300 children were seen in 1000 clinical visits at the Child Trauma Clinic at Texas Children's Hospital. Over 500 children were treated at the Child Trauma Clinic in 1996. Over 300 children have been followed in the Pediatric Injury Center program in 1996; 200 were seen in 300 visits between 1994 and 1995. One year after their initial traumatic event, over 50% of the children seen in 1996 had developed PTSD. The CIVITAS critical incident response team saw 60 children in 1000 visits between 1994 and 1995.

Services Provided

The CIVITAS Child Trauma Program, in collaboration with the Texas Department of Child Protective Services (CPS), has developed critical incident response teams (CIRTs) for working in high-profile crisis-oriented incidents referred to Child Protective Services. The teams assess multidimensional problems, identify areas of clinical need, and establish clinical case management systems. The model was originally used in providing assessment and treatment to the Branch Davidian children. The CIVITAS Child Trauma Programs have implemented various CIRTs models for evaluating a crisis situation, modifying existing procedures, implementing temporary processes for managing the crisis, and ensuring the health and welfare of the children . The CIRTs also have responded to the emotional needs of CPS staff impacted by vicarious and secondary traumatization. CIRTs also were established to provide a proactive, longitudinally oriented clinical approach to address the needs of child victims.

The CIVITAS Child Trauma Programs have established a partnership with the Burnett-Bayland Residential Treatment Center. This center is part of the Harris County Juvenile Justice System following sentencing as juvenile offenders. Juveniles are sentenced for a length of stay ranging from 3 to 9 months and attend an on-site school. The CIVITAS Child Trauma Program has worked with Burnett-Bayland Home staff to screen all youth at time of entrance to Burnett-Bayland Home and prior to discharge, to provide therapeutic initiatives, and to develop therapeutic options matched to the needs of an individual adolescent.

The Healing Arts Project draws from the expertise of artists in Houston's creative arts community to create assessment and therapeutic opportunities for maltreated children. This program has training, service, and research components and utilizes nonverbal and creative arts (dance, drama, painting, sculpture, and music) to help children communicate and begin to heal.

CIVITAS clinicians conduct two weekly assessment/treatment groups for children exposed to domestic violence who are living in the battered women's shelter of the Houston Area Women's Center. These groups provide a structured, predictable, nurturing set of experiences for the traumatized children. The clinicians also seek to develop a model for assessment and intervention that can be exported to comparable settings as well as learn more about the relationships between intrafamilial violence, child maltreatment, and development.

The CIVITAS Child Trauma Programs have collaborated actively with the Pediatric Injury Center of Ben Taub Hospital, a large public hospital in Houston, Texas. This major trauma center serves hundreds of severely injured children. The center follows children immediately after the injury and then monitors their physical, academic, social, and emotional progress periodically for the following 2 years. The longitudinal, multidisciplinary model provides proactive, coordinated care for children who were seriously injured.

Clinical Intervention

Early intervention with traumatized children can ameliorate the intensity and severity of the trauma response and decrease the possibilities of developing sensitized neural systems and persistent hyperarousal and/or dissociative symptoms. A healthy, responsive caretaker who provides support and nurturance can help the child diminish the alarm or dissociative response. Infants, children, and adolescents experience the same event differently.

The Child Trauma Clinic provides a variety of therapeutic services including individual, family, and group therapy, psychoeducation, and pharmacotherapy. The clinic also refers to other clinical or educational sites. The clinic provides proactive, useful, longitudinal care.

The Children's Crisis Care Pilot Project is a collaborative effort between Harris County Child Protective Services and CIVITAS Child Trauma staff. The heart of this program is the integration of traditional functions (initial investigation, evaluation, placement, and ongoing case monitoring) with state-of-the-art methods of assessment and data management This innovative model of collaboration and partnership brings together an academic setting, private foundations, business, and local government.

Principles of clinical work with traumatized children include the following:

1. Don't be afraid to talk about the event.
2. Provide a consistent, predictable pattern for the day.
3. Be nurturing, comforting, and affectionate in an appropriate context.
4. Discuss expectations for behavior and style of discipline with the child and include clear "rules" and consequences if the rules are broken.
5. Talk with the child and provide age appropriate information.
6. Watch for signs of reenactment through play, drawing, and/or behaviors; of avoidance through withdrawal, daydreaming, and/or avoidance of other children; and of physiological hyperreactivity through anxiety, sleep problems, and/or impulsive behavior.
7. Protect the child from potentially retraumatizing activities.
8. Give the child choices and some sense of control in an activity or interaction with an adult to increase feelings of safety and comfort.

Research

In the year following a traumatic event, over 50% of the children who were followed by CIVITAS and the Pediatric Injury Center had developed PTSD. The research study demonstrated a clear neurophysiological result of a traumatic event (Perry, 1993a,b). The CIVITAS Child Trauma Programs are negotiating to create training and research initiatives with the Federal Bureau of Investigation Serial Killers and Child Abduction Task Force, Court Appointed Special Advocates, Texas CPS Training Activities, and the New Zealand Child Protective Trust.

The major focus of research is the brain: how it grows and changes during infancy and childhood, particularly in the face of traumatic experience. There also is an interest in how the brain "stores" experience. Part of the research is to gain an understanding of what part of the brain mediates and/or generates emotional and behavioral symptoms of a traumatic stress reaction. Most of the useful clinical research has not been performed within the conceptual framework of PTSD.

CIVITAS staff members in general, and Dr. Perry in particular, have conducted research on the neurological effects of trauma on children. Recognizing that the brain develops and organizes as a reflection of developmental experiences, when those experiences include fear, pain, threat, and/or terror, the template for brain organization becomes the stress response and a poorly organized, dysregulated CNS catecholamine system. Thus traumatized children are in a persistent state of fear with hyperactivity and anxiety.

Training

The CIVITAS Child Trauma Programs have an Internet web page at www.bcm.tmc.edu/civitas. Information on CIVITAS products and services can be obtained by calling 1-713-770-3750. The CIVITAS Child Trauma Programs have developed educational materials for families, teachers, and others who work with maltreated children; among these materials are videotapes, booklets, and slides.

KIDSPEACE NATIONAL CENTERS FOR KIDS IN CRISIS, BETHLEHEM, PENNSYLVANIA

In 1882, Bethlehem Iron Company President William Thurston founded an interim crisis care facility for children in Bethlehem, Pennsylvania to help 32 children with a staff of 38. Today KidsPeace is the largest not-for-profit children's mental health care organization with 1500 caregivers treating over 2000 children in 25 locations in 5 states.

KidsPeace National Centers and the National Hospital for Kids in Crisis offer broad-range psychiatric services for children, adolescents, and their families in general and trauma services in particular. Treatment aims to help children and adolescents achieve age-appropriate independent functioning through highly individualized treatment plans that are problem-specific, developmentally focused, and time-limited.

KidsPeace has campus-, community-, and family-based treatment programs. It includes an acute care inpatient psychiatric hospital (National Hospital for Kids in Crisis), residential campuses, and specialized community dwellings; diagnostic units; shelters; elementary and secondary special and regular education schools; outpatient clinics; and a child development and therapeutic recreation center.

Mission

The mission of KidsPeace National Centers for Kids in Crisis is to provide intensive and sensitive treatment programs for children, adolescents, and their families and to assist kids in crisis in achieving peace and independence, thus enabling them to return to their communities as productive members of society. The approach is to fit the treatment to the child, not the child to the treatment. The goal of KidsPeace is to restore childhood to the child.

National Hospital for Kids in Crisis

This acute-care inpatient psychiatric hospital for children and adolescents, located in Orefield, Pennsylvania, opened in January 1993. It includes a children's program (5–9), preadolescent program (10–13), and adolescent program (14–18). A special track of treatment is designed for adolescents with concomitant substance abuse and/or addiction problems. The treatment provided by the hospital focuses on crisis management, stabilization, and planning for continuing care over the average stay of 21 days. The program also has a track for treatment of eating disorders.

The extended acute care treatment track addresses the needs of children and adolescents who require inpatient stays of 60 to 90 days. Specialized educational and therapeutic programming and individualized behavior modification systems are part of individualized treatment plans. Clients meet acute medical criteria warranting inpatient hospitalization and a staff-to-client ratio of one staff to three clients.

Dual Diagnosis Program

KidsPeace conducts a dual diagnosis treatment program of 19 beds for teens between 13 and 18 years of age. This program is designed for a moderate length of stay and provides 8 hours of family education, Alcoholics Anonymous/ Narcotics Anonymous support groups, treatment planning, group counseling, and an intensive aftercare program, among other services. This program is located in Saylorsburg, Pennsylvania and is divided into four distinct components including individual and group therapy, educational testing and instruction, medical evaluation and treatment, and recreational activities. Intensive treatment last approximately 6 weeks, followed by a reentry period of 2–3 weeks in preparation for returning to a community setting. Discharge to the family or another setting, if needed, includes comprehensive follow-up services. The emphasis in the program is on individual responsibility and participation in activities benefiting the entire group.

Juvenile Court Related Treatment Programs

KidsPeace offers a variety of programs to the juvenile court population ranging from providing a 45-day comprehensive clinical evaluation with end product of clear recommendations for placement/treatment and comprehensive aftercare placement to specialized residential care for regular juvenile offenders and adolescent sexual offenders. The program also offers transitional residential care in a step-down program after 1–2 months in regular residential care as well as highly structured foster home placements.

Therapeutic Residential Care Programs

This program offers long- and short-term campus and community-based treatment including adolescent residential, preadolescent residential, transitional residential (supervised open residential care transitioning to independent living), and specialized community residential care for children and adolescents aged 7 to 18.

Intensive Treatment Family Program

This community- and family-based program treats children from infancy to 18. The program offers initial out-of-home placement as well as community reintegration and can be accessed as an alternative to failed foster placements. Treatment families are well trained initially and receive ongoing behavior-specific training based on the needs of the children placed with them. Major treatment modalities provided to children in this program include family systems therapy, reality therapy, behavior modification, life skills training, and individual and group counseling.

Family Development Program

This program offers services to maintain the family including one-to-one community-based counseling, short-term crisis intervention and partial hospitalization/day treatment focusing on parenting issues. Most services are provided within the community, home, current placement, or partial hospital site. The in-home counseling service for children 6 or older includes counseling and life skills training for children and teens and parenting and problem-solving training for parents. The family-based service program provides intensive, short-term interventions for families in their homes and in the community on a 24/7 basis to work with family crises.

Crisis Assessment Response Team (CART)

The CART is an emergency service that provides free mobile assessment and evaluation for children and adolescents in crisis, as well as phone consultation. It operates on a 24/7 schedule and is staffed by clinicians who have on-site assessments they can provide when dispatched. The team then recommends appropriate action, taking into consideration the clinical, medical, and financial needs of the client.

School Crisis Assessment Team

This team assists school faculty and student assistance teams in evaluating and referring at-risk students to appropriate treatment resources. The team evaluates clients for biopsychosocial, drug, alcohol, and suicide issues during school hours.

KID-SAVE

KID-SAVE is a national referral network for Kids in Crisis. It assists individual clinicians and organizations in locating appropriate treatment facilities and services within their specific geographic locations in the United States of America.

Kid HelpLine

This telephone service provides information and crisis intervention services 24 hours a day to any individual who calls. Clinicians staff the HelpLine and help callers define problems and then provide options for resolution. They also provide referral assistance.

Treatment Aims and Philosophy

Treatment services are designed to help children and adolescents achieve age-appropriate, independent functioning, facilitating a return to less restrictive environments. The multidisciplinary team creates individual treatment plans for children and adolescents that are child-specific.

Emotional distress in children and adolescents is a dynamic condition and can be changed in a positive manner. Clients have the right to highly individualized treatment plans that address their personal treatment needs and serve as guides for all caregivers in implementing treatment interventions. Treatment plans should be problem-specific, developmentally focused, and time-limited. No single modality fits the variety of needs presented by program clients.

Clinical Intervention

Treatment of children who are traumatized consists of five phases. The first phase of the cognitive–behavioral plan is the introductory phase. During this phase, staff members develop rapport and a beginning therapeutic alliance; trust may be very difficult to establish. The child is encouraged to tell her or his story at her or his own pace in his or her own language, with emphasis on what was the worst part of the experience(s) for him or her. Another important part of the introductory phase is psychoeducation about the process of a posttraumatic stress reaction and/or disorder.

The second stage addresses signs and symptoms of trauma as well as possible coping mechanisms (relaxation, guided imagery). If the child must testify in court once or repeatedly, knowledge of these coping tools can help prevent some level of revictimization. Ventilation (telling the story) with validation of his or her feelings are important aspects of this stage. The third stage restructures and transforms traumatic memory from victim to survivor mentality. Identification and possible correction of schemas and misconceptions is important during this phase of treatment. Helping children to rework and master their stories helps them bring memories under more control.

The fourth stage of treatment is reconnecting with the world. Exposure therapy may be necessary to help them master a situation. The final stage is termination, with an understanding of the dynamics of reexperiencing of the trauma through anniversary reactions and/or trigger reminders. All stages are designed to engender hope in the child and to foster positive coping mechanisms.

The "Spokesfish"

Trusty the Goldfish is the official "spokesfish" of KidsPeace. Created in 1991 to lead the "Stop Child Abuse Before It Starts" campaign, Trusty is a silent observer, present in, yet removed from, the child's world. He encourages others to take responsibility for protecting kids against crisis.

This description is based on a variety of materials provided by KidsPeace; no interview took place.

FAMILY TRAUMA SERVICES, ALEXANDRIA, VIRGINIA

Family Trauma Services, Inc. (FTS) is a private, for-profit mental health agency serving the Washington DC metropolitan area. FTS is licensed by the

Virginia Department of Mental Health, Mental Retardation and Substance Abuse Services to provide outpatient mental health services, intensive home-based counseling, and partial day treatment services and to place children in treatment foster homes in Virginia. FTS also is licensed by the Maryland Department of Health and Mental Hygiene to provide outpatient mental health services and is certified by the United States Department of Health and Human Services as a community mental health center. FTS began providing services in 1993 and has offices located in Alexandria, Virginia, and Prince George's County, Maryland, with satellite programs in Woodbridge and Manassas, Virginia.

Provision of services by FTS is based on the philosophy that traumatic childhood experiences are often manifested in inappropriate acting out behaviors. FTS provides a coordinated, multitherapeutic approach that simultaneously manages and modifies those problematic behaviors while addressing the core trauma issues. FTS believes that youth are best supported within a family context, and that the family is best supported within the community. FTS therefore focuses on empowering families to become less dependent on the system and preserving family togetherness through specialized programs for children, adolescents, seniors, and families utilizing a multitherapeutic approach (e.g., posttraumatic stress disorder treatment, family systems, cognitive–behavioral, and relapse prevention). FTS provides center-based, community-based, and home-based mental health services, including psychiatric assessments, medication evaluations, psychological testing, treatment foster care, individual psychotherapy, group psychotherapy, parent support groups, in-home family counseling, mentoring, and academic tutoring and support.

FTS conducts specialized treatment programs targeted at primary and secondary victims, focusing on sex offenders, PTSD, behavioral disorders, social skills, parenting skills, parent support, anxiety disorders, as well as programs designed to meet the needs of children and adolescents returning to the community from residential placement and/or placement in a correctional facility. FTS currently offers specialized treatment programs for juvenile offenders and for adolescent sex offenders. Tertiary victims also are served through home-based family therapy, parent support groups, and parenting skills training.

A key component of all FTS programs is working with families to help them to develop individualized plans of care. Families and children are viewed as integral members of the treatment team and are encouraged to participate in the treatment planning process. FTS home-based counselors focus on empowering families to take ownership of the treatment interventions. Treatment goals are identified in conjunction with the family and revised as necessary to meet the family's evolving needs. FTS home-based counselors utilize creative, flexible, and culturally sensitive interventions when working with families so as to individualize treatment plans and create solution-focused intervention strategies. Physical contact with clients is made within 72 hours of the case being assigned.

FTS originally split off from a similar home-based program that provided only adolescent sex offender services and established a separate licensed home-based program. Psychological testing, individual therapy, and group therapy were contracted out. Originating from a sex offender focus, FTS expanded to meet the needs of children and adolescents with PTSD and similar symptoms, as well as to meet a variety of other issues such as adolescents transitioning back into the community and home following release from a residential program or correctional facility. Separate services were developed to meet additional needs, including social skills, partial day treatment, and therapeutic foster care. FTS is funded primarily through county contracts for the provision of specific mental health services and by state funds for clinical services.

Staffing

FTS employs male and female licensed psychiatrists, licensed clinical psychologists, licensed clinical social workers, masters-prepared home-based clinicians, bachelor-prepared home-based clinicians, and mental health-related student interns. FTS has found it helpful to hire individuals with professional training in the areas of social work, medicine (psychiatry), psychology, and management. Ethnically, FTS's staff represent a variety of cultural backgrounds and has staff who are fluent in French, Spanish, and American sign language, which has improved their ability to reach various populations. FTS has a consulting psychiatrist on staff who prescribes and evaluates all medications. Counselors provide case management consultation and observe for side effects. Given the seriousness of the problems experienced by the clientele served, FTS does not currently utilize lay caregivers or volunteers to provide clinical services. All new employees, volunteers, and student interns within 10 working days of employment are given orientation regarding the objectives and philosophy of FTS, practices of confidentiality, and critical personnel policies and procedures that are applicable to their specific duties and responsibilities.

A management team is in place to oversee the overall functioning of clinical programs to ensure an adequate level of quality control. All administrative and clinical decisions are approved by that team which is composed of the director and owner of the agency, agency administrator, the senior clinician, program evaluator, and select clinical staff. The primary goals of the management team are to:

1. Monitor services to insure that all applicable standards of federal, state, and local law are maintained, including appropriate certifications, licensure and inspection, and compliance with the federal Fair Labor Standards Act

2. Supervise treatment staff to assure compliance with all FTS policies
3. Supervise the preparation of all required clinical assessments, progress reports, discharge summaries, and evaluation data
4. Monitor service delivery to insure that services are provided with highest standards

Bachelor-level staff is supervised by a masters-level clinician with a minimum of 5 years of experience. Masters-level staff is supervised by licensed clinical social workers with a minimum of 5 years of experience. All clinical staff members are supervised on a weekly basis.

Job security is dependent on the current needs of the agency and the availability of staff. Many staff work in other places and subcontract to do specific work as needed. Some staff work full time for FTS and work in a variety of capacities. The agency is flexible and encourages staff to diversify its skills to be able to provide a full continuum of services. All staff members have a background check on file and are not listed in the Child Protective Services Central Registry. A Division of Motor Vehicles check also is conducted for those staff who operate motor vehicles as part of their job function. FTS staff also complete first aid and cardiopulmonary resuscitation training, and by policy all FTS staff are trained in restraint techniques.

FTS staff members receive ongoing professional development training regarding clinical issues and their individual job responsibilities. Staff providing direct services to the child and family complete a minimum of 40 hours of training annually in related clinical topic areas. By policy all FTS clinical staff attend biweekly group training and team supervision meetings, totaling 36 hours per year. In addition, FTS regularly schedules and facilitates in-house staff training covering topics relevant to the provision of clinical services. Topics have included behavior modification techniques, family therapy, restraint training, client rights, and ethical issues. FTS clinicians are licensed by the Virginia Department of Mental Health, Mental Retardation and Substance Abuse Services, and/or the Maryland Department of Health and Mental Hygiene. Members of the management team work together to help ensure the safety of counselors. As part of staff development training, personal safety issues are reviewed to address issues related to the prevention of violence, personal safety, and self-defense.

Clientele

FTS serves individuals who have experienced trauma in some capacity, either directly or indirectly through witnessing violent actions. Individuals deemed "needy" are those who have been traumatized and are subsequently presenting with behavioral and/or emotional difficulties. Caregivers, siblings, and other individuals involved with primary victims also are viewed as in need of clinical support services. Physical contact with clients is made within 72 hours of the case being assigned. The identified client is viewed as the primary client but is treated as a part of his or her whole environment. Although the services contracted are usually with one member of the family (individual and group therapy for other family members is frequently not included), the home-based counselors address the myriad needs of family members and have flexibility in deciding which family members to include and upon whom to focus.

FTS serves individuals who demonstrate a medical necessity for the service arising from a condition due to mental, behavioral, or emotional illness that results in significant functional impairments in major life activities. Functional impairments may include having difficulty in establishing or maintaining normal interpersonal relationships to a degree that they are at risk of hospitalization or out-of-home placement due to conflicts with family or community; exhibiting inappropriate behavior such that repeated interventions by mental health, social services, or judicial system are necessary; or exhibiting difficulty in cognitive ability to the extent that they are unable to recognize personal danger or recognize significant, inappropriate social behaviors.

The primary populations served are:

- Males and females ranging in age from preschool to 18 years at time of referral
- Children and adolescents experiencing symptoms of PTSD (e.g., depression, withdrawal, flashbacks, psychological distress with exposure to cue, avoidance of stimuli associated with event)
- Children and adolescents with sexual offense convictions or charges
- Children and adolescents who exhibit sexual acting-out behaviors
- Children and adolescents who are or have been at risk of being removed from their homes due to sexual acting-out behavior or symptoms of PTSD
- Children and adolescents returning to the community from residential programs, psychiatric hospitalizations, or correctional facilities
- Children and adolescents who have experienced abuse and/or neglect and who display acting-out behaviors such as physical aggression, noncompliance with authority, school difficulties, social skills deficits, and other significant behavior problems
- Children and adolescents with mild to moderate mental retardation, learning disabilities, or emotional disabilities, who present with sexual acting-out behavior or symptoms of PTSD
- Children and adolescents who are at risk for removal from their home to a more restrictive environment or in need of services to transition from an out-of-home placement in the community
- Children and adolescents in need of services more intensive than outpatient care
- Children and adolescents who are likely to be more successful receiving services in their residence and community

Theory

FTS uses an eclectic model of treatment to meet the wide variety of issues and specific needs of each client and his or her family. Many of the techniques used are cognitive–behavioral. Problem areas and individual and family strengths are assessed and individual treatment goals established. Behavioral modification and management charts are frequently used to teach behavior and are tailored to the unique needs of each family member. Staff are trained in a variety of treatment models and are matched with cases depending on what approach might be most successful. Theoretical principles of informed eclecticism, cognitive–behavioral therapy, and relapse prevention are combined with family, individual, and group therapy principles in designing treatment interventions. FTS does not have a need to utilize debriefing techniques at this time.

Assessment

FTS firmly believes in obtaining outcome measures to assess the outcome of all clinical services. FTS has an evaluation coordinator on staff who monitors outcome measures for all clinical programs to aid in improving service delivery and client functioning. The FTS evaluation coordinator, in conjunction with the FTS management team, conducts evaluations every 3 months to monitor any behavioral, psychological, and environmental/social changes that have occurred in child/family functioning. The primary goals of FTS's evaluation protocol are (1) to determine the impact of specific clinical programs; (2) to establish standards of performance for clinical services; (3) to advise changes in program operations and objectives; and (4) to justify the cost-effectiveness of the clinical program in establishing treatment priorities and allocating available resources. A family assessment is completed within 30 days. This assessment is developed in conjunction with the family and outlines client and family problems and strengths and establishes treatment goals.

To aid in the prevention of out-of-home placements and to meet the therapeutic needs of the family, FTS home-based counselors thoroughly assess the treatment needs of the client and family, including what therapeutic strategies have been successful as well as unsuccessful for the family in the past. FTS counselors assess physical, emotional, behavioral, and social strengths and preferences. This strengths/needs assessment is used as the foundation of the treatment approach and clinical interventions. Emphasis is placed on improving communication skills so as to reduce family conflict, increase the use of problem solving and conflict resolution strategies, and preserve family togetherness.

Treatment and Practice Issues

The treatment goals of the agency are to assess the needs and strengths of the youth and his or her family, to establish individual, family, and client goals, to work with clients toward the completion of those goals, and to coordinate appropriate resources to stabilize and maintain the client within the community. Home-based counseling is provided on two levels. Family counselors will provide family therapy and case management and an additional home-based counselor provides positive social, recreational, and vocational guidance. The client also is assigned an individual therapist and is placed in a specific cognitive–supportive therapeutic group. Examples of treatment goals for the client include:

1. Acceptance of full responsibility for sexually abusive and criminal behavior
2. Development of a clear understanding and sensitivity to the effects of sexual abuse on victim(s)
3. Development of an understanding of the thoughts and feelings that led to offenses and identify preoffense patterns and offense cycle
4. Learning to meet sexual and social needs without hurting others
5. Increasing age-appropriate sexual arousal and decrease deviant, inappropriate, or aggressive arousal patterns
6. Identification of high-risk situations that could lead to further sexual offending
7. Development of an offense prevention plan that other people in his support system will read and agree with
8. Learning and demonstrate responsible day-to-day behavior that includes avoiding high-risk situations

FTS receives referrals primarily through contracts to provide mental health services with local jurisdictions throughout northern Virginia. FTS primarily advertises by mailing or hand-distributing information about FTS to local jurisdictions with whom the center has contracts (i.e., social services agencies, county mental health agencies, and school systems).

Releases of information are signed with all agencies, organizations, and persons involved in the case. All information is subject to sharing among FTS staff working on the case. Personal information is kept confidential if not essential to the ongoing treatment of youth, is not illegal, or does not endanger client or others. The agency director, or his designee, protects the confidentiality of all case records and maintains all case file records in a locked and secured file. Access to these records is restricted to those directly authorized by the agency director.

In times of acute need, FTS home-based counselors are regularly available and on call 24 hours a day. An emergency service is available to back up home-based services. When assessing and responding to intermittent need, clients hours are regulated by the referring county agency who is purchasing services. Services are contracted to meet the specific acute and chronic needs of the population.

FTS has an established transition/aftercare program designed to assist youth transitioning back into the community upon release from correctional facilities or residential placements. This transition/aftercare program works with juveniles paroled from the state correctional facilities as well as children returning home from psychiatric hospitalizations and residential treatment programs. FTS home-based counselors focus on preparing biological families for the child's return home; reintegrating the child successfully back into the home, school, and community; and teaching life skills, conflict resolution, and communication skills. Relapse prevention also is strongly emphasized, and FTS home-based counselors work closely with children and their families on recognizing warning signs that may be a precursor to a relapse. As with all FTS treatment programs, the child and family are involved in the treatment planning process and clinical interventions are needs-driven, family-centered, strengths-based, culturally competent, and community-based. FTS clinical services place a strong emphasis on creativity, flexibility, and the use of multidimensional interventions in order to meet the complex needs of families. FTS offers the following clinical interventions that focus on addressing the core trauma issues, family empowerment and family preservation. Specifically, FTS's services are designed to prevent out-of-home placement, ease the transition from placements back into the home, and maximize resources and the coordination of services. These services include home-based family counseling services, home-based mentoring services, individual therapy, group therapy, case management services, partial-day treatment program, ongoing parent counseling, training, and support, intensive supervision, and 24-hour crisis intervention.

Home-Based Family Counseling Services

FTS home-based services provide immediate, intensive, problem-specific, in-home interventions to the child and family that are needs-driven, family-centered, strengths-based, culturally competent, and community-based. Home-based family counseling is provided by a masters-level clinician under the supervision of a licensed clinical social worker. Home-based counselors focus on individual and family counseling to facilitate the attainment of the specified goals and objectives of the treatment plan. Specific interventions provided by home-based family counselors include (1) support, counseling, and guidance in coping with and addressing specific issues; (2) information, education, and guidance concerning issues of discipline, communication skills, problem-solving, anger management, child development, and coping skills; (3) individual and family counseling to examine core trauma issues and how these issues impact family functioning; (4) family counseling to explore family relationships, roles, and dynamics, and how these impact family functioning; (5) constructing behavior modification programs; (6) empowering the family to locate and appropriately utilize community resources; (7) accompanying clients to appointments relevant to achieving stated objectives (e.g., family assessment planning team, court hearings, and outings as necessary);

and (8) supporting the client's successful participation in school, home, and in the community.

Home-based services are delivered in the context of a treatment team so as to provide multiple levels of service by exposing the family to a variety of therapeutic techniques and styles. Specifically, in-home services are delivered in conjunction with appropriate center-based services, including the availability of individual and group therapy. To facilitate this team approach, home-based family counselors facilitate joint sessions with home-based mentors. In this way, the family sees the counselors as partners working together with the family toward the attainment of identified goals and objectives. Transportation of clients to therapy sessions, community resources, social/recreational activities, and any other needs relevant to the attainment of stated goals and objectives is also included as part of the plan.

Home-Based Mentoring

Home-based mentors are bachelor- or associate-level counselors under the supervision of a masters-level clinician with a minimum of 5 years of clinical experience. Home-based mentoring services include in-home individual and family support, role-modeling, mentoring, academic and vocational support, and participation in family social/recreational activities. Specific interventions provided by home-based mentors include (1) serving as a positive role model for clients to observe and learn socially effective values, attitudes, and behaviors; (2) providing a therapeutic, nonthreatening outlet for clients to explore issues, resolve conflict, and receive positive feedback; (3) helping to link clients with positive experiences in the community such as employment, community service, team sports, and recreational clubs; (4) accompanying clients to appropriate appointments (e.g., FAPT), court hearings, and outings as necessary; (5) independent living skills (e.g., money management, finding a job, health promotion, community responsibilities); and (6) supporting the clients *successful* participation in school, home, and in the community.

Individual Therapy

Children and adolescents enrolled in a specific clinical program (e.g., PTSD, sex offenders) may receive center-based weekly individual therapy as a core component of their individualized treatment plans if deemed necessary. The individual therapy is provided by a licensed clinical social worker and addresses issues related to home adjustment, coping issues at school and in the community, underlying traumatic issues, family relations, issues of loss and transition, personal goals, progress in group therapy, and other significant issues as they arise.

Weekly individual therapy services are delivered in the context of a treatment team so as to provide multiple levels of service by exposing the child or adolescent to a variety of therapeutic techniques and styles. Children and adolescents receiving weekly individual therapy benefit from the one-on-one attention to their specific needs. In addition, individual therapy provides a confidential therapeutic outlet for the discussion and processing of difficult life experiences. Transportation of the client to the individual therapy sessions is facilitated by the home-based counselors working with the family.

Group Therapy

Children and adolescents also may participate in weekly group counseling specific to their therapeutic needs if deemed necessary. The following therapeutic groups are available: adolescent sex offender group, cognitive low functioning adolescent sex offender group, children's posttraumatic stress disorder group, adolescent posttraumatic stress disorder group, transition/aftercare group, social skills group, independent living skills group, oppositional–defiant behavior group, conduct disorder group, and attention deficit-hyperactivity group. The FTS treatment foster care program offers an independent living skills group to clients whose long-term goal is independent living. The independent living skills curriculum addresses the following life domain issues: life skills, financial responsibility, values clarification, impulse control, substance abuse education, decision making, vocational education, self-development, and family relations.

Partial Day Treatment Program

The partial day treatment center for juveniles operates Monday through Friday from 3:00 PM to 8:00 PM. The overarching goal of the day-reporting center is to create an environment in which adolescents can improve their development of social skills, cognitive skills, physical skills, independent living skills, and healthy coping skills. The partial day treatment center functions as a 12-week program in which all of the core program curriculum is covered in a 12-week rotation. Curriculum topics include social skills, life skills, financial responsibility, values, self-development, impulse control, substance abuse education, decision making, vocational education, family values, and relapse prevention.

Participants enrolled in the partial day treatment center are on a level system that corresponds directly to the goals outlined in each participant's individualized treatment plan. Family therapy sessions focus on the adjustment of the family to having a foster child, family relationships, roles within families, and ways family members can support each other.

Intensive Supervision

Intensive supervision services (i.e., daily monitoring of behavior at home, school/employment, and community) also are available for clients who require extensive supervision in order to successfully remain in the community. FTS staff check in with the parents and child by telephone several times throughout the day to ensure that the child is behaving responsibly and appropriately. Staff inquire about school/work attendance, willingness to complete assigned household responsibilities, meeting curfew, personal hygiene, and any other issues that are identified in the individual treatment plan. Careful records are kept to track progress and aid treatment planning.

Crisis Intervention

Home-based family counselors are available to meet face-to-face with clients and their families 24 hours a day/7 days a week. Home-based counselors may be reached via pager after hours or on the weekends. In addition, an additional experienced crisis-intervention counselor is available via pager 24 hours a day/7 days per week. The on-call crisis worker attends a weekly case staffing meeting and is familiar with the clinical issues for all clients receiving services from FTS.

Life, Parenting, and Communications Skills Training

As a part of home-based family counseling, parents receive ongoing clinical training related to the individualized needs of the family during weekly family sessions. Home-based counselors provide individual and family counseling, support, and guidance in the home on a weekly basis. Some relevant topics may include child development and age-appropriate behaviors, parenting children and adolescents who present with symptoms of PTSD; parenting children and adolescents who have committed sexual offenses; parenting the sexually abused child; relapse prevention of all acting out behaviors; transitioning adolescents to independent living; advocating for children and adolescents; crisis intervention and emergency response; utilizing solution focused thinking; competency-based counseling and parenting; interventions for crisis situations; helping children and adolescents transition back into the home and community; strategies for preventing out-of-home placements; attachment and separation issues; special education needs; culture and parenting; issues and skills for working with children who have emotional/behavioral problems; reinforcement, ignoring, and punishment; ABC theory: antecedent, behavior, and consequences; the roles of irrational thinking/cognitive distortions in our actions; giving directives/rules/talking with your children; principles of effective communication: I messages, active listening; establishing a reward system/reinforcement/teaching through encouragement; problem solving and decision making; techniques of discipline: time out/ignoring/praise and attention; techniques of discipline: punishment, natural and logical consequences, designing home programs; anger management; and having fun with your family: recreation and community resources and setting appropriate and realistic goals.

Appropriate social skills, including conflict resolution, mediation, using "I statements," and problem solving, also are incorporated into home-based sessions to maintain and improve good interpersonal relationships. Role-playing techniques and modeling are utilized to reinforce these skills so as to encourage their generalization into a variety of life situations. As with all of FTS's clinical interventions, life, parenting, and communication skills training are tailored to meet the unique needs of the client and family.

Case Management Activities

The home-based family counselor plays the central coordinating role for each client and family. This counselor is responsible for maintaining weekly contact with all FTS counselors working with the family, as well as the parole officer, referring worker, and any other professional or individual involved with the family's treatment. The home-based counselor also helps facilitate and establish relevant community contacts and resources that might be useful to the family. FTS home-based counselors work closely with the family to help them master the skills necessary to make supportive and positive contacts with their community. FTS counselors also work in concert with the assigned community services board case manager to ensure that the needs of the client and family are addressed. FTS counselors are knowledgeable about community resources and are experienced in making appropriate referrals to the client and family.

Medication Monitoring

FTS has a consulting psychiatrist on staff who is responsible for prescribing and evaluating all medications. In conjunction with the psychiatrist, home-based counselors discuss with the youth the name and type of medication prescribed and the purpose and desired effects of the medication. FTS counselors also observe for any side effects of the medication and provide case management consultation with the prescribing psychiatrist.

Training and Consultation

Clinical staff receive ongoing professional development training regarding the provision of home-based services and their individual job responsibilities. Staff providing direct services to the child and family will complete a minimum of 40 hours of training annually in related clinical topic areas. By policy, all FTS clinical staff attend biweekly group training and team supervision meetings, totaling 36 hours per year. In addition, FTS regularly schedules and facilitates in-house staff trainings covering topics relevant to the provision of clinical services. Topics have included behavior modification techniques, family therapy, restraint training, client rights, and ethical issues.

Training is designed to fit the needs of the group being trained, ranging from informative to treatment techniques.

CHILDREN'S CRISIS TREATMENT CENTER, PHILADELPHIA, PENNSYLVANIA

This outpatient inner-city program was conceptualized in 1989 as a new service provided by the larger clinic, in existence since 1971. It specializes primarily in treating children ages 2–14 who have witnessed/survived a one-time catastrophic event or so-called "type I" trauma (Terr, 1991), some of which include witnessing/surviving parental or sibling homicide or suicide, surviving arson fires in which family members perished, surviving a physical assault perpetrated by a caregiver, peer, or stranger, and surviving catastrophic accidents that resulted in physical trauma (e.g., head injury, severe burns, amputation of limbs). During treatment, however, closer inspection frequently reveals that the precipitating event that brought the child to the clinic (e.g., the homicide of a parent) was preceded by a history of exposure to a "litany of horrors." Children tend to be from urban poor, working poor, lower-middle-class, or middle-class families.

The trauma program is physically housed in the Children's Crisis Treatment Center, which provides day treatment, diagnostic/evaluation services, and community programs to young children deemed to be at risk. The trauma program works largely in isolation, functioning fairly autonomously on a daily basis. If and when this larger organization is not secure, though, then the trauma program becomes more vulnerable to cuts or dissolution. Dr. Eileen Cleary, who worked as an intern at the larger clinic prior to completing her doctorate, is director of the Intensive Trauma Assistance Program (ITAP). She was not part of the executive committee of the larger clinic until March 1997.

Mission

The mission of the Intensive Trauma Assistance Program is to offer services to traumatized children when developmental progress has been interrupted or sidetracked through witnessing/directly surviving a catastrophic, onetime traumatic event. The aim is to begin treatment as soon as possible after the traumatic event, before PTSD symptoms crystallize and become part of the child's personality structure. The program's goal is to help these children reconcile the event and return to pretrauma levels of developmental functioning.

Staffing

Since its inception in 1989, the trauma program has been a "one-person band," since the director was also the sole therapist. In 1993, an anonymous donor provided funds for a half-time clerical support staff member. The goal of the program is to add a second clinician.

Funding

The program relies on a variety of funding sources including city grants, state monies for early screening, private insurance, federal programs (e.g., Medicare), and philanthropic donations. The program needs to explore new revenue-generating activities and funding sources so that its existence is not as dependent on funding sources available to the larger clinic. The program came into existence after a large grant from a local foundation.

Theory

The ITAP director is psychodynamically oriented by training, and the primary mode of intervention on-site utilizes this framework to conduct play therapy using trauma-specific play materials. The director draws on family systems theory and the contextual school of family therapy for clinical work with children, caregivers, and family members, the latter who also are frequently experiencing PTSD symptoms and or traumatic grief themselves. The director also turns to cognitive–behavioral techniques to help children with trauma-reactive behavior modification.

Dr. Cleary draws on the "phase-oriented model" of treatment devised by Elizabeth Rice-Smith. Treatment also includes case management including ongoing interdisciplinary and interagency contacts (schools, child protective services, etc.). Dr. Cleary has developed a "survivor bag" technique elaborating and expanding the "garbage bag" technique of Beverly James (1989). Children decorate bags and fill them with inoculation strategies to use in the future and positive things they have learned about themselves. When treatment ends, the children leave the empty garbage bags behind and take full survivor bags with them. Dr. Cleary is writing a manual for caregivers of traumatized/bereaved children.

Service Provision

Treatment is primarily individual and family oriented and is designed to be short term with a projected duration of 6 months to a year. Sessions are generally an hour in length, followed by a 30- to 60-minute family session. Treatment usually begins within a one-calendar-year period after the precipitating event. Most of the children exhibit detailed, graphic recall of the traumatic event at the time of intake. Many factors related to the traumatic event may result in longer periods of psychotherapeutic assistance than initially predicted. For example, if a child has to testify in a homicide trial scheduled a year after the child enters treatment, that child usually will continue in treatment through the time of the trial. The occurrence of subsequent events while the child is in treatment for the initial trauma also will extend treatment length. If the child is referred due to violence experienced in an ongoing situation (e.g., domestic violence wherein the perpetrator remains in the home), the family is referred to appropriate resources.

ITAP's community interventions and environmental advocacy services differentiate it from a traditional outpatient therapy program. The ITAP clinician accompanies the child to court hearings and the trial to provide emotional support and sometimes cofacilitates sessions of the Philadelphia Court School where children learn about the process and procedures of the courtroom. The ITAP clinician provides death notification services to children in the family's home in the immediate wake of a traumatic death and critical incident debriefing following incidents of violence in the community. Many of these cases are high profile and receive extensive media coverage necessitating explanations to children and families as to the parameters and limits of confidentiality. Dr. Cleary generally sees between 13 and 15 children weekly, depending on the case management needs.

Assessment

The initial assessment begins with child and caregiver together. Caregivers may be unaware of certain subjective, inferred PTSD symptoms the child is experiencing. Conversely, children sometimes deny/minimize symptoms out of a sense of shame or concern for the caregiver's feelings. Conjoint interviews help to break the silence and open a supportive dialogue, which elicits comprehensive and accurate information about trauma reactions and symptoms of distress. If sufficient rapport and trust are established initially, the child also is seen individually for a psychodiagnostic trauma-focused play assessment. Child trauma questionnaires, behavioral checklists, drawings, and projective instruments are incorporated into the initial assessment process.

Community Involvement

Dr. Clearly networks with numerous community agencies including the Philadelphia Coalition for Victim Advocacy and others. She has been invited to participate in a citywide child trauma response team, which is being formed. Dr. Cleary has provided training to criminal justice and victim advocacy personnel in Philadelphia and has conducted workshops around the state for school, law enforcement, criminal justice, and mental health personnel.

Trauma-Related Issues

Trauma as a concept has acquired more legitimacy in the recent past. Yet there still is an increasing need to acknowledge and understand its impact on children while building awareness that resilience is something that happens later (Pynoos, 1994). People tend to minimize the deleterious impact of trauma on children. There is a great need to do more outreach in the community with and for children. One such need is the development of a child crisis response team that can go to the site of a traumatic event immediately afterward, to provide critical incident debriefing, crisis intervention, and mental health assessment as well as triage services to affected children and offer follow-up care.

There also is a need to bring trauma-focused services into the community. Many families struggle with more immediate, compelling, and pragmatic issues than obtaining mental health services for their children. These pragmatic concerns, coupled with personal traumatic grief of caregivers, may overwhelm available emotional resources. To ask caregivers to make commitments to attend weekly therapy, to obtain a service whose value may be delayed and not apparent in the short term or which has no value may be asking too much. Child trauma specialists must actively seek ways to meet the clients at their own need stage and offer practical, tangible services to gain trust and credibility. In this way, an effective therapeutic alliance can be built and interventions become convenient and accessible. One of the challenges will be to educate managed care companies about the critical need to reimburse nontraditional, clinically necessary interventions in the home and other community settings. Thus the shape of the "animal" (i.e., trauma-focused psychotherapeutic interventions) needs to adapt to the needs of traumatized children and their caregivers.

THE CHILD TRAUMA STRESS CLINIC, LONDON, ENGLAND

The clinic grew out of evaluation of research results from the sinking of the Herald Free Enterprise (a cross-channel ferry) in 1978. This event brought to the forefront the gradual realization that traumatized children had needs to be met. The organization was created in March 1987 and grew into being part of the Bethlehem Royal and Maudley Hospital Institute of Psychiatry. This national service works with local police, primary health care providers, solicitors, and others to network, obtain referrals, and do insurance claims. The clinic opened in 1997 and is part of the National Health Service, funded as a trust.

Treatments offered by the clinic are predominantly individual therapy, desensitization, exposure-based therapy (up to 8 sessions), very early short-term interventions, and occasionally eye movement desensitization and reprocessing. Clients are also trained in anxiety management techniques. Debriefings, when given on occasion, mainly follow the Mitchell/Dyregrov version of critical incident stress debriefing. In this clinic, research, theory building, and work with clients are well integrated and training provided to professionals about child trauma is unique.

The clinic also is unique because of its social–psychological dimension, its broad approach to trauma, its pioneering work in research, and its long list of publications, which have contributed to the field extensively. The goal is to continue to use knowledge gained from work at the clinic to clarify and improve treatment for children. The work has led to moral support for the clinic's work and generally has changed public attitudes about trauma and its impacts.

Staff

All staff are professionally qualified as clinical psychologists and are supervised and evaluated by Dr. Yule, program director. There is a high level of cooperation between staff and team meetings are held weekly. All staff is part time with two permanent and one temporary staff members as well as a part time secretary. The three clinical psychologists, at the present time, are male and no social worker is on staff. No lay caregivers or volunteers work with the clinic. Staff cooperates with victim support service agencies in the work with children.

Clientele

The clientele of the Child Trauma Stress Clinic (CTSC) are primarily children and their parents and families. These children have been traumatized either directly through deliberate acts of violence or through accidents or disasters. At the present time, the children served primarily are victims of road traffic accidents and/or family violence. All clients are aware that they have experienced "something" that brings them to the clinic for help.

Theory

The primary theory base for the clinic is cognitive–behavioral with elements of social learning theory. Debriefing done by staff follows the Mitchell model. Children may experience severe and chronic post-traumatic reactions; in fact, up to 30–50% may have significant impairment following a major disaster (Yule, 1991). Adults, including parents, often underestimate the extent of these children's emotional distress.

Symptoms of PTSD have an evolutionary origin. From this perspective, posttraumatic stress reactions might be viewed as normal and adaptive reactions that involve both conscious and unconscious processes. A person's conscious experiences of trauma can be deliberately retrieved. Other information is not verbally accessible but can be retrieved in a similar state, often through imagery. In addition, prior life experiences and preexisting schemas about self and the world can influence how a traumatic event is processed. A traumatic event presents the victim with stimulus information that at the time leads to

extreme emotional arousal but is not immediately processed. Some information is deliberately retrievable and some is not available to conscious processing. In addition, the individual forms appraisal cognitions about the information. Event cognitions and automatic thoughts become associated with strong
emotional states that also are subjects of cognitive appraisals. Adaptation to
trauma occurs over time and involves states of mind (see Fig. 11.1) (Joseph et
al., 1997, p. 85). Phenomenological components of the individual's experience
are identifiable in this model.

Service Provision

As soon as a referral is received, within days to weeks to 2–3 years after an
incident, intervention begins. Consultation also is done by phone. In some
cases, when clients are ambivalent about getting help, clinic staff contacts
families to reassess their status on a periodic basis. Initially, child victims and
their families complete self-administered questionnaires (IES, Fear Inventory,
and others), complete a semistructured interview, and spend 3–3½ hours
being tested or giving information. The psychologist in charge of the intake

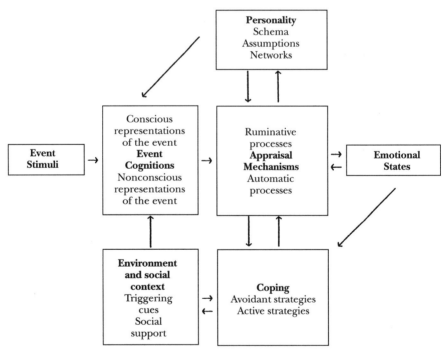

Figure 11.1. An integrative model for adaptation to traumatic stress (from Joseph, Williams, &
Yule, 1997).

process aims to get as detailed a description as possible of all aspects of the trauma and of all persons involved. The objectives of this investigation may be to (1) establish a diagnosis; (2) determine the extent of problems; (3) prepare a report for litigation; (4) advise about treatment; and (5) provide treatment if possible.

The clinic's treatment model, based on Yule's work (Joseph, Williams, & Yule, 1997) suggests that therapeutic intervention helps survivors to:

- Reappraise what happened through reexposure to the event and associated stimuli
- Reappraise the meanings and emotional states associated with trauma
- Reduce emotional arousal in a direct fashion
- Develop helpful coping strategies to deal with emotional arousal
- To review cognitive styles and rules for living, which may maintain symptoms, block reexposure, and determine primary traumatic appraisal (Joseph et al., 1997, p. 119)

Treatment with children first aims to alleviate immediate distress, perhaps using a more guided cognitive and emotional reexperiencing, reenacting, and restructuring approach in a paced, controlled manner. This method helps the child change maladaptive causal attributions.

Community Intervention

Clinic staff offers training to professionals who request assistance as to how to work with traumatized children. The British Psychological Society accredits the training courses because they are conducted by registered clinical psychologists. Dr. Yule works with UNICEF and other nongovernmental organizations and is available to the press to provide information about trauma and lectures to schools and health authority agencies.

THE UCLA TRAUMA PSYCHIATRY SERVICE, LOS ANGELES, CALIFORNIA

The UCLA Neuropsychiatric Institute and Hospital has established a Trauma Psychiatry Service that provides comprehensive care to traumatized children, adolescents, adults, and families. It responds to requests for assistance in the Los Angeles area as well as from communities nationwide that have experienced extreme acts of violence or disaster. Children who have been subjected to sniper attacks, bombings (Oklahoma City), shootings, war, and hostage taking are interviewed through a standard semistructured interview format. This clinical setting at the University of California at Los Angeles is part of the Trauma Psychiatry Service. The clinic treats children and family members together if they have been involved in the same critical incident and also treats children who have been involved in life-threatening situations including a disaster.

Theoretical Basis

The study of traumatic stress among children and adolescents is moving toward a complex developmental psychopathology model. The UCLA Trauma Psychiatry Service has proposed a detailed developmental model of traumatic stress (Pynoos, 1993; Pynoos, Steinberg, & Wraith, 1995) indicating how the interaction over time of many critical factors plays a role in the progression from traumatic exposure(s) to subsequent pathology. The model ascribes a tripartite etiology to traumatic distress, which derives from the child's objective and subjective disaster experience, the nature and frequency of traumatic reminders, and the type and severity of secondary stresses and adversities.

The model emphasizes that outcome measures must extend beyond those of traditional physical and psychiatric morbidity to include proximal and distal developmental disturbances, impact on emerging personality, alterations in self-attributions and schematization of personal vulnerability, interpersonal life, and the function of social institutions, and changes in life trajectory and vulnerability to future life stresses. The ecology of the child influences each step in the outcome pathway and includes child intrinsic factors, parental functioning, developmental cycle of the family, school and peer milieu, and the allocation of resources by the society at large. This model suggests important areas for public mental health disaster planning including types of assessments, primary and secondary preventive interventions, and treatment strategies.

A traumatic experience is a complex experience made of many different moments. In order to understand the trauma experienced by a child, it is important to have a real sense of that child's subjective experience of those multiple moments and the degree of terror, life threat, and extent of loss involved. A traumatic experience includes the objective event, the meaning of that event as it is experienced and reprocessed, reminders of the event and the meaning of those reminders, coping strategies used during the event to address the situation and manage the reaction, and secondary stressors. Traumatic exposure includes both objective (graphic atrocities, exposure to adversity) and subjective (internal threat, degree of upset over behavior during the event) factors Secondary stressors and concomitant changes can lead to comorbid conditions; a greater number of them can lead to more intense psychopathology, including depression and suicidality. Trauma changes a child physiologically and reexposure to triggers can elicit those changes, for example, as heart rates automatically increase or as facial expressions change. Studies have shown that, 5 years after exposure to a traumatic event, basal cortisol levels are reduced and the ability of a child to recover after a challenge to the hypothalamic-pituitary-adrenal axis is delayed One result of exposure is that the child may lose developmental opportunities to proceed in a normal fashion.

When a child's physical integrity is threatened or violated, then the child may direct attention toward fears and fantasies about the nature and extent of harm done. The child may then engage self-protective mechanisms of dissociation or fantasy or others to meet the internal threats and/or pain. At the conclusion of the traumatic moments, the child may make efforts to seek outside help, to aid injured or dead family members or friends, and to separate from significant others. During that time, the child may need and receive medical or surgical care. While this is happening, the child may worry about the safety of others whose well-being is unknown and may experience acute grief reactions after witnessing death or destruction. Some of the disturbances that may occur to the child during this period of time include:

1. Failure of alarm reactions to elicit effective intervention
2. Failure of social referencing to appraise danger
3. Failure of protective shield to prevent harm
4. Inability to resist coercive violation
5. Betrayal of basic affiliative assumptions
6. Failure of catastrophic emotions to protect against harm
7. Struggle over surrender to unavoidable moment(s) of danger
8. Radical shifts in self–object representations

The center also has added to the theoretical and practical understanding of typical reactions in children who have been traumatized. For example, infants utilize alarm reactions to attempt to get aid and assistance. Facial expressions of others are a cue to them that something is wrong. Older children wonder "what if no one comes" if they send out an alarm signal. Children often have fantasies of revenge and retaliation after the trauma occurs. They are concerned with feelings of helplessness and how they might prevent future harm. The symptom presentation and content may vary according to the age of the child, although these also vary with the specific type of traumatic event. In addition, efforts to resolve traumatic experiences can interfere with resolution of more typical childhood tasks including school performance, play, and interpersonal relationships (Eth & Pynoos, 1985).

Issues of traumatic bereavement also are important to consider in working with children. Life changes after trauma frequently involve loss and reminders of the event, which also remind children of the circumstances around that loss.

Assessment

In a major disaster, assessment may take place within a public health approach. The first step of assessment looks at the extent and nature of exposures and the degree of morbidity. This effort is conducted in conjunction with provision of acute services. Another aspect of assessment is conducting rigorous, systematic, periodic screenings of children in the school setting. The initial screening looks at basic exposure information (Where were you? What happened to you? What happened to those around you?). It also includes specific questions about high-risk experiences (life threat, being trapped, witnessing injury, being injured, hearing screams, seeing mutilation, seeing hurt family members or dead family members) as well as questions about the child's subjective appraisal and associated emotions during the event. Assessment also includes a brief explanation about trauma and grief reactions. Teachers and parents can give additional information about the children.

Children receive a variety of assessment measures. Among them are a standard semistructured interview, a posttraumatic stress reaction index, a children's inventory of grief reactions, and a questionnaire designed to assess child's postviolence responses based on parent report. The extent of symptoms appears to be related to the extent of exposure to life threat or witnessing of injury or death. Children appear to exhibit the entire range of PTSD symptoms; children with more severe responses have greater reexperiencing symptoms and greater changes in emotional responsiveness as well as states of increased arousal. These children report intrusive images and sounds rather than flashbacks and reduced interest in activities as well as feeling more distant or alone with feelings rather than feeling "numb." Differences in age and developmental phase contribute to how the child assimilates the traumatic event. Preschoolers are most likely to be regressive with decreased verbalization and cognitive confusion and increased anxious attachment behavior. School-age children are more likely to react to violence with aggressive or inhibited behavior and psychosomatic complaints. Adolescents may become prematurely more independent or increasingly dependent, leading to dropping out of school, marrying early, and changing career choice. Adolescents also may participate in premature precocious sexual activity, substance abuse, delinquency, and reenactment behaviors (Pynoos & Nader, 1990).

Pynoos and Nader (1988) noted that the program employs three self-report inventories: A Posttraumatic Stress Reaction Index designed by Frederick (1985), revised for school age children by Pynoos and Frederick; a child inventory of grief; and the Child Diagnostic Inventory for Children and Adolescents. The PTSD Reaction Index samples children for acute and chronic reactions in response to various forms of violence and allows for comparisons among groups of children with differing degrees of exposure.

Treatment Approach

The UCLA Trauma Psychiatry Program has developed a treatment approach derived from the developmental psychopathology model of traumatic stress (Pynoos et al., 1995). It encompasses a developmental perspective in addressing traumatic experiences, traumatic reminders, secondary adversities, grief and the interplay of trauma and grief, and developmental disturbances. This five-foci approach is used across a spectrum of intervention settings, including individual, group, family, classroom, and community. These foci may be addressed through the selective and integrated use of the following thera-peutic modalities: (1) psychoeducational approaches; (2) social skills training; (3) psychodynamic psychotherapy; (4) cognitive–behavioral therapy; (5) phar-macological therapies; (6) educational assistance; and (7) remedial interven-tions to address developmental disruptions.

Observations have consistently indicated that a number of essential con-siderations must be taken into account in addressing children's traumatic experiences. These considerations include:

1. Traumatic situations involve a convergence of external and internal dangers.
2. Traumatic experiences are *extremely* complex.
3. The organization of memory and strategies of recall of traumatic experiences differ as children focus on different memory anchor points and their meaning, forming an elaborate memory network.
4. Intervention fantasies, which occur during and after traumatic experi-ences, are invariably associated with the experience.
5. Cognitive, affective, social, and neurophysiological development play a role in the appraisal of external and internal threats.
6. Children may engage in self-protective mental efforts to "weaken" certain traumatic details or moments.
7. Children's traumatic narratives typically rely on coconstruction with parents or other adult caretakers, or siblings and peers.
8. New information, further experience, and maturity can lead to re-schematization of a traumatic situation through revised appraisals, new attributions of meaning to aspects of the experience, and new consid-erations regarding intervention (Pynoos, Steinberg, & Aronson, 1997).

Treatment using this five-foci approach was employed successfully in Arm-enia as a brief treatment modality (Goenjian et al., 1997) and in an elementary school-based violence prevention program using a more extended combina-tion of individual, group, and mentorship approaches (Murphy, Pynoos, & James, 1997). Treatment based on this approach currently is being imple-mented in partnership with UNICEF for the school-based treatment of war-traumatized adolescents in Bosnia-Herzegovina.

A traumatic experience for a child is personal and poignant. Children can be helped through individual, family, classroom, group, and/or community intervention. Pynoos and Nader (1988) have observed that

> only during the acute phase after the traumatic event are the incident specific traumatic reminders easily identifiable. With the passage of time, the two most important psychological consequences, the contraction of ego functioning and the dulling of one's emotional life, can result in maladaptive trauma resolution. (pp. 461–462)

In individual treatment, children expand the description and ego construc-tion of the event(s). Individual treatment helps to restore the child's personal integrity. The child is helped to go over the event moment by moment. The child looks at his or her physical reactions, thoughts before the event happened, thoughts after it happened, and wishes/wants he or she would like to see after the trauma has occurred. Part of this expansion is to help children keep a list of traumatic reminders of their individual traumatic experiences. They add to the list over time and their parents/caretakers monitor exposure to the triggers and subsequent responses. Children and clinicians also keep a list of proximal secondary stressors that indicate how their life has changed. These may include changes in school setting, guardians (if parents were killed or injured), homes (if the child had to move), loss of friends, injuries and subsequent medical treatments, permanent disability issues, and loss of money. These secondary stressors also are addressed in treatment as are issues of complicated grief and loss. Reprocessing the traumatic experience and reminders is a skill that children can learn.

Parents and other family members work with clinicians to help reduce the child's feelings of vulnerability and restore a sense of security. Interviews can help to educate parents about trauma and grief. Family therapy can help members gain an understanding of each individual's reaction to the trauma while building mutual support.

When an event occurs, if there is a high degree of life threat, then it is more likely that a posttraumatic stress reaction will occur; if there is a high degree of loss, a grief reaction; if there is worry about another, separation anxiety; and if there are reminders of previous life experiences, exacerbation of or renewal of symptoms may occur. Intervention within the classroom can include enhancement of cognitive functioning through correction of rumors and cognitive distortions, sharing of fears of personal safety and subsequent containment of anxiety, identification of traumatic reminders, and use of the group for support. The classroom also can be a source of support and security through normalization of routines and validation of affective responses. Debriefings and class meetings can be used to help children explore their subjective experiences and to understand the meaning of traumatic responses. Classroom interventions also can help the child integrate the traumatic experience into life experiences and life behaviors. The classroom also is an ideal setting to address issues related to dying and loss through provision of support for grieving.

At the community level, within the hospital setting, intervention begins in the emergency room if children or other family members are brought in for treatment. Intervention begins when a child is hospitalized and helps the child modify an acute stress reaction as well.

In some major traumatic events, intervention relies on the assistance of intervention teams to work with subpopulations of children. These teams include professionals and paraprofessionals with varying levels of expertise and experience. All team members are trained in issues of childhood trauma and are prepared to work in the reality of the disaster setting. These teams may provide acute psychological assistance given directly to children within the classroom setting.

Therapeutic intervention must help the child reprocess the traumatic experience. The intervention addresses feelings of helplessness, helps the child tolerate greater levels of anxiety, and engages the child's abilities to fantasize and take action in constructive ways. Treatment must address the relationship and interplay of trauma and grief, look at the course and risks of complicated bereavement and depression, and deal with developmental disturbances.

Trauma treatment also includes advocacy and social skills education. Children need to be educated as to whom to tell about what happened and what to say. Saying too much can retraumatize, but saying nothing or too little can prohibit understanding of presenting symptoms by others. Reintegration of a traumatized child into the classroom requires specialized and coordinated interventions with the hospital and the school. It is important to minimize traumatic impacts on school attendance and performance. Group work with children who have experienced similar traumatic events can help reduce later symptoms.

As was previously noted, evaluation of the child includes assessments of psychopathology, posttraumatic stress disorder and comorbid conditions, and proximal developmental changes. Evaluation also includes educational testing. Does the child have difficulties taking in visual information because of what that child has seen (e.g., a death or atrocity)? If so, the child may have reading problems and may need additional reading instruction. Screening is initial and periodic over the course of treatment.

The clinic takes a public health approach to treatment after large-scale traumatic events. The most effective intervention strategy for children is school-based treatment using an intervention team. Quick screenings of children at risk can take place in the school. However, classroom interventions have limitations, as do individual/group debriefings. It is not possible to treat intrusive symptoms in a school setting alone because other children may be secondarily traumatized by that treatment (in a group setting). Treatment therefore includes examining objective features of the event, subjective appraisal of internal and external threat, coping strategies used to manage the situation and reactions, catastrophic emotions, ways to gain safe retaliation, reactivity with traumatic reminders, and coping strategies for dealing with and lessening secondary stressors. Each factor is a possible focus for treatment. Treatment is multidimensional and needs to be started early after the traumatic event.

Early Intervention and Psychological First Aid—UCLA

Pynoos and Nader (1988) proposed a procedure for triage and risk screening of children following an extreme act of violence. The number and type of

PTSD-related symptoms correspond most often to the child's exposure. Thus it is important to identify the degree of exposure of the child, the proximity of the child to the event, and the extent of witnessing of injury or death as the first triage step. The second step examines other risk factors including non-exposure-related factors including individual pathology, family response and pathology, worry about the safety of family and close others, previous exposure to and involvement with trauma and/or loss, and familiarity with/closeness to the victim. On-site psychological first aid begins with the establishing of direct, open, mutually supportive relationships with the adults in charge of the site where the event occurred. Interacting with church, school, and public officials is part of this step.

Conducting immediate services on or near the site of the traumatic event provides some degree of initial relief. Whether through the use of defusing (Mitchell model, Everly & Mitchell, 1997) or other models of intervention, the goals of this initial intervention is to help the community restore some sense of control through sharing of experiences and maintenance of normal functions. Often the event occurs at or near a school The school provides an ideal setting for screenings, debriefings, classroom consultations and interventions, and some limited individual treatment. Providing specific help to groups and individuals is part of this response. These groups include administrators, pupil personnel workers who will assist in debriefings, staff members ranging from teachers to clinic aides to playground workers, and students.

Classroom consultation and debriefings allow students to express feelings in a supportive environment, clarify cognitive confusions, screen children for risk factors, promote classroom cohesion and the need to continue the learning process, and encourage help seeking. An initial schoolwide meeting for parents can address questions, educate about posttraumatic stress, and provide a forum for discussions of what happened and what happens next.

SUMMARY

There is a great need for trauma centers designed to help children, teens, and families. Whether outpatient-based or residential, these centers can help survivors cope with and heal from the increasing number of traumatic events that haunt them. As Perry notes in his description of CIVITAS, children's brains are more sensitive and malleable than adult brains and have overly activated neural systems. At the present time, the authors are part of a group of individuals who hope to fund a residential treatment center for traumatized teenagers in rural Virginia. The proposed Germain House Center, under the leadership of Bruce Wyman as executive director and with the consultation of Gerry Eitner of the Masters' Group (www.themastersgroup.org), will eventually implement the assessment, treatment, training, and research paradigms proposed in this chapter.

12

Government-Funded
Trauma Centers

Some trauma centers are primarily government-funded operations. This is particularly true for centers that are connected with military personnel or former military personnel. These programs may service a specific geographic area (e.g., the Veterans Outreach Center serving the Northern Virginia area in the United States) or may serve an entire nation (e.g., in Sweden).

PRESIDENTIAL PROGRAM FOR THE DEFENSE OF PERSONAL LIBERTY, BOGOTA, COLOMBIA

Frida Spiwak Rotlewicz was the victims assistance director of this important program. Her involvement was concerned primarily with victims of kidnapping and their families. An average of 1000 kidnapping cases per year is registered in Colombia, and kidnapping is an extremely complex social issue. A little more than 50% of the cases are attributable to guerrilla groups, which kidnap anyone who has a comfortable lifestyle. They kidnap children, senior citizens, students, and business leaders. Delinquent, isolated individuals do other kidnappings. More than one criminal organization may be involved in one case of kidnapping. One organization may promote the criminal enterprise, another raises funds for the operations, another carries out intelligence tasks concerning the victim, and another negotiates for liberation. Approximately 70% of cases lead to freedom of the victim and only about 4% end in murder. Some cases are the conscription of minors by guerrilla groups into combat and stealing of minors and forcing them into delinquency, prostitution, or putting them up for adoption. In a significant proportion of cases, active members and retired members of the army and police force are involved as participants or perpetrators.

The Presidential Program for the Defense of Personal Liberty was created June 6, 1996, when the president signed Law 282 to give the program permanency. The program therefore initially designed policies and selected priority actions to guide state action in the fight against the crime of kidnapping. Among the initiatives was the creation of GAULA—Groups of Unified Action for Liberty. These groups have specialized units formed by civilian, military, and police members that are assigned to fight kidnapping in their geographical area. The GAULA units are the main source of information for databases about kidnapping.

Mission

The mission of the program is to rescue victims, capture delinquents, decrease impunity, and give attention to families who have had a member kidnapped. The program also includes prevention campaigns and training, technical improvements, and recruitment of professionals for GAULA units.

Service Provision

The major task of the program is to decrease crimes of kidnapping and to deliver trained professionals to combat kidnapping in Colombian society. A major role is to give victims' families informative and emotional support. The program helps families accept their condition and cooperate with authorities during the investigative and rescue phases. The program has prepared an information module broadcast through videos for families who come to GAULA units or to the program's offices. The modules depict the routine development of a kidnapping and ways to cooperate toward liberation.

The Technical Support Division was created to give technical and administrative support to the program. It gathers and systematizes judicial, statistical, and intelligence information at the base and in support of the policies of the program. The division has nine work groups including training, prevention, investigations, coordination and follow-up of GAULA units, and the National Center of Attention to Families, among others.

The program also uses preventive efforts to fight kidnapping. Prevention is a priority goal of the program. Initial prevention activities are targeted to high-risk populations including cattle growers, business people, mining and energy workers, and road engineers. These individuals and groups have been issued general prevention guidelines and have participated in regional lectures and workshops about prevention of kidnapping and extortion. The program is developing a handbook, the goals of which are to increase personal security factors, make recommendations as to the behavior patterns of kidnapped persons and their families during captivity, and help victims deal with handling personal and family situations after liberation of victims.

A major aspect of the program is to provide attention to families of the kidnapped through the National Center of Attention to Families. Kidnapping causes families (and victims) severe trauma. Kidnapping disturbs the entire domestic, social, and working structure of families. The national center's team of 25 psychologists (one for each GAULA unit and for headquarters) are a permanent team tending to the needs of affected families and victims during and after kidnappings. The National Center of Attention to Families offers emotional assistance to help families regain some solidity and structure and avoid disintegration at the program's headquarters, at the regional GAULA, or in their own homes. The program helps families learn to become a support to all its members through the strengthening of tolerance, flexibility, communication, and cohesion. Staff of the program emphasize emotional support and feelings of hope, provide information on the dynamics of psychological trauma, provide counseling during the crisis, and offer continuous follow-up of the families. The program also has developed therapeutic self-support groups.

The program offers families a secure, reliable space to come to find dialogue and credibility. It helps them work through their experiences in an atmosphere of communication and validation. The families are encouraged to have their stories heard, valued, and supported. Thus the program has gathered testimonies from kidnapping victims. The testimonies offer therapeutic support for victims and help in the investigation of future cases through their denunciation value.

The program also has created a national data center to systematize processing of basic intelligence, electronics, judicial, operational, and statistical records. The data center makes it possible to identify organizations, crime networks, and their modus operandi and facilitates the identification and follow up of victims. The data center also condenses information about judicial investigations from the first report to the judicial process and ending up with sentencing.

SWEDISH RESCUE SERVICES AGENCY/KARLSTAD TRAUMA CENTER, KARLSTAD, SWEDEN

When a disaster strikes in Sweden, the Swedish Rescue Services goes into action. This emergency organization serves the inhabitants of the communities and municipalities of Sweden. The Wilhelmsen shipping disaster of September 1989 with 55 fatalities was the impetus for the creation of this organization. There was a lack of preparedness and support for those impacted firsthand by severe accidents and disasters and for secondary survivors. Thus the rescue services developed a course to train teams.

The first course was implemented in 1990, but the program itself began in 1992. By 1996, 250 of 288 municipalities were trained, free of cost, at the expense of the SRSA (Swedish state government). At the time of this write-up, 270 of 288 municipalities have been trained and a new "round" of training of every municipality began in 1998. Municipalities also can buy training courses from the SRSA. The disastrous sinking of the *HMS Estonia* showed the creators of the program and others that the organization had the capability of handling a countrywide disaster.

Mission

The mission is to give the first support to those impacted by a disaster within the first 48 hours after a traumatic event occurs.

Staffing

Course leaders have been in a variety of settings including Ruwanda, Iran, and Armenia and have worked with UNHCR. Some have trained first in military defense, then civil defense, and now crisis support and disaster psychology. There are various levels of persons now prepared to deal with disasters in Sweden. There is the management group at emergency hospitals; this group is linked to the disaster committee and has managerial responsibility for mental and social care in mass accidents. County councils/public health care districts have psychosocial support groups to assist relatives of those killed or seriously injured. Members organize information and support centers for family members and function as support persons for individuals and families. Municipalities have posttraumatic support groups with functions similar to hospital's psychosocial support groups. Psychosocial support teams of the national defense support the networks at military units. Committees work with eight community segments: social services, fire and rescue, schools, church, police, medical care system, and voluntary organizations. Laypersons are used as support persons for families and individuals during emergencies.

Theory

When a disaster occurs, 20% of those involved who survive will be helpless or need help and take flight; 50% will look on and not know what to do; and 30% will do spontaneous work to help out before official help arrives. The model for training is a wellness model that needs to be introduced to Swedish citizens between the ages of 12 and 14 through adulthood. The theoretical basis is to provide education to preteens and older persons so that they can become more spontaneous in their willingness to intervene. The normal period of mourning after a disaster is 1 year; however, some persons become stuck in their traumatic stress reactions and need help to work through what happened.

Services

The service began to educate municipalities and develop support groups in 1992, training 250 of 288 municipalities. A Swedish law passed in 1995 stated that all municipalities have total responsibility for crisis defense. Thus the

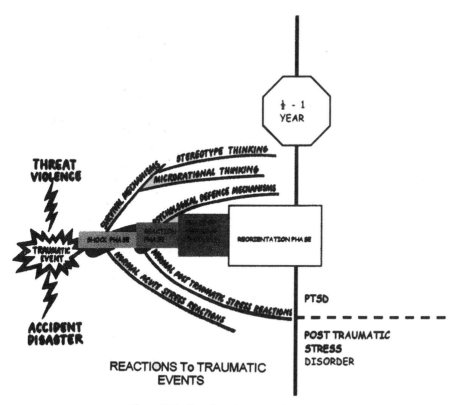

Figure 12.1. Reactions to traumatic events.

Swedish Rescue Services Agency began to develop training courses for munici-palities, schools, and hospitals to educate persons about trauma, PTSD, and trauma response (see Fig. 12.1). The service cooperates with the National Board for Health and Welfare. The government pays employees for their work. The service also conducts support groups, for example, in shootings or in the aftermath of the *Estonia* disaster. The service has developed 10 courses and trains about 50 municipalities a year. Every municipality is entitled to 5 days training for five persons at a certified SRSA rescue school. Services provided range from a onetime event to a one year support group. Figure 12.2 illustrates the multileveled service provision system.

The Karlstad Crisis Support Center

This center was created in 1997 to provide treatment to trauma survivors within a 48-hour postevent period. As consultant Lars Osterdahl noted, the trauma center has been a success and "many, many people have gotten support

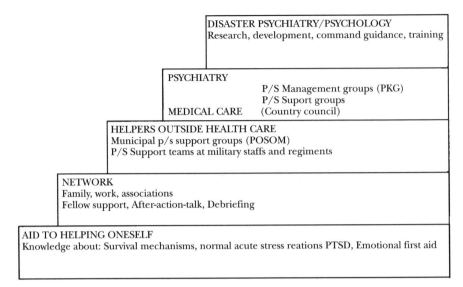

Figure 12.2. Ladder of psychosocial support: Prevention activities to prevent future mental distress.

and help this first year" of its existence. This center has trained laypersons to work in the center. It is open Monday through Friday to give anyone with an acute life crisis caused by accident, death, crime, violence, loss of job, or other circumstances some assistance. Anyone who thinks she or he needs help can walk in for that aid. The center works with persons from Karlstad county and two other counties.

A program that has been developed is a crisis training and treatment program for peer supporters (students) at the local high school. This program provides 30 hours of training in four separate phases. The first looks at rights of students, attitudes, violence, and attitudes to foreigners and similar topics (8 hours). The second provides lessons on drug problems, violence, racism, and mob situations (6 hours); the third, first aid training (10 hours); and the fourth, crisis intervention training (8 hours). The goal of this program is to train students who want to help in various situations including accidents, violence, and drug-related situations so that they can provide emotional first aid after the event happens. The students are from the Karlstad school system.

THE NORTHERN VIRGINIA VETERANS CENTER, ALEXANDRIA, VIRGINIA

The Northern Virginia Veterans Center, part of the Readjustment Counseling Service, under the auspices of the US Department of Veterans Affairs

Health Care Administration, is one of 204 veteran centers in the United States. The Vet Center programs were established in 1979 by congressional mandate initially to address the needs of Vietnam veterans. The objective of this center and fellow centers is to provide counseling services to veterans and their families for war-related issues within the community. The center was opened in May 1986. It also does outreach to community agencies, military installations, veterans' facilities, and veterans' service agencies.

Mission Statement

The mission of the Vet Center is to provide readjustment services to traumatized war veterans and those veterans who were sexually traumatized/harassed while serving on active duty. The philosophy is to provide the highest-quality service possible and to act as an access point to refer veterans to other services as warranted (within the Department of Veterans Affairs). The philosophy is "veteran helping veteran."

Staffing

The center has five staff positions. Team leader is Bob Tecklenberg, whose primary job is administration. Other staff members include an office manager, drug and alcohol counselor, two clinical social workers or a clinical social worker and a psychologist. The focus for staff hiring is mental health and generally staff are veterans themselves. As federal employees, they are part of the US Civil Service. The center also uses volunteers to assist with clinical work and clerical duties. Interns from several local universities also provide limited services. Staff members receive support and direction from the Department of Veterans Affairs and one of the seven regional managers. Staff members meet weekly in team-building meetings and also try to do social activities together and participate in training programs.

Clientele

The primary clientele of the Vet Center are veterans from the combat theaters of World War II, Korea, Vietnam, Grenada, Lebanon, Panama, the Persian Gulf, and Somalia. Since 1992, an additional client group comprises men and women veterans who were sexually harassed or traumatized while on active duty. The secondary client group given services are family members of veterans. Veterans with specific trauma-related issues receive services on a priority basis and the majority of veterans receiving counseling at the present time are Vietnam War veterans. These veterans have extensive input into their treatment planning because of the community-based nature of the program. The veteran population of Northern Virginia is between 100,000–200,000 veterans of which approximately 90% is male; 60%, white; 30% African American;

and 10%, Hispanic or Pacific Islanders. The veteran population is aging and, through mortality, is shrinking. There have been no major wars since 1973; however, the conflicts that have occurred have generated some need.

Theory

The model of trauma on which services are based is an eclectic model. Much of the work is didactic and depends on the particular expertise of the clinician and needs of the client. Much of the work done is based on cognitive and behavioral theories.

Assessment

Intake assessments are done for clinical and drug and alcohol issues; however, assessments for medication needs are done by medical center professionals. After the initial assessment is made and treatment plan is devised, reviews of those plans and follow-up assessments take place every 6 months, unless an earlier review is indicated. Many veterans can be dually diagnosed with substance abuse and depression coexisting with PTSD. Part of the assessment process includes a psychosocial workup.

Clinical Services

The center provides individual and group counseling, psychotherapy, advocacy, and system intervention. Clients who need medication are referred to the nearest VA Hospital. The treatment plan for a veteran may include a period of inpatient care and aftercare. The majority of services are provided at late and very late postevent time periods. Services for family members include family counseling and groups for significant others. Veterans are primary in developing the treatment plan. The principal mode of long-term therapy for veterans is group psychotherapy.

Much of the work done is crisis intervention, both in person and via the telephone. Staff are trained to handle clients in crisis. This work is basically client centered wherein clients are encouraged to engage and ventilate while focusing on their issues. Staff members help clients to get to a protective setting, if appropriate. The center offers clients the opportunity to get better and to get healthy. It also offers clients an opportunity to get information and a way to access the Veterans' Administration system.

Community Services

The staff members of the center participate in a variety of outreach projects. They give presentations to a wide range of community groups, military personnel, mental health providers, educational institutions, and veterans' service organizations. They develop and present public service announcements and do public education. They participate in "stand downs" for homeless veterans (organized resources, colloquia) and are actively involved in developing programs to combat homelessness. Staff members also offer consultation to various agencies concerning Vet Center clients.

THE NATIONAL CENTER FOR WAR-RELATED PTSD, HEIDELBERG, VICTORIA, AUSTRALIA

The National Center was founded by Professor Philip Morris. He initiated and developed the work of the center and resigned as director in April 1997. Associate Professor Mark Creamer, a clinical psychologist, is deputy director. The center responds to the clinical challenge of treating the 12% of Australian Vietnam veterans who suffer from chronic PTSD as well as veterans from other eras and Defence Force personnel. The center opened in June 1995 after funding was obtained from the Department of Veterans' Affairs. The center has academic affiliation with the University of Melbourne and is located at the Austin and Repatriation Medical Centre, Heidelberg, Victoria, Australia.

A key mandate of the center is to work with the Australian Defence Forces (ADF) to improve early recognition, prevention, and treatment of traumatic stress reactions in military personnel. As a consequence of this mandate, the ADF and the center have run a 2-week intensive course on traumatic stress for military personnel likely to come into contact with individuals who have experienced traumatic events during their military service, whether overseas or in training exercises.

Mission

The mission of the National Center for War-Related PTSD is to work to advance knowledge about PTSD, improve treatment of the condition, and prevent the disorder. The goals of the center are to facilitate the development of effective treatment services; train health professionals in recognition, assessment, and management of PTSD; educate the general and veteran communities, defense forces, and health professionals about PTSD; encourage and direct research into PTSD: implement strategies designed to prevent PTSD; and collaborate with international agencies with similar objectives.

Staffing

The staff of the center consists of a professor/director, a deputy director, a manager, and a secretary. Advisors include a clinical reference committee (made up of senior academics and clinicians) and an advisory committee (for administrative oversight).

Theory

Chronic PTSD is associated with disturbances in adrenergic, dopaminergic, and opiate neurotransmitter systems as well as alterations in the hypothalamic–pituitary–adrenocortical (HPA) axis and thyroid function. The mechanisms of kindling and behavioral sensitization have been proposed to explain the chronicity of PTSD. Drugs that act on these neurotransmitter systems are being tried in the treatment of PTSD. No one drug class seems to have a primary role in PTSD. PTSD is an anxiety disorder and benzodiazepines are often prescribed. However, they do not seem to impact the core features of PTSD. Therefore treatment may include using different drugs to address differing aspects of the condition. The following drugs might be used for different symptom clusters:

- Intrusion: monoamine oxidase inhibitor phenylzine, tricyclic antidepressants (including clomipramine), and selective serotonin reuptake inhibitor (SSRI) venlafaxine.
- Avoidance: SSRI antidepressants (venlafaxine), valproate
- Numbing: SSRI antidepressants (venlafaxine), valproate
- Hyperarousal and irritability: SSRI antidepressants, propanolol, clonidine, and benzodiazepines (clozepam)
- Insomnia and nightmares: benzodiazepines, cyproheptadine
- Impulsiveness and anger/rage: lithium carbonate, carbamazepine, valproate

When using these or other psychotropics, it is important to be aware of potential drug interactions and watch for side effects. When medication is stopped, symptoms often return at their previous intensity.

PTSD is frequently a chronic condition. When that occurs, it is rare that it exists in isolation. Many patients have comorbid illnesses, including depression, alcohol dependence, and other anxiety disorders including panic attacks or agoraphobia. Adequate fitness is important to deal with the stress that is part of PTSD. Exercise is part of a preventive approach for physical illness and helps to combat aging. The average veteran benefits from a daily routine of exercise that the veteran enjoys, that focuses on "quality" not "quantity," and is specific to the veteran's needs. As fitness improves, so do motivation, desire, self-discipline, esteem, and confidence. The ideal exercise routine includes three weekly 30-minute sessions of aerobic exercise (brisk walking, swimming, cycling), stretching, and use of weights.

Assessment and Evaluation

One of the first tasks of the center was to develop and implement an assessment and evaluation process to monitor progress of veterans completing accredited treatment programs. Principles guiding this effort included ensuring that selected instruments covered a broad range of functioning. Second, protocols needed to be as brief as possible to maximize response rates and compliance. Third, both objective, clinician-rated measures and patient self-report data were included in protocols. Finally, attempts were made to ensure that data were comparable with overseas programs, particularly those in the United States, while maintaining an Australian focus.

Protocols for interviews included coded identifying information, demographics, and occupational and financial information, combat experiences, other life traumas, diagnosis, problem definition and management plan, alcohol use, medication use, family functioning, symptom severity, legal problems, anger issues, general functioning, life satisfaction, use of health services, and satisfaction. These areas are covered at pretreatment and if appropriate at 6-, 12-, and 24-month intervals after entry into the program.

Services

Current programs have cohorts of six to ten patients progressing through treatment together for a 8- to 12-week period of time. The program combines group and individual therapy in exposure-based treatment models. The program also includes alcohol rehabilitation, medication management, stress and anxiety management, healthy living skills training, social skills training, anger management, physical conditioning, and assistance for partners and families. In 1996, a day hospital program for World War II veterans and a treatment program for peacekeepers with PTSD were given. Long-term follow-up treatment is provided by Vietnam Veterans counseling services, local practitioners, psychiatrists, and counselors.

The center collaborates with the Australian Defence Force to provide treatment for personnel suffering from PTSD and assists with a comprehensive psychiatric assessment of personnel before their discharge. The center has conducted a dot probe study investigating the way veterans pay attention to things around them that can be associated with Vietnam. The study found that veterans with PTSD are more likely to focus on Vietnam-related words than neutral words than are veterans without PTSD. An additional study examined the association between intrusive memories and avoidance and dissociation. A general tendency toward dissociation, as well as reported dissociation during time in Vietnam, were strong predictors of current PTSD.

Training

The national center has a key role in providing education and training. The center conducts a variety of workshops including those discussing assessment and evaluation of PTSD and treatment of PTSD, as well as presenting teleconferences and teaching a course offered through the University of Melbourne. These workshops are of interest to clinicians, clinical directors, and program coordinators of PTSD treatment programs, as well as other mental health professionals. The assessment and evaluation workshop trains clinicians in the comprehensive assessment of PTSD and associated comorbid-ity using instruments that form the basis of the center's assessment protocol and evaluation questionnaire. The treatment workshop provides participants with an overview of individual and group treatment approaches as well as medication management. The center also maintains a library of books, video-tapes, and treatment manuals in the Austin and Repatriation Medical Centre Health Science Library. Tapes from the center's 1996 and 1997 annual confer-ences are available. The annual conference, in conjunction with the Australian Society for Traumatic Stress Studies, focuses on the nature and treatment of traumatic stress disorders in veteran populations.

Research

The national center is conducting or has conducted a variety of research studies: a treatment study investigating EMDR (individual sessions), stress management interventions (group format), and writing therapy (group for-mat). The study aims to investigate which treatment works for what veteran, if any, and then seeks to determine what predictors lead to success.

A positron emission tomography (PET) study has been gathering infor-mation about the brain activity involved in attention and memory processing in PTSD. Using PET scans and magnetic resonance (MR) scans, studies of brain regions involved in attention and memory and the phenomenology and neurophysiology of traumatic memories have begun. A study of treatment of alcohol problems using naltrexone, a drug that acts as an opiate antagonist, also is being conducted. This drug blocks the effects of natural morphinelike substances released by the brain when alcohol is consumed and thereby re-duces the pleasurable effects of alcohol. Three sleep studies also are being conducted using sleep questionnaires and sleep logs. These studies look at relationships between PTSD severity and sleep disturbance, between reexperi-encing phenomena and sleep, and at the efficacy of using commercially avail-able sleep retraining and dream reprocessing therapy interventions to im-prove sleep and reduce primary symptoms of PTSD. Another study is a neuroendocrine study using blood samples. In this study, the growth hormone response to clonidine is blunted in subjects with high levels of PTSD symptoms. Results suggest that central alpha-adrenergic receptors are down-regulated in PTSD. The national center also is collaborating with the Australian Defence Force to measure the effect of selected interventions to prevent PTSD in the military.

SUMMARY

Although all trauma centers need governmental support of some kind, at some level, few are actually funded in total by national governments. In the

United States, the largest group of centers that offer services to traumatized individuals as well as those without a PTSD diagnosis are the Veterans Outreach Centers and inpatient programs at VA hospitals. Yet their services are being cut tremendously as inpatient programs are being shortened in length of stay or eliminated entirely, as positions are being cut, as services are being revised and "managed." In many of the countries where programs are desperately needed, governmental resources are tapped to the maximum and funds are not available. Any monies for trauma centers therefore must be solicited from humanitarian organizations, governments of more affluent countries, or private foundations. Macedonia, for example, was overwhelmed by the masses of Kosovo refugees who poured across the borders. Perhaps the Swedish Rescue Service Agency model best shows how to utilize government resources in a preventive manner. Studying it in depth and seeing how it can be adapted to less affluent countries will be a future challenge to organizational leaders in the field.

13

The Experts View of What Trauma Is and How to Treat It

This volume has presented a diversified approach to the treatment of trauma. Many of the directors of the comprehensive trauma centers described in this book discussed their views of the "state of the trauma world" at the present time. These views differ, to say the least. In fact, many of their perceptions of the existence, intensity, and frequency of traumatic events are in direct juxtaposition. In spite of these contrasting views, the respondents offer insight into the current state of trauma in the world today. The various respondents are cited at the conclusion of their statements.

WHAT IS THE STATE OF TRAUMA IN THE WORLD TODAY?

The field of traumatic stress, as an established field of interest and inquiry, is a growing field. More practitioners are learning about the role of trauma in psychopathology and the role of trauma-oriented treatment in healing (SSTAR). Traumatolgists and others are beginning to examine the basic nature of good and evil and the role of trauma as it impacts the masses. On one hand, the field tends to overemphasize psychopathology; on the other, it underemphasizes resilience, prevention, and the power of community (Harvey, Victims of Violence) as well as the natural healing resources of the individual and the environment (Slovene Foundation). Many clinical psychiatrists do not understand trauma; many clinicians do not know how to listen to clients, take good social histories, or understand the research about trauma, let alone recognize the cultural aspects of the diagnosis or treatment (Bell, ITRI). Some languages do not have nomenclature to describe trauma as a concept or recognize the "self" as an entity rather than part of a collective.

To be sure, PTSD as a diagnostic descriptor is inadequate to describe all things trauma-related. PTSD as a concept does not describe the impacts of cumulative trauma, community trauma, or intergenerational trauma. PTSD as

301

a diagnosis is inadequate to describe all things and the definition of PTSD is an evolving growing, changing creation (Chester).

One of the major areas of concern in the field of traumatology is that of "turf" issues. Many persons fight over access to survivors of disasters or traumatic events. Practitioners descend en masse to the site of a traumatic event to "offer" their services. Whether or not they are trained to do critical incident interventions is immaterial. They are there. They have come to offer themselves to the "cause." For many, their offers of help are financially motivated or motivated by a desire for fame and prestige.

One of the major concerns in the trauma field is that of funding. How do trauma centers justify their existence? From what resources can a center find financial support in a world of limited resources, a world in which agencies fight for funding in order to survive (Bergmann)? It is particularly difficult to treat massive trauma with limited resources (South Africa). As Colin Ross notes, the denial of the role that trauma plays leads to a decrease in financial resources for its investigation, prevention, and reduction.

Another area of concern is how to ensure that traumatologists receive assistance to resolve compassion fatigue. There is a lack of resources for practitioners to obtain support. In fact, many "trenchers" do not take good care of themselves (Porter).

The field is also being driven by popular thinking rather than scientific thinking (Laub), and is not trying to examine the efficacy of treatments based on research. The media has glorified the world of violence. As a field, the media does not tend to show the realistic, actual impact of violence and trauma and does not portray their real effects.

What are some other trends in the field? There seems to be a "coming together" of biological and clinical components as more and more clinicians as well as researchers recognize the impact of trauma on biology. In fact, there is a greater repository of knowledge about how trauma affects the biology of the brain (Gaston).

The world today is a very stressful place. Even though the symptoms of trauma are more widely recognized, treatment of trauma is still in the Middle Ages (Ticehurst, Tinnin). Treatment of trauma tends to be fragmented, particularly as more persons get involved in the field (Schubbe) and as nonprofessional groups converge to question the validity of the work done (Cosentino).

THE INCIDENCE OF TRAUMATIC EVENTS

Massive psychic traumatization is the unified currency of the 20th century worldwide (Laub). There is a greater recognition of the existence of trauma (Becker, Poijula) and the world is becoming more traumatic and violent (Porter, Harvey). Many respondents believe that trauma seems more visible (Yüksel, Turkey; Sweden), that knowledge of its existence seems more evident

(Ross, Homewood), even though the public perception of PTSD can be very negative (Vet Center). Trauma is omnipresent (Teter) and the world is becoming more aware of its harsh reality (Homewood). Perhaps people are beginning to realize that things that cause victimization are bad for the species (Wilson).

Richards believes that multimedia coverage of traumatic events makes them seem larger and more frequent; however, it does appear that the frequency of mass terrorism and violent attacks is escalating, particularly in the United States. In Germany, the frequency of occurrence of violence, particularly violent acts by foreign criminals, is increasing, as is the quality of violence. There are even more incidents of hostage taking and attacks against witnesses (SIAM). Some experts believe that traumatic events are not really more frequent (Tinnin, Becker, Shalev, Mikus Kos); others believe that it is difficult to tell whether they are more frequent (Teter, Homewood); still others believe that events are more frequent in occurrence (Ross, Sweden).

Tunnecliffe is among the most verbal about his views of increased incidence. He says that there is an increased recognition of trauma as a (potentially) serious debilitating problem. There is an increased reporting of traumatic incidents, an increasing number of trauma groups who want recognition and the right to speak, a destabilization of family and community supports, an increased amount of occupational mobility and social change, and an increase in the numbers of activities that contribute to the greater incidence of trauma (crime, arms sales, drug traffic).

THE INTENSITY OF TRAUMATIC EVENTS

As people become more aware of the role trauma plays in everyday life, they can see that trauma appears to be more intense at the present time (Chester). Massive traumas are very visible (AMCHA) as the world shrinks. Other respondents who believe that trauma now is more intense than in the past are COPIN, Homewood, Cosentino, and Ross. The staff of the RCT believes that trauma is more intense in some areas and less intense in others. Yet others say that trauma does not seem to be more intense (Becker, Tinnin, Shalev).

THE THEORY OF TRAUMA

The paradigms describing trauma are changing and the language to describe trauma also is changing (Chester). However, the knowledge base on which treatment is built is not receiving enough attention (South Africa). The state of continuous trauma in the world, a world in which no place is truly safe, a world in which there is a continuous fear of retraumatization, leads to crisis response rather than time for prevention or development of theory. Yet the key to survival and service in this field is primary prevention (Turner).

As Bloom notes, understanding the effects of trauma and how to treat them is at an early stage of development. There is enormous professional and social resistance to the implications of what trauma means. Pearlman agrees that knowledge of trauma is still in its infancy while the work of treating trauma is becoming ever more global and international. In many countries, treatment of trauma and the theory of trauma are separated from mainstream therapy and psychiatry. Shalev adds that the field, since it is so young, is still ideologically driven rather than being pragmatically driven. If treatment is to be successful, it is necessary to understand what turns individuals into healthy survivors (Wilson) rather than hopeless victims. Furthermore, if the theory and knowledge base of trauma is to be accepted, it needs to be directed more to the average, everyday person who has had something horrible happen in his or her life.

THE TREATMENT OF TRAUMA

The work involved in treating trauma is becoming more credible as it has been reality tested to a greater degree (Turnbull). The standards on which treatment is based are becoming more scientifically based (Cosentino). Vet centers have made significant contributions to treatment, as have other centers. Yule believes that the practice of trauma treatment has become a huge industry involving a great deal of money.

Tinnin has written that trauma treatment does not have to be prolonged with numerous difficult to manage emotional abreactions. The belief that trauma must be relived in order to be healed is mistaken. On the other hand, treatment cannot be completed within five or six sessions as determined by managed care. The impact of managed care on trauma treatment, according to the staff of Benjamin Rush Hospital, is cutbacks in programs and layoffs. Standards of treatment for PTSD, disorders of extreme stress, not otherwise specified (DESNOS), and other trauma-related symptoms are not clear and those that do exist are not widely adopted (Blythe). In many instances, there are insufficient capacities and time for intense treatment of PTSD (Mikus Kos) and the range of treatment approaches for non-Western, non-industrialized nations are narrow (Bell, ITRI).

CHALLENGES FACING THE FIELD OF TRAUMA

Perhaps the biggest challenge to the field is to set some type of standard of treatment and develop a model of treatment, based on research and theory that can be applied to different populations of survivors (BNMO). If and when this occurs, then it would be necessary to train those who work with trauma in an integrated, formal way (Poijula).

For some practitioners, a major challenge is learning how to deal with an aging population. Is there a different way to treat survivors who are soon going to die and are in the later stages of trauma? Some of these survivors have never acknowledged their traumas previously; others have acknowledged them but have not sought treatment (AMCHA).

A third major challenge is how to get money to treat survivors, particularly in underdeveloped countries or in situations in which there is massive traumatization. It is important to make information about and treatment of trauma available and accessible to greater and greater numbers of survivors (Mikus Kos). In many instances, there is a lack of government funding for both education and treatment of trauma (Sweden). Health care organizations continue to place limitations on treatment sessions as they try to stretch the health care dollar in the mental health field. Shalev also notes that finding funding resources to treat acute trauma as well as do preventive work with those who are acutely traumatized so that they do not develop prolonged PTSD is a challenge.

Additional challenges include how to keep up with the burgeoning literature of trauma and the present research as well as how to determine which types of treatment are reputable and which disreputable as statements of miracle cures in a minimal number of sessions blossom, and how to do the work on a daily basis (Bryant, Wilson). Trauma treatment can become political, particularly when the traumas involved have political ramifications (e.g., domestic violence) (Moore). Teter believes that dealing with the social and political contexts of trauma and the rise of repression as a response to social problems is actually the second greatest challenge to the field (the first being funding). A further challenge is to try to prove the scientific validity of the realness of trauma and the effectiveness of posttraumatic treatment (Homewood) in a world in which most people who are providing treatment to trauma victims are not familiar with the trauma model.

In many cultures, it is still a stigma to seek help for psychological problems, particularly those that might be related to the workplace (SIAM). If institutions and professionals do not accept the diagnosis, if the false memory movement can have such a following, if society seeks to deny and minimize the existence and impact of trauma, then the challenge is to help all those groups realize that an external experience can be connected to a specific psychiatric disorder, PTSD (Schubbe).

THE NEEDS OF THE FIELD AT THE CLOSE OF THE 20TH CENTURY

The needs of the field are many according to the respondents to the research protocol. Rather than creating a narrative to describe those needs, it seems more feasible to list the most significant needs:

1. The most important need is money: money to do the research, to do the work, and to create comprehensive trauma centers (COPIN, Bergmann). In order to obtain funds, it is necessary to convince those

persons who allocate and raise funds that trauma-oriented treatment is important, as are research, prevention efforts, and education (SSTAR).

2. There is a need for a change in belief systems, particularly about the politics of trauma in general and violence in particular (Moore). The field needs to take a stand on issues of violence (Bloom).

3. There is a need to do research on psychotropic medications for chronic, complex PTSD patients who have sleep disorders, as well as problems with hyperarousal and self-soothing (SSTAR).

4. There is a need for public awareness and public recognition to combat the muteness and fragmentation in the field. There also is a need for scholarly research and the need for dialogue and collaboration among various groups and treatment centers (Laub).

5. There is a need for quality training and teaching about trauma (Gaston).

6. There is a need to delineate which approach(es) to treatment is (are) effective, when that/those approaches should be used, with whom, and in what combination (Gaston).

7. There is a need for greater collaboration and communication between clinical researchers and clinical practitioners and a need to find a balance between biological research and other types of research (Harvey).

8. Bell points out the need for the development of therapeutic approaches that are consistent with multicultural differences. The trauma profession needs to enlarge its cultural horizons and become more multicultural, perhaps through conducting culturally competent treatment outcome research (Chester).

9. Patients can help design treatment protocols and can help to develop a standardized protocol of treatment that can be applied to all settings and all types of patients/clients.

10. There is the need to increase the knowledge base on which trauma treatment rests. This base needs to have constant updating so that it can serve as a basic fund of knowledge as to "what one has to know" (Bloom). This knowledge base also would serve as a permanent source of information (Mikus Kos).

11. Trauma workers need to have ways to receive help for compassion fatigue and vicarious trauma that are nonstigmatizing, readily available, and without excessive costs (e.g., within a nationally funded rehabilitation system) (Poijula).

12. There is a need for research in all areas of trauma (Porter, RCT). This research should be multinational and multilateral with international monitoring (RCT). This research could help develop effective intervention/prevention strategies (Richards) and would have the financial backing to study how proven educationally based protocols could be applied to other populations immediately after a traumatic incident (acute stage) and over the long term (prolonged stage).

Another research need is to conduct good therapy outcome studies that identify what makes healthy survivors (Wilson).

13. It is important to link the fields of traumatic grief and trauma in diagnosis, research, and treatment (Poijula).

14. There is a need to investigate and understand the usefulness of mind–body approaches to the treatment of trauma and undertake the creative study of these approaches in a scientific way (massage, aromatherapy, Reiki, and others) (Becker).

15. There is a need to develop ways to provide help to elderly victims who have kept silent for most of their lives and who need to talk about what happened to them in an accepting environment that has an atmosphere of safety and gives them the control they need (AMCHA).

16. There is a need for a broad, consistent certification for traumatologists, responders, and debriefers (Bloom), such as that provided by the Association for Traumatic Stress Specialists (ATSS).

17. All trauma organizations need to respect one another and network with one another in an atmosphere of cooperation, professionalism, and respect for cultural differences (RCT).

18. There is a need to establish standardized protocols and practices to deal with complicated cases of PTSD and DESNOS (Yüksel).

19. There is a need for public education about trauma. The world needs to know about psychological trauma and torture if it is to progress toward health and maturity and overcome denial, avoidance, and victim blaming (Lubin).

20. Children often are the unacknowledged victims of trauma. There is a need to give more attention to treatment of children (Becker) and to develop a child crisis response team that can respond immediately to situations involving children. This team would provide critical incident stress debriefing and management, assessment, and triage. There also is the need to bring trauma-focused services into the community as well as to convince managed care companies to reimburse nontraditional, clinically necessary interventions for children in the home and in the community. In other words, there is the need to adapt the shape of the "animal" to the needs of traumatized children and their caregivers (Philadelphia).

21. There is a need for lobbyists to work on behalf of the trauma field in all areas of research, practice, and funding.

22. The government needs to pay for free, public education about how to help oneself should a traumatic event occur. This education about acute stress, emotional first aid, and building of support networks constitutes preventive intervention (Sweden).

23. There is a need for free treatment that can be offered to *all* trauma survivors within 48 hours after an incident occurs (Sweden).

24. There is a need for ongoing support groups that can be offered free to

survivors of severe trauma. These groups would meet for an extended period of time if necessary (Sweden).

25. There is a need to provide services to victims of workplace violence. This type of violence is growing by leaps and bounds (Blythe).

26. There is a need to focus on health, not pathology (Wilson).

27. There is a need to establish comprehensive trauma centers around the world; these centers need to be funded for extended periods of time (a 5-year minimum) (Turnbull). These centers could have satellite centers that would be based at local health clinics or schools (South Africa).

These needs are not the only ones in the field. Others come to mind. There is a need to establish the efficacy of critical incident stress debriefing as one means of intervention after a traumatic event in such a way that stops the present attack against it. There is a need to separate trauma theory from personalities. In many instances, the question of efficacy of theory has become more of an attack against individuals than an investigation based on scientific methodology. There is a need to create a network of credentialed, certified professionals who have *earned* their certification, not bought it. The most important need, though, is a network of comprehensive trauma centers throughout the world that provide treatment to all persons at no cost or minimal cost in an efficient, culturally competent manner. It is our hope that this volume will help lead the way to the creation of that network.

14

Trauma Center Directors Describe the Ideal Trauma Center

The concluding question in the research protocol asked respondents to describe their conceptions of the ideal trauma center. This chapter summarizes their ideas, attitudes, and suggestions. Most are identified by their author. We offer their suggestions as a prologue to the final chapters, which describe our own conceptualizations of a comprehensive trauma center.

PHYSICAL ENVIRONMENT

The physical environment of the ideal center is more than a building. It includes land that can be used to grow gardens and allow displaced trauma survivors to reconnect to their homes and gives a sense of community (Chester). The type of population served also determines the location of this center (Bergmann).

The ideal center must have a good location and good equipment (Poijula). Any setting must be safe in its accessibility (well-lighted, for example) and have a physical layout of spaciousness, privacy, and nurturance [Stanley Street Treatment and Resources (SSTAR)]. It also may have sleeping facilities. It definitely has community rooms for social gathering, rooms in which to hold meetings, and rooms to tape and view oral histories (Danieli). It has a library, pool, sauna, and workout facilities (Richards). It also is located within (and treats within) a cultural context. In other words, if a center treats a specific ethnic population, then it must be located in an area that is accessible for that group (Perren-Klingler). As a community-based center, it is self-contained and freestanding, no matter its actual physical base (e.g., in a university) (Richards). It is not part of, nor is it entangled in, a large bureaucratic system. The center also has adequate secretarial support, as well as adequate space. The level of support and space allows for collegial interchange and other self-care provisions (South Africa, Harvey). Ideally, even if there is one primary location

309

for a center, that building serves as hub of a trauma network (Wilson). This network may consist of satellite centers that are community based. The model on which a center is built is a human resource development model that is a dynamic, developmental organizational model (Niles).

FUNDING OF THE IDEAL TREATMENT CENTER

The ideal center has a secure funding base, whether governmental or private in origin. If the funding base is governmental, that base does not impact the independence of the center's decision making (Oulu). Having a long-term secure financial commitment allows the center to treat complex PTSD and do extended research (SSTAR). The minimum financing term is 5 years. A 5-year period of time also allows for greater job security, treatment innovation, and eliminates constant worry and struggle for survival. A well-funded center allows for access to services by all at no or reduced cost. In this way, the center is not dependent on ever more restricted third-party payments by insurance companies. Other sources of support are companies and organizations. The well-funded center also has a secure legal standing and legitimate status. This status allows for a greater independence in decision making.

STAFFING

The ideal center, whatever its actual structure, follows independently set professional guidelines that are trauma-based, espouses a high level of ethical standards, and has highly competent staff members. The ideal center has a professional team of at least eight to ten persons; this team includes clinicians from different professional backgrounds and disciplines (Oulu). The actual staffing patterns of centers may vary, depending on the traumas involved, the culture of the environment of the centers, and other factors.

In this center, staff members are well-trained, dedicated, responsive, culturally aware and representative, optimistic, and committed to a strengths perspective of treatment (Poijula). They also have a good sense of humor and are open to spiritual components of care [International Trauma Recovery Institute (ITRI)]. The large majority (if not all) are trained in trauma, are knowledgeable about the recent literature, understand the role of substance abuse in trauma, and also understand the role of pharmacological intervention (SSTAR). These individuals, from leadership through support staff personnel, are sensitive, empathic, and have a strong knowledge base (Vet Center). All staff members, if possible, are certified professionals (Niles) who have done their own healing (the Meadows). They constantly participate in extensive standardized training (Benjamin Rush) and believe in a team-based model of treatment. Leadership in the ideal center is not autocratic; instead, it tends to be more decentralized, following a network model (Sanctuary). At least some staff members have language capabilities to speak the language of clientele.

If the center utilizes non- and paraprofessionals to provide some level of psychosocial intervention, those individuals also are well-trained. Legal and vocational services or referrals also are provided, depending on the staffing of the center. Teams ideally are multidisciplinary and consist of health-related, social, educational, and legal professionals (Slovenia). Teams do not have counterproductive competition.

THEORY BASE

A strong value system underlies the theory base of an ideal treatment center. Among those values are respect, humility, resiliency, and recovery (Harvey). The ideal center has an open-mindedness to various perspectives about treatment and speaks the language of trauma. Any theory base is scientifically grounded, allows for cultural differences, and accepts the client–patient as partner in the process.

The theory base is the foundation on which models of prevention, intervention, and follow-up care are developed (Wilson). It also is the foundation for publication of theory-based literature.

Contributors to this volume have various thoughts about that model:

- It is holistic with a mind-body approach to treatment.
- It espouses nonviolence (Sanctuary).
- It determines effective models of treatment and debriefing (Turner).
- It utilizes an interdisciplinary approach (South Africa).
- It is essentially biopsychosocial (Becker).
- It has a global perspective.
- It recognizes the importance of prevention.

ASSESSMENT

In the ideal center, assessment uses a trauma-based protocol that includes measurement of dissociation. Assessment also uses a variety of approaches including physiological and psychological. Assessment varies from being formalized, using standardized measures, to being informal and information-gathering in scope. Some assessments may be forensic in nature. An extremely important part of any assessment is a comprehensive life/trauma history, if clients recall their own histories. If clients do not recall their own histories, helping them construct life lines with primary and secondary traumatic events depicted can be helpful. Assessing how clients describe themselves and the language they use also is important. Client narratives, as subjective recountings of trauma, can give information that objective paper-and-pencil assessments miss.

Assessment is done as early as possible after a traumatic event occurs and is redone at intervals to measure change (and treatment effectiveness). Assessment and evaluation advance clinical work, provide feedback about client progress to staff, inform the community about the successes of the center, and can (through demonstration of successful trauma resolution) contribute positively to fund-raising efforts. Assessment based treatment plans are realistic and concrete (Slovenia).

SERVICE PROVISION

According to the experts, the comprehensive trauma center (CTC) ideally offers a continuum of services for its clientele of children, adolescents, adults, families, work places, survivor groups, communities, and even nations (Ross, Poijula). These services range from defusing, debriefing, and other crisis-oriented services to services for complex PTSD (Turner). As Teter noted, these services are responsive and individualized. They are respectful of clients and are theory driven and based on research findings, if at all possible. They are provided across the life span and across traumatic events (Danieli).

A major focus of the work of the center is prevention (Turner). Perren-Klingler stated that a center provides both primary prevention and secondary prevention (through critical incident stress debriefing) and helps develop prevention plans and strategies for a number of situations and client groups. These preventive programs are proactive and broad (Wilson).

Services are designed for intervention with acute stress disorders (SIAM), posttraumatic stress reactions, posttraumatic stress disorders, and disorders of extreme stress. The types and amounts of services provided for each of these conditions is determined by a needs assessment (Perren-Klingler). Yule stated that the ideal center must respond to acute referrals within 24 hours.

Treatment provision in the ideal CTC respects clients as coequal partners and focuses on their cultural strengths (Chester). Clients therefore are involved in planning and delivery of those services in an ethnically, racially, and culturally responsive manner (Teter). Treatment includes individual, group, and family counseling. Simultaneous treatment for PTSD and chemical dependency also is part of the treatment protocol (Wilson). Thus, service provision is multidisciplinary (Lubin). Treatment relies on eclectic methods ranging from education about trauma and trauma memories, to expanded use of expressive therapies (SSTAR), to creative therapies including movement therapy and body-oriented therapy (Sanctuary). If possible and if needed, the center has a day treatment program for individuals with more chronic needs (Ross).

Services, if at all possible, are provided at a low-cost, if not a no-cost, fee schedule, unless there is insurance reimbursement or governmental provision for payment for services. Some services may be provided by volunteers; others, through peer counseling and peer support (Niles).

Once treatment has dealt with the traumatic events themselves, then the focus can change to one of resocialization, [including resocialization so that a client can get off disability (Ross)], social support, and referral (Sweden). Ross stated that part of this process is pain management, preparing for work, and affect regulation. The center may provide space for a drop-in program so that clients can just "hang out" (Danieli). Support groups may include goal setting, planning, grief work, anger management, problem-solving, and other foci. If possible, the center has facilities that encourage recreation and exercise (weight room, gym, pool, sauna) (Benjamin Rush Hospital). Services also include community-based outreach (Poijula) and creation of community-based programs. These include health-related services, work-related services, and informational services (Perren-Klingler).

RELATIONSHIPS WITH OTHER AGENCIES

The ideal trauma center maintains cooperative relationships with other local and international agencies and programs (SIAM, Wilson). The center also builds and is part of a local and international network (Poijula) because trauma work is becoming increasingly global and international (Pearlman, ITRI). The ideal trauma center therefore interfaces with and is known within its local, national, and international communities (Cosentino). It connects with sister organizations (Turner) and maintains a high positive profile through excellent public relations (Moore). Public relations building occurs through involvement in consortium and coalition building (Richards), advocacy, and community action (Harvey). Ties to grass roots activities also help build awareness and recognition of the role and functions of the center (Harvey). As the ideal CTC provides training to the community, it builds some of that awareness. Thus, the ideal trauma center gives constant attention to networking with and education of other organizations and larger systems within its environments (Lubin).

TREATMENT SERVICES

The ideal center provides biopsychosocial–spiritual interventions to help traumatized individuals, families, groups, and communities overcome the hindering impacts and effects of exposure to traumatic events. Treatment is broadly based as well as innovative and uses expressive techniques and physiotherapy to supplement problem-oriented therapies. Services are provided to a survivor's family as well as other components of the survivor's social environment because trauma does not happen within a social vacuum (Croatia). The common features of service provision in all trauma centers should be comprehensiveness, accessibility, affordability, cultural and social appropriateness, and cooperation with other services (Slovenia). In order to provide good treatment, clinicians collaborate with primary health workers, teachers, volunteers, and staff members of other organizations.

When working with trauma survivors in general and refugees in particular, treatment provision aims to reduce suffering and prevent further traumatization, supports and develops natural support systems, and helps the survivor establish structure, daily routine, and a sense of normalcy. Treatment combines individual and group work with social activities and advocacy in an outreach-oriented manner (Slovenia). Treatment also aims to increase the survivor's abilities to cope with what he or she has experienced.

ADVOCACY

A major component of service provision by an ideal treatment center is advocacy. The center has the duty to make individuals, groups, and societies aware of trauma and uses that awareness to stop violence (Turkey). The center offers education for peace, procures official declarations of attribution of responsibility for torture victims, and helps with redress—seeing through governmental intervention and national and international levels (Switzerland). Center staff also participate in cathartic programs at national and international levels.

The ideal center provides information to the public about the extent and causation of trauma. Center staff members create and participate in demonstrations, memorials, commemorations, and celebrations. The center helps people remember old symbols and also helps them develop new ones (Teter). Staff members are visible at the community grass roots level. They are pro-human rights, understand the political aspects of trauma treatment, and stand by their social commitment (Teter). The comprehensive center must deal with the political realities of the environments around it (Niles), recognizing that trauma is intimately linked with societal norms (Lubin).

The center also works to increase awareness of the mental health needs of traumatized individuals, families, groups, and communities. Center staff members work with the media and may themselves publish leaflets, brochures, manuals, videos, journal articles, and other works. The ideal center holds public lectures and participates in public forums, organizes local conferences, networks with other agencies, and encourages staff members to participate in and present at various professional conferences (Croatia).

TRAINING

It is important that the ideal trauma center takes a broad role to provide trauma training on a variety of levels. Center trauma experts train each other (or obtain training from outsiders). Staff members often offer workshops throughout the center's country or throughout the world (Pearlman) and may maintain a speaker's bureau (Danieli). Center staff members train community leaders about trauma. They also train indigenous peoples about trauma, service delivery, and mental health. Staff members may train para-professionals to act as support group leaders (Ross). The center initiates the building of a professional support network to serve as a catalyst to increase awareness of the mental health needs of its care providers (Croatia). In other words, the ideal center becomes an important educational center (Sanctuary). The center may even offer accredited courses as well as continuing education units (Richards, Harvey).

Training modules developed by the center are flexible and allow the curriculum to be tailored to the specific need profiles of each particular training program. The ideal center offers culturally specific and culturally sensitive training programs that are locally based and can serve large numbers of service providers from a variety of institutions and organizations. The center also develops exchange and partnership training programs with other institutions and experts (Croatia).

RESEARCH

The ideal trauma center has a large research arm (Ross). Objectives of the research are to expand the database on which trauma intervention is based (Wilson) and publish research-based literature. Staff members should support the center's research efforts and in the ideal center willingly participate in studies. Having a 5-year funding base allows staff to conduct outcome studies and do longer studies on the impacts of trauma and various treatment methodologies. The ideal center is able to give evidence of good research, is open to new studies, and seeks to become an international research center (Bryant, Harvey, Yule).

Research may examine how symptom reduction can be achieved through stabilization by a present-centered treatment focus that strengthens clients' skills (Homewood). Furthermore, research can examine how programs can reduce the frequency and intensity of PTSD symptoms through that stabilization and present focus. Other research studies might focus on evaluation of the program's theoretical and practical approach (Sanctuary and the therapeutic milieu), vicarious traumatization (Pearlman), the value of debriefing, and comparisons of various treatment methods. Ideally, the center will develop its own research protocols and scales.

CONCLUSIONS

These ideas are offered by many of the respondents to the study. However, they do not examine the various functions, roles, and components of the ideal CTC in detail. The last two chapters therefore describe our ideas of what constitutes an ideal trauma center in Western as well as in non-Western environments.

15

Constructing the Ideal Trauma Center

Reflections, Recommendations, and Realities

INTRODUCTION

The venture begins with an idea—a vision. There is no comprehensive trauma center in your community or region, yet there appears to be a need; significant numbers of trauma survivors exist around you. But is that need real? And if it is, what do you do next?

The blueprint for developing a comprehensive trauma center (CTC) ideally flows from a needs assessment that defines the groups at risk or in need of services, identifies the extent of problems of those groups, designs a means to reach and interact with the groups, selects and adopts a service delivery system, and links the center's program to other institutions, facilities, and organizations (Galano & Neziek, 1986). A needs assessment may mean you must design and implement a community survey, conduct interviews with key informants and leaders, host a series of community forums, analyze existing service usage and waiting lists, and look at the extent of traumatic events that have occurred in your immediate environments. It is important to have data from multiple sources to determine whether there is an actual need for a CTC. Discovering gaps in service provision and problematic areas of service delivery through a survey can pave the way for justification for the creation of a center. If the CTC you seek to create has grown out of a specific traumatic event (e.g., a disaster, war, or large-scale crime), then the need may be more obvious to a greater number of individuals, groups, organizations, and political entities.

317

THE BUSINESS PLAN AND SERVICE DELIVERY PLAN

If your needs assessment determines that the need for a CTC truly does exists, next comes the creation of your business plan or action plan. What must be included in your plan? Elements to include are the mission statement, principles and objectives of the center; the organizational components of the center including management and leadership and flow chart of proposed structure; the target markets, marketing goals, revenue and profit goals; competitive resources that might prevent obtaining those goals; services that are going to be offered; financial considerations and needs; and operational factors.

Establishing a service delivery plan leads you to ask what types of victims will the center serve? What will be the needed physical design? What types of services will be available? Will there be a 24-hour answering service or will staff members carry beepers and/or answer crisis calls directly? Will they respond to crises within a 24-hour time period? Will there be crisis counseling that involves emergency referrals to medical care, shelters, and other facilities? Will staff members do death notifications or accompany law enforcement to provide emergency intervention when a death notification occurs? To what extent will staff provide advocacy and counseling? Will they help clients with applications, claims, and disputes? Will they provide information and referral services? All these issues must be considered before any initial decisions are made, before the organizational structure of the CTC is established, or before the duties of center personnel are defined.

THE INITIAL CONSIDERATION: PHYSICAL SAFETY IN A CTC

The "buzzword" of a CTC is "safety first." The CTC must be a safe haven that is consistent, predictable yet flexible, boundaried, and committed to the client's healing. The physical environment and construction of a comprehensive trauma center is an extremely important aspect to take into consideration. The actual physical setting of the CTC has at least one of six basic functions; it is designed to

1. Provide shelter and security to trauma survivors
2. Facilitate social contact between survivors and providers
3. Provide symbolic identification
4. Enhance task attainment (the work of trauma resolution)
5. Heighten pleasure
6. Stimulate growth (Steele, 1973)

Everything within that setting needs to convey self-efficacy and self-worth of clients and staff as well as the worth of services offered. New, nontattered magazines that deal with normal, nonpsychological topics need to be available. Furniture that also is new, with soft, culturally congruent colors (e.g., red is the color of life for Native Americans; for others, it symbolizes blood and death) must be used. Furniture needs to be arranged in curved or angled formats with backs to walls to not replicate any trauma setting that might have had rigid, square furniture arrangements. The center has adequate lighting (with no shadows) as well as adequate heating and cooling facilities and a cleaning service that tolerates (and cleans up) food debris, since the ideal program in some manner includes food and eating. Because many trauma survivors are extremely intolerant to noise, the center has a quiet atmosphere; noise is muffled by high-quality carpet and good padding.

It is important to have some space within the CTC that allows clients to come together in a normal setting to give each other support and community. One possibility is a community area that also is a crafts center, includes some space for children to play, and has space for groups to meet. The CTC needs to be accessible to persons by public transportation. It also is especially important for clients who have handicapping conditions to have access (Hanna & Ritchie, 1992). In addition, good parking facilities with good lighting are essential. The ideal center has land available for gardening, recreation, and (perhaps) also has a Ropes course.

It is important that the setting of the CTC is predictable and ordered. If a client is used to a certain room for a session, then that room needs to be available consistently. Furniture and accessories remain the same, unless the client is prepared ahead of time for a change ("we will be getting some new furniture next week, Mrs. J"). When a new client enters the office in which therapy is to occur for the first time, it is important for the therapist to observe that client's scanning process. What objects catch the client's eye? What objects might trigger the client? Does the client want to have doors/windows/blinds open or closed? Does the client need to have a safety object placed in the room (picture, rock, or other object)?

Safety and Perpetrators

Safety and security are of supreme concern to staff and clientele of the CTC. Part of safety for victims is *not* to be near their perpetrators, if those perpetrators seek or are ordered into treatment and come to the same facility. It is important, therefore, for the center to take a brutally honest look at who is seen and when. Victims of intentional malice do not need to be retraumatized when treatment seeking.

Talking about what happened during a traumatic situation may be a direct threat to a perpetrator. Therefore anyone who works in a trauma center can be viewed as a threat by a perpetrator who does not want the victim(s) to speak. This includes even the receptionist who is the first-line contact. Everyone in a trauma center who deals with victims of intentional malice, terrorism, and attack needs to have self-defense training and take part in drills. Liaisoning with local law enforcement for support and training in self-defense strategies and responses (e.g., if a hostage situation should occur) also is important.

There may be times when safety escorts for staff and clientele are necessary. Hiring a security consultant to check out potential dangers and make recommendations also is a possible avenue of response to these situations. Decisions to consider would include who has keys, how locks are installed, how many exits to have, whether to have "panic" buttons and, if so, where.

Personal Safety of the Clients

The CTC, in working with persons who have been severely traumatized or persons who have disorders of extreme stress, needs to establish policies and procedures for handling potential suicide ideation, threats, and attempts as well as self-mutilation. What levels of self-destructive behavior will be tolerated or accepted? How much mutilation is acceptable, if any? What is the protocol for hospital admission (when is a client hospitalized)? Are there hospitals more suitable and more aware of how to treat trauma survivors? What training has been given to local hospitals in terms of treatment protocols for trauma survivors, for example, for torture victims, rape victims, and others? Have CTC staff members conducted in-service presentations or trainings to help change those facilities, with the aim of making a more appropriate "fit" between their services and the survivors who come to them? The ideal center has considered and answered all these questions. Consideration for the maintenance of personal space boundaries of traumatized clients is essential. Making sure that center procedures and physical arrangements do not directly intrude into personal space of clients includes making sure that there is no overcrowding in waiting rooms or meeting rooms, that offices have adequate space, as do hallways and entrances/exits. Personal space, according to Brown and Yantis (1996), operationally is approximately a 4-foot area around the client or client group. However, that personal space expands and contracts based on the individual's psychopathology (Cavallin & Houston, 1980). Trauma survivors with PTSD tend to need more personal space (Brown & Yantis, 1996). Negative reactions to intrusion of personal space include lowering eyes, assuming a rigid posture, turning away from others, and leaving the situation. Intrusion of personal space may cause anxiety in a trauma survivor because it decreases personal control and the identity of the individual. Decreased personal control can lead to increased anger and episodes of violence. Therefore, as a potentially preventative strategy, it is important to be aware of and ask permission to enter the physical space of clients.

Safety and Boundaries

The CTC physically recognizes and respects the personal space of those who use it without crowding, intruding, or causing discomfort. Many persons diagnosed as PTSD-positive have need for more personal space and consistently respond with greater psychophysiological reactivity to personal space intrusions (Brown & Yantis, 1996). Nesbitt and Stevens (1974) viewed personal space as a device used to control the intensity of stimulation from others. Intrusion into the personal space of a trauma survivor by a caregiver, support staff member, or even another survivor can evoke anxiety, decrease personal control, and suggest threat that leads to a potential rage reaction (Bullock-Loughran, 1982). Research has shown that increased personal space protects individuals from personal aggressive impulses, increased anxiety, and insecurity (Cavallin & Houston, 1980).

Setting appropriate, safe boundaries is a transcendent aspect of constructing safety. Violating a client's boundaries misuses the power of the therapist and breaches the core intent of the therapeutic relationship, which is to empower the client to heal. It is important to teach the client what to expect and what not to expect (Peterson, 1992). Personal needs of the therapist must take a backseat to the needs of the client. It is never appropriate for the client to take care of the therapist or to make the therapist's decisions.

One boundary issue is the issue of touch. Touch and physical contact may or may not be acceptable, allowed, or appropriate. It is up to the entire CTC leadership team and staff to discuss how touch is to be used or not used within the cultural framework, ethical code, and other environments of the center. Establishing policies about appropriate touch (a hug, handshake) with the client's permission therefore is important. What touch rituals might be acceptable or permitted? Touch needs to be professional, social (a handshake), and based on the absolute "say" and permission of the client (without threat).

Safety and the Client–Counselor/Therapist Relationship

Berg (1994) noted that it is important to learn many things about clients to help them work with their traumas. It is important to get the client to answer questions as to:

1. What is important
2. What makes sense
3. What constitute his or her problem-solving strategies
4. What constitutes his or her successes and failures in coping with the traumatic event(s)
5. How she or he views the trauma and its impacts
6. What she or he is willing to do and what she or he refuses or is unwilling to do
7. What are his resources in his or her family, among the neighbors, and within various organizations and groups to which she or he and others in the family belong (church, social groups, civic groups) (p. 54)

Although the client is the "expert" on his or her own traumatic history and reactions to that trauma, it also is important to explain trauma and traumatic reactions to that client without using jargon, using language that "fits" the client's style and ability. If a client is concrete, use concrete language. If a client has a visually oriented learning style, ask the client "What do you see?" If the client has an auditorially based learning style, use hearing-oriented words.

The ideal relationship between client and therapist/counselor/case manager, according to Gordon and Edwards (1995), is person-focused, humanistic, patient-centered, empathic, and compassionate. This relationship is collaborative and recognizes that

1. Each participant in the center (whether employee or client) has unique responsibilities.
2. That relationship is consensual and not obligatory.
3. There is a willingness to negotiate aspects of the relationship.
4. Each party derives some benefit from the relationship (Quill, 1983).

A major component of this relationship depends on active listening skills of the therapist who responds to a client's communication by "feeding back" the staff member's understanding of the sender's message. According to Gordon and Edwards (1995), active listening has numerous benefits, among which are fostering catharsis of troublesome feelings, facilitating problem solving, reducing fear of feelings through acceptance, keeping ownership of a problem with the client, and diffusing strong feelings.

THE MISSION OF THE CTC

If you are considering developing a CTC, it is essential to begin with a vision that leads to a destination. That destination, the vision converted into reality, is the mission statement. It contains the fundamental creed and philosophy of the organization and paves the way toward creating a tangible facility. It contains the essence of the CTC's value system, purposes, and priorities. It is the heart of the commitment of the center and presents the CTC's face to the world.

The mission of a CTC therefore is presented in a clear, articulated statement of direction, philosophy, and goals. That statement takes a salutogenic point of view, stressing wellness, states the population served by the CTC, and respects cultural differences. The mission statement of a comprehensive trauma center ideally is succinct and clear. Examples of one- or two-sentence mission statements include the following:

• The mission is to give the first support to those impacted by a disaster within the first 48 hours after a traumatic event occurs (Sweden).
• The mission of the Sanctuary program is to provide a healing environment for survivors of trauma. The program is designed to be a temporary refuge and retreat within which significant life change is encouraged, supported, and directed (Bloom).

- The goal of the center is to help survivors learn to cope with their experiences and prevent long-term posttrauma consequences for themselves and their families (Bergmann).
- The mission of the program is to restore control and a sense of independence to persons who have experienced a loss of control and loss of independence after traumatic events. The main strategy of the mission is the cognitive and emotional processing of traumatic memories (Turnbull, Ticehurst).
- The mission of the center is to treat trauma patients within the context of general care and the general framework of psychology and psychiatry. The mission also is to provide good care to survivors of trauma and their relatives and to do good research to improve knowledge (Shalev).
- The mission statement also can be somewhat longer. Two examples of a longer mission statement are provided by the Homewood Hospital and Benjamin Rush Hospital programs:

    The mission of the (Homewood) program is to offer a safe haven wherein healing can occur through specialized therapy within a community in which survivor helps survivor. The community creates a warm, secure environment for recovery. The mission also is to provide excellent inpatient care and to serve patients to the best of the program's ability in a client-centered manner while focusing on safety and empowerment. The goals of the program are helping patients to create physical, emotional, and relational safety; to examine patterns of revictimization and traumatic reenactments; to reduce symptoms; to modulate affect; and (at times) to "metabolize" trauma.

    The mission of the Trauma Recovery Program is to provide a safe, therapeutic, structured environment for people to address psychological trauma caused by overwhelming life experiences. The goal of the hospital is to help each ... patient regain health and ability to function in normal daily activities, giving them the tools they need to enjoy a better life by teaching them healthier ways to resolve future problems. The focus is on the "person" rather than just the "illness."

Perhaps one of the most detailed, comprehensive mission statements is that of the International Trauma Recovery Institute (ITRI) in Arizona. It is included here to give an example of the entire continuum of mission statements that could be developed for an ideal center.

- ITRI is dedicated to the prevention and amelioration of the effects of traumatic stress in individuals, families, the workplace, and community settings. ITRI also is committed to assisting communities, regions, and countries who are in the midst of rapid development and industrialization, as well as assisting in efforts to reduce the turmoil that commonly accompanies relocation and reunification. ITRI offers consultation, development, and implementation of specific negative-reaction-reducing plans and appropriate treatment options. Their services are designed to aid assessment, resource provision, and recovery in a prompt, knowledgeable, skillful manner while taking into account culturally differing worldviews, social systems, expectations, relationship dynamics, religious practices, and political and historical factors. Central to a successful recovery is the goodness-of-fit between the social-cultural-community context of the trauma and the selection and delivery of services.

The mission of a CTC, according to persons who responded to a question at several International Society for Traumatic Stress Studies (ISTSS) presentations, is to build optimal wellness and help clients who come to the center achieve or return to some measure of autonomy. The mission statement, including philosophy, goals, objectives, values, ethical standards, and directions for intervention, is generic in focus but specific as well. It has a tone that emphasizes restoration, wellness, and reduction of further chances of victimization. It also acknowledges and respects cultural differences.

FROM THE MISSION COMES ...

The philosophy, goals, direction, directives, and objectives of the center all flow from its mission. If the mission is to restore clients to their prior status (before trauma), that mission may not be realistic. Perhaps a more realistic mission is to help clients reduce future revictimization, whether by person, event, or system, or is to build optimal wellness in its clientele. Ideally, one aspect of the mission of a CTC is to provide a safe environment for doing the work that needs to be done. The mission is guided by a code of ethics as a reality check for the work that is done.

What else is included in a mission statement? The mission statement may include clear, definable targets of the work of a CTC. It may include a statement about a "common enemy" of the center (e.g., fighting crime or injustice) or it may propose that the center is a model for service provision. In other words, the mission statement contains the purposes or aims of the center and its guiding principles.

RIGHTS AND RESPONSIBILITIES STATEMENTS: A SAFETY-CREATING TOOL

Part of the literature developed by a CTC is a description of the center's services, expectations, fee schedules, and similar operational components. Policies for availability of staff (in terms of return phone calls, response time to emergencies, numbers of sessions, 24-hour response procedures, and backup policies) are included in this statement. Also included are policies about confidentiality and informed consent, limits to confidentiality (suicide threats or attempts, child abuse, duty to warn/protect), adjunctive collaborations and contracts, termination policies, and use of hospitalization. Courtois (1995) suggested the use of a "rights and responsibility statement" to outline the CTC's therapeutic orientation, ways of working with trauma survivors, and mutual rights and responsibilities regarding many of the above-mentioned aspects of treatment. Other topics that might be included are the use of treatment plans, payment policies, insurance issues, use of medication, and how medication usage is determined. Specific informed consent forms for use of more "novel" techniques of treatment such as eye movement desensitization and reprocessing (EMDR) and thought field therapy (TFT) may also be included.

THE CULTURE AND CLIMATE OF A CTC

The ideal trauma center has its own organizational culture. Culture, as was stated in Chapter 2, is the character or personality of the CTC (Schneider, 1994). A CTC's culture includes the basic assumptions, shared values, and shared beliefs that guide the way the members of the CTC function within the organization, whether toward clientele or toward each other. Kurstedt (1997) wrote that culture "is the collective shared feeling of or belief in the organization and what it stands for ... culture questions are we questions" (p. 1298). Any CTC has at least four cultures (Schneider, 1994): (1) the culture of control and decision making; (2) the culture of collaboration and is people driven, based on trust and actual experience, and is the culture of the team; it is dynamic, participative, and focuses on the immediate realities within the center; (3) the culture of competence; and (4) the culture of cultivation. The cultivation culture looks at possibilities and creative options. It, too, is people driven and nourishes self-expression in staff members. It is a catalyst for growth and change. It is possible to build a cohesive culture in the CTC. Figure 15.1, modified from Ivanevich and Matteson (1995, p. 38) is a visual representation of that process.

Climate is "the individual's feelings, attitudes, and perceptions of their current relationship or alignment" with a CTC, according to Kurstedt (1997, p. 1298). Climate questions are "I" questions. The ways that the staff members describe a CTC are indications of the climate. Symbols of that organization describe both culture and climate. They include a logo that is simple and recognizable, certain components of language (jargon, slang, humor, slogans) as well as certain narratives (stories, legends, myths), rituals, rites, and ceremonies.

Each comprehensive trauma center described herein has its own culture. Within those cultures are the power culture (who decides and determines what happens); the role culture (the structure, order and control mechanisms of the CTC); the achievement culture (who is successful, competent, commit-

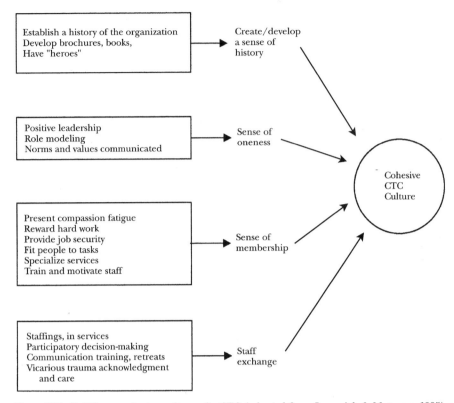

Figure 15.1. Building a cohesive culture of a CTC (adapted from Ivanovich & Matteson, 1995).

ted); and the support culture (what are the relationships within and outside of the CTC, the elements and sense of belonging, mutual caring, or connection). Ajdukovic (1997) echoes these statements by noting that "... trauma does not happen in a social vacuum Nor does it heal apart from ongoing social processes" (p. 33).

As Mink, Owen, and Mink (1993b) have noted, to a great degree culture is the unwritten rules that define the workscape. The ideal workscape is productive and those rules support and encourage high performance. The high performance workscape has six essential processes:

1. A shared vision, purpose(s), and goals hold the organization together; purpose of the organization and actions of the leadership are consistent and reflect the organization's mission and vision.
2. All staff members, to the greatest degree possible, trust and accept one another, working toward accomplishing the shared purpose.
3. People with expertise and the work that needs to be done are more important than are structure, status, and position. Staff members identify with the organization and their personal positions.

4. Staff members at all levels focus on performance in a climate of shared learning and constant searching for improvement.
5. Supportive management identifies and reduces constraints that interfere with accomplishment of the organization's goals.
6. Staff members know what is expected of them, seek to improve their skills, use them autonomously in the "right" way, and use feedback to improve performance.

The authors continue to describe the 12 pillars of a high-performance climate that exists within an ideal comprehensive trauma center or other organization. This pillars create a performance-oriented environment with staff involvement, self-management, commitment, and personal/professional empowerment by staff members and clients:

1. Shared vision for the organization of ultimate purpose(s)
2. Shared values and processes to achieve the goals
3. Shared goals that are important, specific, and constant with values
4. Focus on what is really important within the CTC
5. Desire for productivity and meaningful accomplishment
6. Support for accomplishment
7. Competent staff members "hired for quality, trained for excellence" (Mink et al., 1993b, p. 59)
8. People work together in teams with trust and mutual acceptance as well as creative use of differences; the leader is the coach of the team, key to setting standards and making use of the talents of individuals
9. Leadership enables everyone on the team to contribute fully.
10. Provision of accurate feedback as to how all staff members are doing (their behavior) in relation to their performance goals
11. Each staff member is free to contribute to team goals and functions within the CTC in a flexible, creative, responsive manner, based on the needs of the clients
12. The efforts of staff members lead to their desired, valued outcomes

FUNDING OF THE CTC

Once the CTC has a mission, then it must obtain resources for its creation. This is probably the most difficult part of the entire process—finding the money to fund a CTC. Where are the most viable sources of funds? Grants? Private corporations? Government programs (e.g., revenue from slot machines)? United Nations funds? Philanthropic donations? Consideration of funding must include start-up costs, salary considerations, and costs of materials and goods (e.g., furniture, electronics), security system, rent/mortgage, insurance, and consultants' costs (e.g., attorneys, accountants). If the center is nonprofit, what is the source(s) of money? Does it come from the government (and at what price?) or from donations? Can the organization get grants or donations? Are corporations willing to help fund the organizations? Can clients pay for services either directly or indirectly (through goods, services, or insurance moneys)?

The ideal trauma center is funded for a minimum of 5 years at a time so that positions and research operations can be stable over that period. It also has multiple sources of funding and a secure funding base for both the short and long term. If the trauma center is a nonprofit or not-for-profit organization, it is able to apply for grants and donations. If the center is for-profit, it may have a not-for-profit component as well. In developing countries, there often will be no private pay or insurance reimbursement to pay for the services. Use of volunteers and acceptance of some type of "in kind" donations may be necessary. Funding issues are a major challenge to the ongoing work of a CTC. From where does the money come? How is money raised? Is it donated, obtained through grants, paid by clients (through self pay or third party payment), paid by government organizations or other sources? What services are given without expectations of pay? Are in-kind services/donations accepted (time, materials)? Giving away too many services or too much professional time can lead to resentments. Taking financial support from other agencies and organizations can set up the wrong expectations from clients as well as place expectations on the center (e.g., if a certain drug company gives a grant, the expectation may be that the company is acknowledged as a sponsor of a training or that the medication the company manufacturers is preferentially prescribed to clients).

Funding seems to be a major issue for all trauma centers. Ideally, the center is funded by the government either directly as part of the health system (Turner, Traumatic Stress Clinic), through a university (Bryant, Post Traumatic Stress Disorder Unit), or through dependable insurance reimbursements (the Swiss Krankenkasse). Third-party payments have become less reliable; funding from private foundations and individual donations is competitive to obtain, and moneys from research grants often are limited. The Traumatic Stress Institute/Center for Adult and Adolescent Psychotherapy (TSI/CAAP), for example, receives 80% of its funding from clients (including from their insurance companies); the remaining 20% comes from royalties, forensic fees, and speaking and consulting fees. International organizations including the United Nations can provide some funding to certain activities of trauma centers [the Rehabilitation Center for Torture Victims' (RCT) work with torture survivors].

THEORY BASE

The theory base of a comprehensive trauma center is a viable, inclusionary theory base. It operates upon the DSM-IV and ICD-10 frameworks, acknowledging the disorders of extreme stress not otherwise specified (DESNOS) classification. It recognizes that these definitions offer working hypotheses about trauma. The comprehensive trauma center operates from a biopsychosocial view of the person, group, organization, or nation.

What do the various centers say about the theory base they use? Soili Poijula of the Crisis Center in Oulu, Finland writes that the model used by her organization is integrative and includes belief, affect, social, imaginative, cognitive, and physical components. Debriefing, based on Mitchell/Dyregrov/Ayalon models (Everly & Mitchell, 1997), is used frequently to prevent unnecessary aftereffects of exposure to trauma, to accelerate normal recovery, to normalize reactions of rescuers, to stimulate emotional ventilate, to stimulate group cohesion of rescuers, and to promote the gaining of a cognitive grip on the situation. This method is used in early crisis intervention. Not all centers believe in or espouse the Mitchell model; among those that do are Moore, Turnbull, SIAM, Yule, Perren-Klingler, and Cosentino. Turner notes that debriefings done by his center are "not quite Mitchell" and use a salutogenic process offered as an early intervention designed to normalize the response to a traumatic event occurring in the previous 2 months. Debriefing is followed by six to eight sessions of treatment. Bergmann has developed a debriefing model that is one component of an overall approach to crisis and organizational intervention.

Dr. Sandra Bloom, in her description of the theory base of the Sanctuary model, lists a number of trauma-based assumptions. Rather than repeat these here, the reader is referred to the description of that program (see Chapter 8, this volume). The acronym SAGE stands for safety, affect management, grief, and emancipation, the four steps of recovery.

The majority of centers rely on a cognitive–behavioral theory of treatment as a primary means of intervention (Chester, Ross, Turner, ITAP, Yüksel, Benjamin Rush, BNMO, Yule, Tunnecliffe, Jagellonian University). Colin Ross expands that theory base to include "cognitive systems and psychodynamic principles." The theory base leads to a nonevent treatment approach that is systems-oriented with healing elements of treatment lying within the process and structure, not at the content (what happened) level. This systems approach also draws on family systems theory and the contextual school of family therapy (ITAP). Turner also notes that the major focus is on modifications of cognitions–schema; clinical work is more exposure-based with a primary emphasis on cognitive restructuring. The theory base recognizes that dealing with the meaning of a traumatic event is fundamental. Ways to deal with that meaning include reframing, giving testimony, and building understanding. Richards uses an educational ergonomics model that is essentially cognitive/behavioral.

One theoretical principal that guides the work of what was Chester's center is "Qa Tutsawinavu," or a state of mind that is unintimidated by fear from any source. This state of mind and philosophy helps people come to positions of inner strength to deal with adversities in a proactive way. Other theoretical principles used by various clinicians and centers are casework theory, stress response theory, disability management, and crisis intervention. Theories of prevention also are important in designing treatment strategies, interventions, and training programs.

The theories of trauma espoused by different centers lead to stage models of treatment (Becker). For example, Rousseau at the NECTR has a four-stage model that includes (1) denial and (2) a vague awareness of the traumatic event; (3) awareness, leading to resolution as the experience gets integrated; and (4) concludes with emergence when the past is left behind as the past and the survivor emerges as a whole, energized self. Courtois' and Turkus' stage-oriented model at The Center also has four stages: pretreatment assessment; early stage safety and stabilization; middle stage trauma resolution; and late stage self- and relational development. The theoretical framework encompassing these stages is based on pacing and timing. Niles uses a trauma critical stage intervention model (TCSIM) that is developmental, cybernetic, and holistic and provides constant feedback analysis and evaluation. The model has stages of integration, disintegration, and reintegration. In this model, intervention is based on diagnosis of level of traumatic reaction as well as stage of personality reintegration. The model also integrates Western personality and organizational development theories with Eastern natural law developmental perspectives.

Homewood Hospital echoes many CTCs by describing the model of intervention used as predominantly eclectic, incorporating medical, cognitive–behavioral, spiritual, contextualistic, and psychodynamic theoretical principles. It also uses theoretical models of complex PTSD (disorders of extreme stress) and the therapeutic milieu model of Sanctuary; this latter model recognizes that social wounds require social healing. Some centers (e.g., Bell's ITRI, Wilson, Perren-Klingler) recognize the importance of culturally relativistic models and the influence of culture, geography, and economic/political/historical contexts as they impact client(s) and system(s). As Perren-Klingler notes, a social–cultural contextual understanding of trauma is very important as is a model of community prevention.

Perhaps one of the most important theoretical bases of the comprehensive trauma centers described in this volume is the biopsychosocial model. This model is essentially a social work model that recognizes the interconnection of all aspects of the survivor's self and life (Turnbull & Ticehurst; Ross, Perren-Klingler, SSTAR). Another extremely important theoretical base is the constructivist self-development theory (CSDT) as developed by McCann and Pearlman (1990) and further expanded by Pearlman and Saakvitne (1995). Rosenbloom and Williams (1999) have operationalized this theory into workbook format. The CSDT is a relational psychotherapy model based on clients' strengths and resilience and has as its core the aspects of self, individual identity, self-esteem, inner experience, and worldview.

CREATING THE STRUCTURE AND MODEL OF THE CTC

Our research has found that there are many ways to structure a CTC, just as there are many organizational models to describe those centers. The structure of the CTC is formally stated and informally implemented, as was noted in Chapter 2. The six primary components of structure are:

1. Reporting relationships and locus of power and influence
2. Methods of communication (staffings, meetings, reports, memos, brochures, chapters in journals, books, research as formal methods; rumor, networks, gossip, chatting, and sharing as informal methods)
3. Decision-making procedures to solve problems including regulations, policies, pressure, gathering of support
4. Accountability systems including formal performance reviews; measurement of "successful" treatment; financial accounting; informal collusion between staff to cover up incompetence
5. Norms including formal rules of conduct (flex-time, work hours; comp time; dress codes if any) and informal norms (expectations for unpaid overtime, staff relationships)
6. Reward systems of formal rewards of compensation, benefit packages, recognition programs; informal rewards of positive feedback or recognition

The center may be a central provider organization with a leader or leaders who set policies and procedures and make strategic plans (e.g., Gaston). In this structure, the founders of the organization have the control over the primary location and any community-based offshoots. In other instances, the leadership of the CTC is dispersed laterally through committees and teams.

The ideal center, though, uses a more lateral structure because it builds a deeper investment in and commitment to the CTC. In that ideal center, all staff members respond similarly when they complete the following statements:

1. The environments within which our center exists view it as _____ .
2. Staff members of our center give their first priority to _____ .
3. Our center treats individuals, groups, communities by _____ .
4. Decision making in our center is made by _____ .
5. Jobs/tasks within our center are assigned by _____ .
6. Motivation to do a competent job is a result of _____ .

Some centers are limited liability companies (TSI/CAAP) or practice networks of partners (Perren-Klingler) whose liability is limited to the investment in the firm. All members of the networks are involved in the management of the organizations and their structures are flexible. Income passes through the organization to the practitioners who are not salaried. When the practice consists of independent contractors, each individual assumes risk for his or her work and is not an employee per se of the center. That individual is responsible for his or her own insurance, equipment, and tools of practice. While this structure allows for flexibility, there is little control over persons who participate in the company, unless they sign some type of contract under a leader or leaders with these self-employed practitioners. An advantage of this type of structure is that a larger geographical area can be served and that more types of practitioners can be included in the network.

A workable structure for a CTC is a centralized group practice with satellite offices at more remote locations, for example, as exists in South Africa. All clinicians are actual employees and generally are salaried. Some are based at the central location and others at the satellite centers that cover a wider geographical area. This organization offers multiple types of services and also has a not-for-profit component to conduct research, do training, and publish.

Figure 15.2 is one model of an organizational system that is adapted from

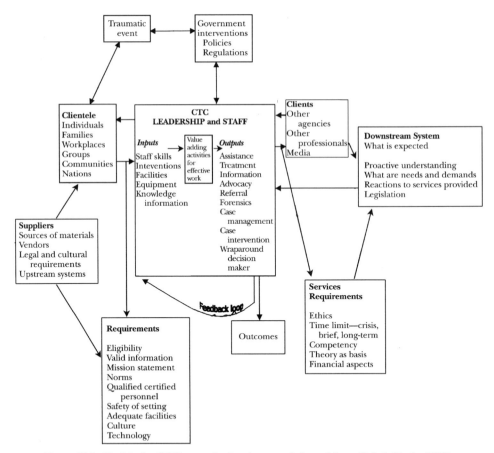

Figure 15.2. Model of a CTC's organizational system (adapted from Sink & Tuttle, 1989).

Sink and Tuttle (1989, p. 167). This model is a fairly comprehensive way to look at "generic work" of a CTC that includes the various components of input (clients, demands from the traumatic event, requirements for service provision, policies), the role of leadership and staff , and the outputs (with accompanying feedback). However, this diagram does not look at the specific "types of work" of a CTC. For that reason, another model that depicts how work gets done in a CTC is by Ivanevich & Matteson (1995, pp. 301, 308). This diagram is shown on page 16 of this volume. Still, this diagram also is not specific to a CTC.

The model for a CTC that we have created is based initially on a model designed by Kate Garay (TRIARC model) (Figure 15.3). She described it originally as a "thriving beyond trauma" model that included a variety of professional activities. But systems and events impact all of these activities.

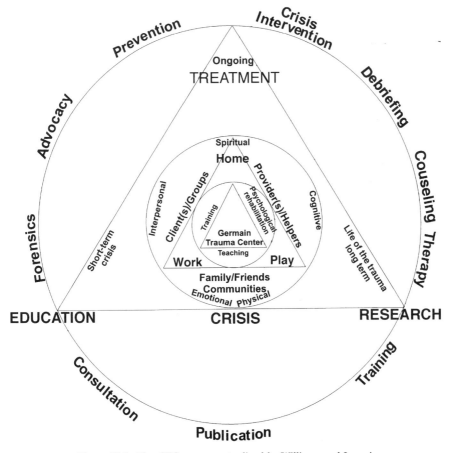

Figure 15.3. The CTC as conceptualized by Williams and Lurmi.

Within the inner circle of the model are the three major areas of healing: cognitive, emotional, and physical. The cognitive and emotional components form the psychological segment of the biopsychosocial model and the behavioral area mentioned is the social area. Even if a traumatic event appears to impact on the psychological aspects of self, it also impacts the body and ultimately the survivor's relationships and interpersonal activities. This model was originally designed to describe intervention within the context of a hospital setting; however, we have expanded it to apply to all settings and all types of interventions (Kate Garay, personal e-mail communication, 8/15/96).

One additional model needs to be considered, and that is the global model for counseling centers developed by Pace et al. (1996) (see page 6 in this volume). The model developed in their article looks at targets of intervention ranging from individuals to institutions. We expand those targets to include nations, for example, in the case of a major disaster that impacts an entire country. We also expand their threefold purposes (remediation, prevention, development) to four: remediation, prevention, development of theory, and development of strategies and techniques. Finally, we expand their methods of intervention from three to four: debriefing/defusing/crisis intervention, direct service, consultation/training, and research. This cube is a more complex way to envision the functions of a trauma center than are some linear models.

In our final version of the model, we have an overlay page which looks at the contexts of the CTC (Fig. 15.4). This overlay is like a flower. The stem is the core processes of the center which undergo change and growth. The five petals include theory, culture, organizational dynamics, and processes of technology, stakeholders, and traumatic events. They are what drives the service delivery of the center.

The authors suggest that centers take a collaborative approach to determine the needs for various interventions, involving client groups needs and expectations, with the allocation of resources made on the basis of those expressed needs. Thus service provision would be flexible and accommodating. The center also takes on consulting and training role and a research role. This model is quite similar in content to what we envision as functions of an ideal trauma center.

RIGHTS TO SERVICE

Whatever the structure, though, it is important to remember that mental health services of the CTC are provided within a consumer-rights-based world. Each client of the CTC is entitled to competent trauma treatment and intervention from skilled individuals. As Haas and Malouf (1996) reported, competence includes both declarative expertise (knowing the "what" of trauma treatment) and procedural expertise (knowing the "how" of trauma treatment). They continue that credentials are not a guarantee of compe-

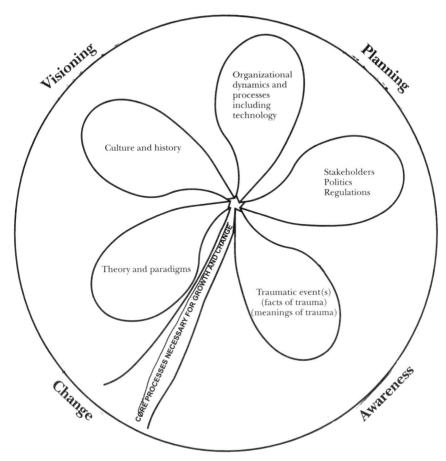

Figure 15.4. The context of a CTC (Williams, 2000).

tence. A competent practitioner recognizes personal limitations as well as strengths; has appropriate education and training; is willing to have his or her work examined by peers, acknowledges error when appropriate, and consistently seeks to "deepen ... clinical craftsmanship" (p. 22).

The relationship between client and therapist/counselor/case manager is service oriented in the way it defines roles, responsibilities, duties, and limitations of all participants (Woody, 1988). However, it does not discount the role of intuition in practice and decision making. Intuitive decision making has four stages: (1) preparation: getting ready to be creative; (2) incubation: letting the subconscious do the work; (3) illumination: waking up in the middle of the night and shouting "I know what to do; I've got it"; and (4) verification: working it out in a linear fashion (Rowan, 1986, p. 33).

Rowan (1986) also describes the most likely paths to intuitive decision making:

1. Keep the problem continuously in mind.
2. Redefine it frequently.
3. Consider a number of alternatives simultaneously.
4. Maintain a childlike view that is unsophisticated.
5. Rely on nonverbal imagery while pursuing trial-and-error thinking.
6. Distinguish between real and imagined obstacles.
7. Use a zigzag or obscure route when needed to reach the objective.
8. Expect setbacks; the road is generally slippery.
9. The key element is timing and knowing when to act.

PERSONNEL ISSUES IN THE CTC

Any personnel of a CTC must be committed to caring for traumatized individuals, families, groups, communities, and/or nations. Therefore, personnel in a comprehensive trauma center need to have had experience with trauma that includes professional education, training, and (probably) self-taught knowledge beyond that gained in a professional program. At least a majority of professional persons on staff need to be licensed with corresponding accountability and credibility. Ideally, all professional staff members also are certified as Certified Trauma Specialists or Certified Trauma Responders through the Association of Traumatic Stress Specialists.

Staffing of the CTC is a major focus for all concerned. At least one licensed professional is on staff and all are certified. Ideally, all are licensed as well. Staff members include forensic specialists, body workers, psychologists, psychiatrists, clinical social workers, and others. Ideally a psychiatrist is on staff or is at least available for referral; he or she knows the biochemistry of trauma. If the center does not have a physician on staff, it is important to educate local physicians about medications and management of traumatized patients. Center staff needs to be aware of medications that are suitable for trauma survivors as well as the side effects of those medications.

Total team triage is important if the center is to provide optimal services to clients. This process uses the person best suited to serve a client as the lead in treatment provision. That person is the one best suited to work with a particular trauma (e.g., hostages, torture survivors, rape victims), a particular gender or ethnic group, or a particular culture. If the center works with various nationalities and language groups, it is important to have staff who can serve as representative mirrors of that cultural group as well.

Many centers have a dynamic leader who is well known in the field of trauma. For example, Colin Ross is medical director, creator, and owner of his institute, as are Laurie Pearlman, Mary Harvey, Larry Bergmann, John Wilson, and others. The majority of his clinical staff are licensed and certified by their specific boards. Larger centers have their own psychiatrists and employ a variety of professionals from differing specialties and educational backgrounds. These individuals ideally work together as a team and are given ample opportunities for self-care through case conferences, staff meetings, supervision, retreats, and other activities designed to help mitigate compassion fatigue and vicarious traumatization. Staff members ideally do not work in isolation. As Pearlman notes at TSI/CAAP, a major goal is to build a community of professionals within the workplace. With this goal in mind, it is important to recruit staff members who fit the goals of the specific center and are able to work together efficiently and cooperatively with commitment.

The Team in the CTC

The key to successful service provision in the CTC is the team. Mink et al. (1993b) define a team as "a group of people who coordinate their efforts to achieve a goal they perceive to be important to the members of the team" (p. 99). As Guns (1996) writes, the "essence of a team is its members/interdependence. Each team member needs the others to get the work done ... interdependence builds collaboration" (p. 58). Hall and Hord (1986) discuss the characteristics of effective team operation. They include:

- Continuous, informal contact with other team members
- Complementarity of roles among team members
- A shared common view of the goals of the center
- Open, ongoing planning
- Professional collegiality
- Sharing of knowledge and competencies

In order for the team(s) within an ideal CTC to function in the most optimal manner, the following requirements must be met:

- Team members work together harmoniously.
- Each team member functions at his or her highest level.
- The team assesses its progress regularly through feedback.
- The team solves problems in a productive manner, using the feedback that is given.
- The team makes adjustments in operating procedures as needed (Mink, Esterhuysen, Mink, Owen, 1993a, p. 133).

Mink et al. (1993a) add to that list the following norms of effective teamwork:

- Trust occupies a central role in team behaviors and activities.
- Team members accept each other's uniqueness as a strength.
- Team members can let go of past events and focus on the present.

Team members also must have three different kinds of trust: self-disclosure trust (mutual sharing), contract trust (making and keeping agreements), and safety trust (read each other's intentions). In the ideal trauma center, work gets done efficiently, within the existing power structure.

The Use of Volunteers: A Personnel Issue

A major consideration for the leadership and staff of a CTC is whether or not volunteers have a place in the service delivery system. If volunteers are part of the structure, these individuals need to be recruited to fit into specific "slots" in the CTC. Volunteers, as well as paid staff, sign contracts as to hours to be worked, duties, and benefits received. The contract designates the individual(s) responsible for overseeing volunteer programming, provides a written job description, sets training requirements and standards, includes a method of evaluation, deals with insurance issues, and specifies volunteer responsibilities (e.g., maintenance of confidentiality, ethical practice, limits of job duties).

Volunteers are able to fill many roles in the day-to-day work of a trauma center. They may be used to market services, to corroborate the need for services, or to build bridges with other service organizations and populations. Volunteers also may function as peer counselors, as is the practice in the BNMO. They may take an active role in fund-raising for the CTC, may have direct service provision duties, particularly in case management, may perform crisis interventions or staff the hotlines (when trained), and may be included in all training events offered to paid staff members.

If the CTC is to utilize lay caregivers and volunteers, specific policies about liability and confidentiality need to be determined concerning their responsibilities and liabilities. In addition, these individuals need to be given extensive training.

Preventing Compassion Fatigue: Issues of Self Care

Staff members participate in regularly scheduled supervision (weekly), in-service presentations (monthly), and debriefing sessions (as needed). They take responsibility for professional and personal growth and have been warned of the inevitability of compassion fatigue and vicarious traumatization. Therefore the management and leadership of the CTC is committed to the prevention of compassion fatigue and proactively work to lessen its impact through internal, day-long retreats, external retreats at a retreat center on a biannual basis, social activities, and provision of membership in a local exercise facility for all staff members.

Staff retreats can help to create a mood of positive change within a CTC. A successful staff retreat begins with the involvement of staff members. With a high degree of staff involvement, nothing at a retreat is a surprise or shock (Richards, 1998). Retreats can provide everyone who works in the CTC with an opportunity to examine what works, what does not work, and how to improve the latter.

Successful retreats have an agenda that is planned and is mutually supported by leadership and staff, as well as volunteers if they are included. A successful retreat focuses on only a few items, including review of the CTC's mission, innovative visioning for the future, and determining how to monitor progress. The retreat is held at a location that is creative, comfortable, and private.

The successful retreat begins with a meeting that reviews and adopts the mission of the CTC. The meeting sets the tone of the retreat, establishes ground rules, and stimulates collegiality. Another function of the retreat is to clarify responsibilities and set new directions for the CTC. The retreat concludes with an evaluation of the progress of the CTC toward meetings its goals, as well as an evaluation of the retreat itself.

Staff members function as a team and consult regularly with each other and network with persons outside the CTC whenever indicated. They have common values regarding intervention with victims of trauma as well as expertise in the field. They understand and respect each other's professional training, perspective, values, knowledge, roles, and expertise while articulating their own roles, expertise, values, knowledge, and perspective. They design service plans and procedures that support collaboration and teamwork. Team-building activities are built into meetings, retreats, staffings, and trainings. These activities are designed to develop respectful communication strategies, emphasize team goals, encourage interaction and interdependence of staff members, and recognize the need for flexibility (Quick, Quick, Nelson, & Hurrell, 1997).

Additional training to combat compassion fatigue and vicarious traumatization also is important to develop and utilize regularly. Perhaps one such way is to provide all staff free memberships in a local gym as a "perk." Another way is to have a staff support group. Requiring ongoing education is a third.

It is important that the norms of the center legitimize self-care and combating compassion fatigue/vicarious traumatization. As Catherall (1999) notes, norms clearly supported by leadership and management accept the existence of compassion fatigue as real and legitimate, treat that condition within a systems context, seek solutions to problems of compassion fatigue without assigning blame to personnel, and encourage open communication among staff members. The ideal center has norms, which are extremely tolerant of individual innovation and creativity, role flexibility, and an environment that tries to catch staff members "doing something right" (p. 85).

Practice Style of Personnel

Any staff member who works within the CTC needs to have a style of practice that exudes safety. What are some of the components of that style? The ideal therapist/counselor/caregiver is empathic and reflective; nonjudgmental, genuine and "real"; congruent in affect and behavior; respectful of the client's capacity to heal and grow; able to use appropriate self-disclosure; and warm. The caregiver uses appropriate timing and pacing of interventions; these interventions include gentle "pushes" when needed and confrontations when appropriate. The competent caregiver is present with the client, follows through on promises, respects boundaries, and is committed to the job she or he is doing. The caregiver expects to be tested and is able to admit mistakes. That individual accepts a client's perceptions as that individual's personal reality, a reality that is real to the individual. Ethical values guide the work of that individual as he or she enters into a collaborative relationship that views the client as capable and competent.

The caregiver who works in a CTC helps to create a "trauma membrane" that is a buffer for clients' overwhelmed egos. The therapist/caregiver functions as a role model, nurturer, mentor, liaison with various systems and agencies, challenger of inappropriate/ineffectual beliefs, teacher, comforter, listener, mediator, and confidant, among others. The caregiver also recognizes the sources of his or her personal and institutional/organizational power in working with trauma survivors. Some of that power is assigned by society to a mental health professional, no matter her or his licensure or the "letters" after his or her name. Some of that power is assigned by virtue of the caregiver's knowledge and expertise. Other power comes from the persona/self of the caregiver (Markowitz, 1992).

Ideally, any staff member of a CTC is a self-identified helping person. What makes an individual a true helping person? A helping person is a growing, living, becoming individual who is creative, expressive, and able to search for alternative ways to define a problem, and once the problem is defined is able to help the trauma survivor identify new, alternative ways to attempt to solve it The helping person is open to life's experiences, holds a wealth of knowledge, and has a curiosity that is never satisfied.

In a report to the state of Maine (Jennings & Ralph, 1997) by 127 survivors of trauma and 122 professionals who responded to a needs assessment conducted by the Department of Mental Health Mental Retardation and Substance Abuse Services Office of Trauma Services looking at what is needed to ensure safety in the relationship between client and professional, survivors noted that it is of the utmost importance for the therapist to establish a relationship and some level of trust before asking questions about the trauma.

LEADERSHIP AND MANAGEMENT

In the ideal trauma center, leadership/management is collaborative and team based. Leaders turn to the real trauma experts, the victims and survivors, to help in decision making as to service provision needs. Programming also is team based in order to lessen staff polarization. The ideal CTC has a leadership and management staff dedicated to individual and organizational health (Budman & Steinbarger, 1997) As Quick et al. (1997) noted, the health organization is adaptable, flexible, and productive. The healthy CTC adjusts activities to enable its people, structure, technology, and tasks to work in harmony through an active process of planned change.

An ideal leader in an ideal CTC "walks the walk and talks the talk" of the center's mission statement: Allegiance to the mission is something the leader preaches, teaches, and loves. The leader has vision for the future and designs that vision to fit with cultural values and expectations and with the mission and goals of the center. The leader has a good understanding of how things get done and designs an appropriate structure and teams to fit that structure. The leader also is aware of how the CTC fits within larger systems and environments as well as within the day-to-day life of those it serves (Jamieson, 1996).

The leader works with others to develop a marketing plan that takes into account the position of the CTC in the environments in which it exists. The leader recognizes the needs of target communities and helps the organization develop strategies to address those needs. This situational assessment leads to the recruitment of appropriate staff and also looks at the role of competition. The leader also is aware of how the public perceives the CTC. She or he then helps to design strategies to project a specific public image and message that builds referrals and develops professional relationships with therapists, hospitals, managed care groups, governments, and others.

Leadership/management equals decision making. No one decision-making style is appropriate in all situations; the ideal leader is flexible and changes style to fit the situation. The main focus is the problem to be solved and the situation in which that problem occurs (Ivanevich & Matteson, 1995). The ideal leader is trustworthy and builds trust within the organization. That trust develops because the leader is competent and honorable She or he has integrity, speaks truthfully, makes commitments and keeps them. The ideal leader is enthusiastic, dedicated to the work of the CTC, and perseveres to meet goals. He or she also is able to make decisions and follow those decisions with action plans. The ideal leader knows his or her organization well, both formally and informally, and supports the strengths of others. She or he keeps no secrets, has no hidden agendas, and hires persons who have more skills than him- or herself (Cox & Hoover, 1992). Cox and Hoover (1992) describe these strengths of the ideal leader:

1. He or she builds affection by gaining knowledge and respect and by caring for her or his staff, clientele, and the work process itself.
2. He or she attracts allegiance by having a vision that is communicated to others and draws on the vision of those others; that vision stimulates the imagination of and includes the dreams of staff members.
3. He or she develops purpose and meaning through communication of the vision.

4. He or she builds trust by positioning her- or himself in a collaborative
   position with others to carry out the vision while surrendering self to
   the strengths of others.
5. He or she generates confidence by accepting responsibility for failure
   and giving others recognition for success.
6. He or she promotes growth and improvement within the CTC by
   dedicating self to a healthy passion for learning as an individual and as
   an organization.

The ideal leader also is a successful coach who supports and encourages trust within the workplace (Mink et al., 1993b). The effective leader/coach has a guiding vision for the CTC and shares that vision with all team members in a passioned manner. The ideal leader knows self and the environment/context in which the CTC operates. This leader understands the vision of the CTC and has an overall sense of purpose. Ideal leaders trust themselves and operate from their own intuition. These leaders are able to get others to trust them by being constant in purpose and intention, open to sharing facts and feelings, competent, and having integrity.

The style that a leader uses depends on a variety of things. Among them are the value system of the leader, the definition of the leader's job, the confidence that the staff has in that leader, the leader's need for certainty or ability to tolerate uncertainty, the habitual style of the leader, and the personal contribution that the leader has made and is making to the organization (Vroom, 1964).

Leadership also is communication that is designed to bring about results (Ritti & Funkhouser, 1987). A strong leader has healthy self-regard and the ability to convince others to follow certain courses of action in order to make a decision work. Schein (1985) notes that the essential function of leadership is the manipulation of culture.

The ideal leader gets the attention of the followers of a CTC (whether present or potential) through visioning and providing meaning for the vision through communication incorporating ideas of empowerment, intimacy, liberation, and enabling. Followers, that is, staff members, claim the vision of the leader(s) as their own. The leader draws out that vision from everyone in the employ of the CTC or who volunteers services. The leader also builds trust by positioning self and the CTC in a way that enhances reaching the vision. The ideal leader gains staff members:

- Attention through visioning
- Meaning through communicating
- Trust through positioning
- Confidence through healthy understanding of success and failure (Bennis & Nanus, 1985)

She or he discovers, builds on, utilizes, and integrates the strengths of those others into work performance The leader shares power with followers as a steward, giving staff members freedom, resources, and support to make decisions and take action within the policies, limits, procedures and realities of the CTC. Thus the ideal leader:

- Builds affection, gains knowledge, and gains respect
- Attracts allegiance through visioning and listens to the dreams of team members
- Develops purpose and meaning
- Communicates his or her vision and the mission of the center
- Generates confidence and accepts responsibility for success and for failure
- Builds an environment of safety
- Promotes trust

The leader of a CTC may be a solitary individual who contracts with other professionals, supervises them, trains them, and then refers clients to them for a certain percentage of fees earned (e.g., Gaston, Traumatys). Leadership may rest with a group of persons who have expert power (based on special knowledge, skill, expertise) and legitimate power (the staff of TSI). To a degree, then, needed qualities, characteristics, and skills required in/of the leader(s) are determined, to a large degree, by the demands of the organization itself and the situation in which the center functions (Fiedler, 1967; Hale, & Hyde, 1994; Hall & Herd, 1986; Hersey & Blanchard, 1978; Hogan, Curphy & Hogan, 1994). Thus, leadership may be situational, dependent on the multifaceted nature of the CTC itself and the environments in which it functions (Walsh & Donovan, 1990). The most successful leaders, according to Hallam and Campbell (1992), communicate clear mission and sense of purpose for the CTC, identify available resources and talent within the personnel of the CTC and volunteers, develop that talent, plan and organize the interventions/activities of the CTC, coordinate work activities, and obtain extra resources when needed. They build teams and resolve conflicts among team members when they occur.

According to Kurstedt (1997), there are certain characteristics most people associate with "leader" and "leadership." A leader has consistent and dependable integrity and a high standard of personal ethics. A leader is patient and has courage. A leader is a change master, a catalyst, and a transformer (p. 1424); a facilitator, enabler, and agent of change, "obsessed with the mission and vision of the organization," and goal oriented (p. 1424). The leader is competent and knows the work and the workplace intimately and:

- Focuses on the importance of good communication
- Has high ethical standards
- Has a high level of energy
- Reframes issues
- Develops backup contingencies

- Is patient
- Has a true sense of inner security
- Takes risks and sticks with a risk until a result occurs
- Learns from failures and is humble about success
- Is committed to hard work
- Is appropriately intimate with staff, clients, and environments
- Surrenders self to the strengths of others
- Has imagination and creativity and uses them creatively, sometimes unorthodoxly
- Has a desire to help others grow and succeed (p. 1426)

Mink et al. (1993a) believe that one of the most important characteristics of a leader is trust. Trust includes competence, intentions, reliability, and honest disclosure. As a change agent, leaders have a variety of knowledge competencies (trauma theory, administrative knowledge, training strategies, change processes, self-knowledge), skill competencies (listening, teaching, counseling, coaching, diagnosing), and attitude competencies (maturity, open-mindedness, humanism) (Lippitt, 1982).

MANAGEMENT IN THE CTC

Leadership is not generally the same as management. However, depending on the size and diversification of staff in the CTC, it may not be possible to employ a business manager or staff manager to oversee the "business" of the CTC. In many ways, a leader is a manager. Gardner (1994) notes that there are five aspects of leadership that might be considered as managing:

1. Planning and priority setting
2. Organizing and institution building
3. Keeping the CTC system functioning
4. Agenda setting and decision making
5. Exercising political judgment

If it is possible, a CTC needs to have a business manager to oversee the operational aspects of the day-to-day "workings" of the center. This individual would be in charge of the technological aspects of the center, as well as financial and budgetary aspects.

The strategy that seems to be best suited to a CTC is total quality management (TQM). The major aspects of TQM, according to Swiss (1992), are the following:

- The survivor group (individual, community) ultimately determines the quality of work provided.
- Services are given in an error-free environment.
- All staff members work toward improving the quality of service-delivery.

- Service inputs, processes, and outputs are continuously improved.
- The culture of the CTC shows commitment to quality improvement.
- TQM relies on process management, survivor feedback, performance measurement, teamwork, and decision making that is data driven.

ETHICAL PRACTICE IN A CTC

The ethical codes and principles to which the caregivers adhere guide any work done within a CTC. These codes may be part of professional licensure (e.g., as a social worker or psychologist) or as a certified trauma responder [e.g., as a member of the Association of Traumatic Stress Specialists (ATSS)]. Professional codes of ethics and the specific ATSS code that relates to work with trauma victims help to stabilize practice so that professional efforts are less likely to be undermined.

Values lie at the foundation of ethical practice. Values to which ethical trauma practitioners ascribe include:

- Persons working in a CTC belong to an organization that cares for people within that organization and within the clientele of that organization.
- The CTC seeks to do no harm (nonmalficience).
- The CTC seeks to promote human welfare and acts to benefit others (beneficence).
- The CTC provides fair and equal treatment and/or services (justice).
- The CTC fulfills commitments and keeps promises; it is faithful to the client (fidelity).
- The CTC staff strives to model empathic, engaged, responsive interaction with a high degree of professionalism.
- The CTC staff engages in acts intended to assist in the normative healing processes of trauma recovery through multiple levels of interaction.
- The CTC staff is sensitive to and respectful in interventions with persons, families, groups, communities, and nations who have experienced trauma.
- The CTC staff acknowledges that human beings as individuals or in families, groups, communities, or nations can be overwhelmed by traumatic events and may display acute and/or traumatic stress responses.
- The CTC serves people as ends, not means.
- The CTC staff shares power with clients.
- The CTC staff respects autonomy of the client(s).
- The CTC provides information about or direct access to scarce resources.
- The CTC provides clients with flexible choice making.

- The CTC promotes the common good.
- The CTC staff is truthful (veracity).

General ethical standards recognize that the primary obligation of all persons working under the auspices of a CTC is the physical, emotional, and spiritual safety of the client/patient (whether individual, group, family, community, workplace, organization, nation). If safety does not exist, no beneficial services can be provided by the CTC and no healing will occur.

Staff has the ethical responsibility to assume an advocacy role with these client groups. Corresponding interventions may include taking action to obtain informed consent, maintaining confidentiality, and avoiding actions that might retraumatize, to the greatest extent possible, within the limits of the law.

The CTC, as a client-centered organization, holds the welfare of the client paramount. Each staff member acts in a manner that upholds the honor, integrity, future promise, and potential of his or her personal profession, sharing expertise when indicated. Thus, each staff member functions *only* in those areas of practice, research, training, and/or assessment in which she or he is proficient, competent, and qualified, whether by license, certification, education/training, and/or experience. All actions taken by any staff member, at whatever level of interaction with a client or client group, are designed to contribute to the normative healing process of trauma recovery. Each staff member is responsible for follow-through in order to deliver services in an ethical manner. If services cannot be delivered as they have been promised or contracted, then it is the responsibility of that staff person to advise the client and modify interventions accordingly or provide alternative services. Staff members must place the needs of the clients above themselves.

In addition, staff members seek to be culturally sensitive, operating within the cultural norms of the population(s) they are serving, to the fullest extent possible. Each staff member is accountable for identifying and maintaining a heightened awareness of personal ethnic, gender, sexual, religious, or spiritual biases, so that the staff member does not compromise the performance of providing care to trauma survivors in any venue.

Staff members also have the ethical obligation to share information and knowledge about trauma and its impact with victims, colleagues, organizations, communities, and nations in order to promote healing. When staff members conduct research about trauma and its impact, that research takes place only when safety of respondents is assured to the highest degree possible. Research that compromises the well-being of a client group is in violation of those ethical responsibilities. Staff members also are obligated to protect and be accountable to any client group that becomes research subjects. Each staff member also has the ethical responsibility to obtain education on a continuing basis, working toward the advancement of his or her profession.

A very important ethical component of trauma work for staff members of a CTC deals with staff member self-care. Staff members have the ethical responsibility to self-monitor their capacities to do the work of trauma recovery, research, training, and/or assessment. Staff members are made aware of the impact(s) of secondary trauma on themselves and their colleagues through appropriate training, supervision, and consultation. While leadership of the CTC (through supervisors, managers, and others) is responsible to ensure that vicarious traumatization is identified and addressed, staff members also have the ethical responsible to monitor each other's performance, in a helpful, non-judgmental way, ensuring awareness of each other's need for self-care. (These ethical principles are adapted from the Code of Ethics of the ATSS).

SERVICE PROVISION IN THE CTC

An ideal CTC offers a broad range of tightly integrated services. Service provision is well coordinated and there are formal, written guidelines for triage and treatment planning as informal but well-known ways of "getting things done." Ideally, these services are provided under the unifying perspective and model of trauma. Trauma theory and practice guide clinical decision making, program development, and service provision.

Service Provision to Whom

But exactly who are the clientele of a CTC? There is no one answer to this question. The clientele of a center varies. Clients are traumatized; the type of trauma experienced determines the type of client. If two local families involved in a major automobile accident, clients would be survivors, witnesses, rescue workers, hospital staff, and/or others. If, was there a major flood after a hurricane, entire communities could become clients.

The client groups served by the various trauma centers interviewed also varied widely. Clientele in the Homewood Hospital Program generally were in their 30s and 40s and were 80% female; most had chronic PTSD (approximately 90%) and comorbid diagnoses ranging from major depression to dissociative and mood disorders, among others. About 50% of Stanley Street Treatment and Resources' clientele were male and many of them were substance abusers. Clients entering the Sanctuary program were admitted to treat acute symptoms that require hospitalization as intervention. Many of the primary victims served are abuse victims or domestic violence victims. The large majority (65%) of clients are chronic in their symptomatology, distant from the original traumas. The Northeast Center also treats a majority of clients who have experienced sexual, physical, and/or emotional trauma.

Many of the centers have veterans as their primary client populations (BNMO, Vet Centers, Porter, COPIN); others, primarily deal with sexual abuse survivors (Becker, Turner, Lubin, Ross, Yuksel in Turkey) as well as survivors of assault, crimes of violence, and state violence (Turner, RCT, Switzerland,

ITRI, South Africa, among others). Many clients in a number of centers exhibit symptoms of complex PTSD (Turner, the Center, Harvey). Only a few centers primarily treat children and their families/caretakers. Centers who treat Holocaust survivors generally do not do work with acute stress (Danieli, AMCHA) and many survivors have comorbid disorders of depression, anxiety disorder, and personality disorders. This is due primarily to the advanced age of many of these survivors. Elderly survivors (average age 65) are also the clientele treated by the center in Poland: survivors of political persecution during the Stalin period.

Some of the centers deal with clients with work-related issues (Blythe, Posen, Reinecke) or clients who are referred by EAPs (Bergmann). Moore describes the clientele served in his center most aptly by stating that they "represent the demographics of the geographic area."

One aspect of service provision may focus on facilitation of social functioning through provision of psychosocial support. This level of intervention is designed to strengthen the coping mechanisms of trauma survivors, to facilitate access to social opportunities and networks, provide support while survivors regain control over their lives, and to some degree recreate a social network through the CTC. Supportive psychotherapy often focuses on problem solving, learning social skills, and advocacy.

Other services may focus on grief and resolution of loss. In this aspect of the service provision system, survivors receive comfort, protection, and consoling. They are encouraged to share their experiences and feelings, recognize and accept their suffering and pain, and link with others who have similar levels of suffering and grief.

Competency Building

Competency building is a central feature of treatment in a CTC. Competency-based treatment techniques are oriented toward skill development and improvement of the quality of life of trauma survivors (Hunter, 1995). Hunter and Marsh (1994) noted common competency-based psychological interventions include empowering clients, teaching clients about trauma and its consequences, identifying strengths as well as deficits in skills, teaching of new skills, modeling adaptive behavior, and integrating interventions that are psychological, psychosocial, interpersonal, educational, rehabilitative, biological, and even spiritual with social issues related to housing, transportation, employment, medical care, social support, and income (Hunter & Marsh, 1994). According to Berg (1994), three rules govern competency based, solution oriented treatment:

1. If it ain't broke, don't fix it.
2. Once you know what works, do more of it.
3. If it doesn't work, don't do it again; do something else.

More about Service Provision

In this ideal world, the psychological treatment that the CTC provides is flexible, not always brief, operates from a perspective of strengths of the clients, and utilizes a developmental perspective. Clients are triaged to appropriate service providers who respond to individual (group, team, family, community) needs using a continuum of care and culturally relevant, appropriate interventions. Case management by treatment teams coordinates service provision and evaluates treatment compliance. Treatment is given promptly. The CTC also has links to other resources and service providers so that specialized interventions are available.

Availability is the first key to appropriate treatment provision. Services needed by survivors must be available to them. Second, these services must be accessible whether at the CTC itself or from satellite centers or mobile-based treatment units. Staff members in the field may seek out survivors, interview them, screen them for PTSD, refer them to the center or to more appropriate institutions, and work with local leaders to plan wider-based interventions. These interventions might include provision of debriefing sessions, assessment of health and treatment needs, provision of medication, and supervision of other field workers. Third, the services must be adaptable to fit the circumstances, culture, and survivor groups. Fourth, the services must be appropriate to the groups who need them.

If treatment is based on the value of empowerment and views the client (in general) as competent enough to make choices within a collaborative relationship that constitutes a joint venture between center staff and client(s), then the client helps to set goals and helps the therapist select appropriate treatment procedures and options. The client recognizes that she or he needs help to solve problems and seeks out that help from various staff members.

COMPREHENSIVE SERVICE

To be comprehensive, services offered by the CTC range from prevention to provision of emergency aid and on-site crisis intervention, to availability of a 24-hour hotline, to short-term counseling, to long-term intervention. The center provides referrals to other agencies, organizations, and individuals when staff members recognize that the center cannot provide the type of service needed.

As a subspecialty, the CTC may have protocols in place to intervene when there are traumatic workplace incidents. Perhaps the CTC contracts with an organization to develop critical incident stress management interventions, in a preventive fashion. Should an incident occur, then the organization/ workplace is ready to provide competent response and service. The CTC may train managers, supervisors, union officers, CEOs, employment representatives, and others on workplace violence and help these individuals develop policies and procedures as well as crisis response plans. CTC staff members may educate organizational leaders and staff about domestic violence, terrorism, or crime impacts and responses.

Some individuals within a CTC must be trained to work with media. These individuals may lead forums for journalists about ethical reporting, including ways to respect victims and protect their identities. These individuals may help to develop debriefing protocols for journalists, as well, and may be the media spokespersons when a traumatic event occurs (Office for Victims of Crime, 1998).

Center staff members may use additional techniques to help clients. The staff member may choose to normalize any acute or posttraumatic stress reactions the client is having. For example, the staff member may praise the client, even if that praise is for sitting in the session and not getting up to leave. The staff member may opt to make home visits. The staff member may use reframing to help the client see what has happened in a different light as a way to find meaning from the disaster or attack or other traumatic event. As Berg (1994) notes, "Reframing is ... usually a positive interpretation of ... behavior that gives a positive meaning ... and suggests a new and different way of behaving" (p. 174). Reframing a crisis as an opportunity to bring about some type of change is an example of this technique. A crisis event may provide an opportunity for learning about oneself or for trying out new ways of coping.

Thus, treatment may be conducted within a continuum of options ranging from crisis intervention to possibilities for respite are or retreat, from drop-in socialization groups to topic-focused or trauma-focused support groups to day treatment, and in some cases to residential care for crisis or long-term intervention. While this treatment takes place, a variety of alternative therapies including art therapy, sand tray work, exercise therapy, bodywork, music therapy, and others may be incorporated into the protocol.

The key to effective treatment is a healthy environment based on all the principles and techniques of safety that have been previously described. Treatment is coordinated among all team members and is individualized to fit the survivor (whatever the individual, group, family, nation, etc.) within that team context. As the Maine Trauma Advisory Group Report (Jennings & Ralph, 1997) noted, essential to recovery is:

- Stabilization and structure
- Consistent therapeutic intervention
- Collaboration among all treatment team members (and outside consultants or agencies)
- Well-trained, mature staff members who are caring, empathic, consistent, appropriate, expressive, accepting, self-revealing, and willing to care

PREVENTION

In an ideal world, the CTC has opportunity to conduct many prevention-oriented activities. According to the definition of prevention written by the Fairfax–Falls Church Community Services Board (1998), "Prevention is a proactive process that creates and reinforces conditions that promote healthy behaviors and lifestyles." Prevention-focused activities of the CTC attempt to help people acquire or enhance skills that increase resiliency and coping as well as those that reduce factors putting individuals, groups, communities, and nations at risk for acute stress reactions and posttraumatic stress reactions or disorder. Prevention helps these individuals and groups examine aspects of their emotional, social, physical, and spiritual lives and also works to improve conditions in the environment(s) of the center as a whole. The work of prevention falls into six strategies:

1. *Environmental:* This strategy looks at compliance issues and works to establish or change laws and norms, written and unwritten community standards, codes, attitudes, legal/regulatory initiatives, and service/action-oriented initiatives.
2. *Information dissemination:* Communication from the CTC to its many audiences about trauma, acute stress, coping, resilience, and other topics can occur through brochures, public service announcements, information clearinghouse activities, library facilities, resource directories, health fairs, and other activities.
3. *Education and training:* These are major functions of a CTC. Two-way communication and interaction take place in workshops, small group sessions, communication groups, training sessions, and others.
4. *Creation of alternatives:* These activities are designed to improve self-esteem, coping, and resilience and lessen the potential impact of traumatic events. Among activities held at a CTC are recreation programs, drop-in programs, workshops, community forums, trips, sports activities, and others.
5. *Problem identification and referral:* One important task of a center is to identify clients who are at high risk and assess how to help those individuals prior to the occurrence of a traumatic event. The center might conduct screenings for stress, depression, and need for services. The center might hold staffings, be the focal point for wraparound service planning, offer consultation, and/or conduct family/group/community interventions.
6. *Community-based process:* The final prevention effort of the CTC is one of enhancing a community's ability to provide appropriate treatment services when needed. The CTC serves as a focal point for the planning, organizing, collaborating on, and coalition building of necessary

networks and resources. The center itself can function as the catalyst for building these networks and also serve as the location for meetings of professionals, community leaders, interested citizens, groups, and others.

Therefore the preventive services offered by a CTC grow out of these six aspects of prevention. These services, too, are adapted from the Fairfax–Falls Church Community Services Board's (1998) plan.

1. Increase individual and family knowledge of healthy lifestyles, warning signs of stress, acute stress reactions, and posttraumatic stress reactions, and available resources through information dissemination and education and creation of new materials.
2. Provide education to increase problem-solving and decision-making skills and to promote attitudinal change through education.
3. Enhance services available to needed groups/communities/individuals considered to be at-risk through creation of alternative programs and activities.
4. Provide consultation, education, and information about trauma and all its aspects through problem identification and referral.
5. Increase community involvement and linkages to organizations, businesses, faith communities, and other community groups through service planning and processing and community-based process.
6. Develop awareness and knowledge of prevention programming with decision makers, officials, media, and the general public through media efforts, videos, service boards, and other activities.

ASSESSMENT

While gathering data for research usage is important and while the CTC has a mission to further knowledge, the process of data gathering is *not* paramount if it has a negative impact on persons being served. Safety and trust are more important issues to consider at intake than is gathering a mass of factual information. While it is important to obtain a comprehensive biopsychosocial history and personality assessment of trauma clients, immediacy in data collection is not always the best policy. For example, during periods of extreme crisis requiring immediate attention and intervention, obtaining a thorough history might not be possible, let alone feasible or practical. Still, professionals need to ask clients questions about trauma histories in a routine, standard manner that does not imply pathology or convey negative reactions.

As part of its protocol, the CTC can decide what types of instruments to administer and when. Perhaps sending home a packet of trauma-specific tests after several sessions is indicated. Asking trauma survivors to "tell their stories" is a way for them to take one step backward from themselves. This technique for data gathering may be indicated when a client is extremely retraumatized through revealing details as to what happened. In others instances, though, stepping back may be a distancing measure for both client and staff member.

If the center has video equipment, taping a life history interview that includes a client's traumatic experiences may be a valuable tool for data gathering and treatment planning. The client can be given this tape to watch later as a measure of progress or as a trigger for further exploration of what happened. Clients also may make trauma lifelines on freezer paper, a trauma "Torah" that can be unrolled to a specific time of life or event. On this lifeline, clients place pictures, words, phrases, and events related to their own traumas and the traumas they secondarily experienced through others.

Assessment recognizes and examines the biopsychosocial components of the individual. History taking must be comprehensive, looking at military history, abuse history, relationship history, and others. It is composed of both objective evaluation and subjective self-evaluation and recognizes that an individual's PTSD is person/phenomenologically driven.

Carlson (1994) recommends that the CTC take a systematic approach to assessment. Intake interviews always ask about the traumatic experiences of the interviewee. The questions use standardized formats with neutral wording and do not lead the respondent to particular answers. The assessment also includes self-report measures, structured interviews, standardized psychological tests, and physiological measures. All data-gathering results are presented in understandable language at the level appropriate to the client, taking cultural issues into consideration. The goal of assessment is to lead to the creation of an appropriate treatment plan. Data gathering also may lead to research studies that are by-products of therapeutic interventions.

Centers interviewed use a variety of assessment processes and protocols. SSTAR has a lengthy structured intake interview that includes a questionnaire to identify PTSD symptoms as well as other materials and a detailed history of trauma-related experiences. The assessment packet helps team members establish diagnoses and comorbid conditions. Sanctuary also uses a standard clinical interview coupled with trauma-based tools, scales, and measures. Some centers have computerized assessment programs to generate scores that can lead to diagnoses (Becker). Some use rating scales and structured questions initially, saving testing for a later time (Shalev). Tinnin administers a test battery that leads to the creation of a "trauma profile" and a subsequent individual treatment plan. Repeated assessments monitor progress (Tinnin, RCT, Ross, Ticehurst) and can be used to evaluate treatment outcome. Many of the instruments used by centers are the same: The Beck Depression Scale, Mississippi Civilian PTSD Scale, SCID, DES, IES, SCL-90, State–Trait Anxiety Scale, Harvard Trauma Questionnaire, and others.

TREATING TRAUMA SURVIVORS

Treatment in a CTC is not a static response but a flexible process that uses a variety of techniques, procedures, and strategies designed to fit the phenomenology of the client. Treatment is person driven, carefully selected, and fits the mission of the center. In other words, preferences of clients for specific types of treatments are taken into consideration when a treatment plan is developed. All treatment is based on principles of safety as well. The length and timing of sessions help to provide stability and safety when they are predictable and set ahead of time. Identifying and utilizing the therapeutic window (Cole & Barney, 1987) helps guide treatment. This window is the period of more moderate distress that exists between intrusive recollections of a trauma and periods of intense denial and avoidance. It is the zone during which work on resolution of the trauma occurs, the time period when that work is *not* blocked by escape mechanisms or immobilized through extreme intrusions, thoughts of or attempts at self-destruction, and hyperreactivity.

A major area of consideration is work of any type on memories of the traumatic event. Inherent in this process is the identification of a safe place for the client (in reality, preferably) as well as grounding methods (should state-dependent trance or escape behaviors/cognitions occur), and safe persons who might assist the client in times of extreme distress. Knowledge of a variety of memory-enhancing (flooding, in vivo exposure) and memory-controlling (EMDR, TFT, TIR) techniques by a variety of CTC caregivers is essential (Williams, 1994).

Treatment efficacy can be examined within a framework of remission of symptoms. How quickly are traumatic reactions resolved (speed)? Do the symptoms come back (durability) and to what degree? Does a specific treatment technique have side effects (is it tolerable) and are there positive expectations that derive from its utilization (acceptability)? What are the expected benefits from a specific intervention? How reliable is the outcome from that intervention?

Guidelines for treatment protocols need to be written by at least a team (subset) of staff members and then are distributed among all center staff for consideration and discussion with clients. They also are presented in case consultations and training sessions. These protocols also may be distributed to clients in written form (perhaps in a brochure).

Treatment of trauma is a stage-based process that must be timed and paced to fit within the client's ability levels. The aim of treatment is not to overwhelm or incapacitate the client; it includes establishing safety, teaching skills that mitigate retraumatization, education, and resolution of present crises. If a client is involved in a legal process or is having difficulties with memory-based issues, it is important that the therapist audiotape, videotape, or take process notes of the session.

Furthermore, treatment is conducted within a continuum of options ranging from crisis intervention to possibilities for respite care or retreat, from drop-in groups to support groups to day treatment. Treatment includes traditional models of intervention (individual therapy, family therapy, group therapy), as well as advocacy, consultation with agencies (e.g., schools, courts), mobile capacities, home visits and possibly home-based programs, referral, holistic methodology (bodywork, nutritional counseling, medication management), and more nontraditional models (TM, TIR, rewind, and others). Trauma work also includes art therapy, sand tray work, exercise therapy, music therapy, and others.

If possible, treatment interventions use a "strengths perspective" (de Jong & Miller, 1995), which recognizes that "all people and environments possess strengths ... (and can) improve" the quality of their lives (p. 729). Clients are more easily motivated when a strengths-based perspective is used and is consistently emphasized. Discovery of strengths rests on cooperative exploration and looks at survival, not at victim blaming. Strengths-based treatment rests on formulation of goals that are:

1. Important to the client
2. Small and achievable
3. Concrete, specific, behavioral so that progress is accessible
4. Based on beginnings not endings
5. Realistic in the context of the life of the client
6. Want something to be present rather than taking away something (de Jong, & Miller, 1995, pp. 729–730)

It also is important in this process to identify or reidentify the source(s) of meaning in a client's life (clients' lives). According to Ebersole (1998), among the most important sources of meaning are:

- Relationships and an interpersonal orientation (family, friends, spouse, love relationship, combination or the above)
- Service: a helping, giving orientation to people
- Beliefs, whether religious/spiritual and/or social/political
- Materialistic possessions
- Growth: self-improvement, self-understanding, reaching goals, developing talents
- Physical or mental health
- Life work from a job or occupation
- Pleasure, happiness, contentment, experiencing each day as fully as possible
- Psychological rewards of respect, success, prestige

One possible type of intervention with survivors is advocacy. As an advocate, a clinician helps the client change behaviors, attitudes, values, policies, and laws, as well as fight for him- or herself when in conflict with another agency or individual because of those factors. As an advocate, the therapist may help the client seek system change or program change. Advocacy, according to the National Organization for Victims Assistance (1993), is risk taking; it sends understandable messages, helps clients to explore options, and assists victims to act on choices and to change others' minds. The advocacy process is challenging, assertive, and adversarial. It involves taking action in a clear way with confidence and conviction using tact and timing.

Maxims for Providing Trauma Treatment

Fontaine and Hammond (1994) proposed 20 counseling maxims for beginning counselors. Some of these maxims are appropriate for treatment provision in the CTC. They have been modified to fit that setting and structure:

1. Trust yourself, your reactions, and your intuition but use the information you gain from your observations with care and tact; it may not be appropriate to share with the client (if the client is rude, unattractive, etc.).
2. Take a risk and try something new that might seem to fit; use an alternative technique or method.
3. Be open to all sources of information; actively challenge your impressions.
4. Self-monitor your own responses to a client, particularly any strong emotional responses you may have. Be aware of countertransference.
5. What is good for one client/group may not be good for another, even when each has experienced the same traumatic event (each has a different history, perception, meaning to and of the event).
6. When discussing the traumatic event(s) be concrete and get specifics about it, ask about the context of the traumatic event, and look for conceptual themes and patterns.
7. Pay attention to the structure of treatment: timing, pacing, openings to address issues, bridges between past/present, trauma and life experiences.
8. Share your perceptions of and insight about the trauma and the client with that person as feedback.

Looking at Services Provided by the Various Centers

Rather than describe the various aspects of service provision by name(s) of center(s), this section describes principles of treatment espoused by one or more treatment centers. These principles also can serve as general guidelines for the ideal center:

1. Treatment occurs within the context of the therapeutic milieu.
2. Psychoeducation is a vital tool of treatment.
3. Treatment is tailored to the needs of each individual client, whether a group, individual, organization, community, or family.
4. Treatment occurs in stages/phases. The first phase gathers informa-

tion, takes a trauma history, begins to establish an alliance, addresses avoidances, deals with retraumatizations. The second phase involves a detailed inner and outer world examination of the event and its meanings, addresses emotions, lessens and attempts to modify (if not eliminate) PTSD symptoms, helps the client accept the traumatized self, and integrates the trauma-based information. The third phase helps the survivor work on new defensive, cognitive, and behavioral patterns. The final phase helps the survivor move beyond the trauma to be a thriver, finding purpose, goal, and meanings for life.

5. The earliest stage of treatment establishes multimodal safety. The goal is to help the survivor(s) reestablish a sense of safety and predictability as they begin to improve biological, psychological, and social functioning.

6. Treatment also includes the provision of, or referral to, direct medical services.

7. A major focus of treatment is on the prevention of further traumatization.

8. The most frequent approach to treatment used by the centers is a cognitive–behavioral approach. Cognitive therapies help clients correct specific cognitive distortions.

9. Treatment looks at exploring the impact of trauma on past and present, skill building for stabilization self-support, and case management.

10. Experiential treatment modalities help clients develop awareness of self, recover traumatic memories, and work through emotions.

11. An essential component of treatment is provision of appropriate medication at limited to no cost.

12. Treatment needs to have a spiritual (and, at times religious) component that addresses healing through metaphor and ritual.

13. Treatment often includes construction of a time line or a narrative history that is taped, drawn, and/or otherwise formalized.

14. Treatment may be done within short-term or long-term models; however, brief therapy models try to treat trauma within a 6-session format), but are often unsuccessful.

15. The general goal of treatment is to help clients create physical, emotional, and relational safety within the here and now as well as challenge problematic behaviors that may be linked to past traumatic experiences and interfere with healthy living in the present.

16. Treatment includes advocacy work.

17. Treatment includes early crisis intervention when possible.

18. Treatment includes focused crisis therapy.

19. Treatment includes posttrauma therapy, when appropriate. This type of therapy helps clients understand and integrate traumatic memories. Treatment helps clients reappraise traumatic exposure through reexposure to the event and associated stimuli and reappraise meanings and emotional states associated with that trauma.

20. Treatment includes help for the helpers.
21. Treatment may utilize more "experimental" treatment methods including EMDR, TIR, TFT, Rewind, and others.
22. Treatment includes grief work and mind–body approaches.
23. Treatment for dually diagnosed clients includes appropriate interventions or referrals.
24. Transmission of hope is crucial in the treatment process.
25. An overall goal of treatment is to help survivors live lives in the present, rather than continuing to experience the present as an extension of the traumatic past.
26. Critical incident stress debriefing is not treatment.
27. Treatment must be culturally appropriate and fit the client's traditions, geography, and political situation. Central to recovery is a goodness-of-fit between the sociocultural–community context of trauma and selection and delivery of all trauma-related services.
28. Trauma treatment occurs within a biopsychosocial–spiritual–relational context.

CRISIS INTERVENTION

Crisis intervention is immediate, person-to-person assistance. The CTC needs to be a crisis-prepared organization. The central thrust of crisis intervention is engagement in a problem-solving process with the goal of developing a plan to alleviate specific problems through specific behaviors (France, 1996). The comprehensive trauma center ideally has 24-hour crisis availability for its clients, whether through beeper, phone contact, or mobile crisis unit. The phone number(s) must be available and well-advertised (Smith, 1985).

A center also is not immune to its own crises and has its own crisis intervention plan developed. In other words, the CTC has its own emergency management plan to prepare for, mitigate, respond to, and recover from a crisis event. Should the center be the victim of a hostage situation, a natural disaster, or a violent act toward staff or clientele, if center staff have predetermined roles for action, less damage may occur (Pauchant & Mitroff, 1992). This is a dynamic process, according to FEMA (1998), and includes planning, training, conducting drills, testing equipment and response protocols, and coordinating responses. This plan, kept in a manual and available for immediate access to all staff members, would include an evacuation plan, hazardous materials plan (in the case of a terrorist attack), risk management plan, and debriefing plan. The plan ideally is short enough and simple enough to be understood easily during the crisis and is tested periodically to see if it works.

Why is there a need for such a plan? A comprehensive trauma center is an at-risk facility: at risk for facility-based as well as community-based emergencies. These emergencies could be related to fire, severe weather, natural disaster, terrorism, location (proximity to other facilities or transportation routes that might have disasters), human error, or human response (a threat of violence or violent act by a disgruntled employee or client), among others. The emergency response plan of the CTC is designed to spell out how the center responds to any or all of these emergencies and determines action to be taken by staff members and clientele. This plan is submitted to staff members for review and revision and is not formalized until it can be adapted by all. Staff members need to be trained so that the plan becomes integrated within its operations and procedures (FEMA, 1998).

Should the entire staff of a CTC be traumatized, then it is essential to have identified individuals or groups who can come in to defuse and debrief center staff. These individuals may be from local Red Cross chapters, National Organization for Victims Assistance, or the American Psychological Association.

During a crisis, traditional approaches to delivering services may not be effective. The general population who has experienced a disaster may not be accustomed to using mental health services or may be resistant to coming to a center. Any staff members who are working with specific disasters or events need to visit the site or that disaster to see what people have experienced and to get a personal sense of what the situation is. Services need to be offered at numerous locations and times, including weekends and evenings and in schools, churches, community centers, synagogues, and others. Services also need to be given as early as possible after the event has occurred. When a disaster strikes, the center needs to make itself known to the public, to the governmental agencies, and to other trauma resources (Smith, 1985).

Task division in a crisis also is important. Does the leader of a CTC assume the role of service coordinator or is another staff member better suited to organize responses, troubleshoot, or problem solve? Identification of who makes up various teams and who offers various services is important. Who relates to the media? Who develops public service fliers, press releases, or helping brochures (or are they generally available in a standard format that can be modified)? Who organizes staff responses into crisis teams or connects with other community groups to organize crisis teams? Who designs the research and gathers research materials? Who begins to administer the materials? Who performs clerical tasks? Is there a need for more telephone responders, more persons with computer skills? The CTC should seek outside help if necessary. It is extremely important to keep the unique characteristics of the crisis in mind when answering all these questions: that is, the language and cultural needs of the target group(s), the impact on children, the location, and the impact on the larger community.

The Mobile Crisis Team

Does the CTC want to have a mobile crisis unit that could offer outreach services? If so, certain questions need to be answered. What level of staff availability is needed to have a team on call, around the clock, 24/7 coverage by beeper or phone, and for what types of emergencies? What types of services call in the mobile crisis team: debriefings or defusings, assessment, or triage? The event might be a serious accident, a natural disaster, a line of duty injury or death, or an organizational traumatic event. If the event is not within the scope of the team, team members must have resource information so they can then contact other agencies that are trained. These agencies also have been trained to know when to call in the mobile crisis team.

Zealberg, Santos, and Puckett (1996) noted that mobile crisis teams are a preferred method of response to communities of disaster victims needing emergency psychiatric care. These teams assess emergency mental health needs, do on-site evaluations, offer defusings and debriefings, and work within previously established disaster protocols and within designated lines of power. Members acknowledge and respect the authority of law enforcement, emergency medical services, fire and rescue, natural and local political groups, and mental health organizations, among others.

Disaster Intervention Services

A CTC offers disaster intervention services. The CTC is in an ideal position to coordinate the efforts/interventions of a variety of agencies. The center can serve as a hub for referral, advocacy, and service provision. Personnel can offer in-service trainings to a variety of agencies prior to the need for intervention services. The CTC offers phone consultation in time of disaster as well as walk-in and outreach services. Staff members of the CTC can go to areas that have been damaged and canvass neighborhoods to identify those in the greatest need. Staff members can help to organize support groups for discussion, ventilation, validation, debriefing, rumor control, and triage of services.

A major part of disaster intervention is to assess survivors' needs for referral, hospitalizations, stabilization, and services. A major aspect of assessment looks at the individual in terms of his or her thoughts (looking for confusion), perceptions (looking for sensory distortions and hallucinations), emotions (looking for severe reactions), behavior (looking for unusual and/or disturbing actions), and relationships (looking at sources of support). Referrals are made for food, clothes, housing medical care, emergency assistance, money, legal assistance, business relief, funeral arrangements, and others.

A large number of survivors may necessitate "24/7" availability of staff members. A major part of these services can be offered through around-the-clock telephone service by trained personnel, through consultation with walk-in clients, and through outreach. The latter services are best offered as a team. Outreach teams may have a need to carry weapons or have weapons at their disposal, carry educational materials and reference information, and must carry appropriate identification.

LESSONS FROM REFUGEE CENTERS

Kos and others (1998), in work with Bosnian refugees, recognize that the major goals of a center are to prevent new stressful and harmful influences; to normalize, organize, and structure the lives of those who have been traumatized so they can maintain independence, normal social functions, and human dignity; and to strengthen capacities to cope.

If a center must deal with large numbers of survivors and if that center has only limited resources, traditional clinical models of mental health service provision do not work. The most important services that can be offered become caring for material needs, raising funds, and advocating. Mental health providers must collaborate with primary health workers, teachers, volunteers, various groups who "show up" to help, shelter staffs, and governmental employees.

In this situation, one of the most efficient models of service provision is the mobile mental health team that goes out to where survivors live, are being temporarily housed, or go to school. This model does not separate mental health services from other service provision activities (health, education, social services) except if a group or individual needs intensive psychological intervention for PTSD. These visits include group meetings with survivors in their native language. Trauma workers reach out to the survivors rather than expect those survivors to come to the workers. It is extremely important that groups do not compete counterproductively to provide these services.

Kos et al. (1998) continue that the main objectives of treatment of trauma survivors are:

- To reduce suffering and prevent further traumatization
- To support and develop natural support systems
- To help establish an environment that enhances recovery and normalcy
- To establish structure and daily routines
- To support education of children
- To work toward reconstruction of the social world of the survivor
- To increase coping capacities
- To provide opportunities to avail oneself of therapeutic help
- To conduct population-oriented outreach activities
- To introduce an ecosocial mental health approach
- To combine individual work with social activities and advocacy so that victims/survivors are empowered and work as partners with mental health personnel
- To prevent the occurrence of long term psychosocial disorders, including PTSD
- To use concrete circumstances, needs, and characteristics of the survivor population as reference points for service design

- To consider the social and cultural context of service provision and use methods and techniques that are culturally appropriate and acceptable
- To form multidisciplinary teams of health-related, social, educational, and legal professionals
- To make all plans realistic and concrete as well as flexible
- To make sure information about all programs is widely dispersed to improve utilization
- To monitor and evaluate service delivery on a continuous basis
- To start fund raising efforts for relief efforts as soon as is possible
- To make sure those in charge of service delivery are educated in trauma and are given adequate training and support
- To conduct research only when indicated to be nontraumatizing and in an informed manner
- To inform authorities responsible for funds about needs and activities on a constant basis

CASE MANAGEMENT STRATEGIES

The focus of case management is provision of a continuum of care. Case management includes case finding, assessment, care or service planning, coordination, follow-up, and reassessment (Netting, 1992). Case management uses a holistic body–mind approach and requires extensive cooperation among CTC staff and community resources. Staff members of the CTC, as case managers, may act as service brokers, may arrange for services for clients and link them to services within local environment(s), as well as provide clinical care. The process of identifying, coordinating, and providing needed resources across the continuum of care, professional disciplines, and (perhaps) treatment locations (which may include home visits) is called "care mapping." The care map has collaboratively set, shared goals of practitioner(s) and client(s), addressing needs for support, treatment, and identification of environmental resources. Partnerships are developed as consensual relationships in response to the shared goals.

Case management is an ongoing process. According to Kier (1995), citing other case management authorities, the tasks of partnership building are alliance, accompaniment, agreement, action, and accessibility. Alliance building is the cornerstone of case management. Providing education and communicating effectively with clients are essential aspects of this task. Staff members have multiple contacts with the client(s) in order to gather information, conduct assessments, and gain an understanding of the trauma and its impacts.

Accompaniment is the coaching mechanism used by a case manager to assist the client(s) to negotiate services offered by a CTC, as well as services received within the community context. Accompaniment encourages the client(s) to use self-help and support groups, if available. Agreement is the task of identifying goals for treatment (as for training and research) and then achieving consensus on those goals. Action is the behaviorally oriented task that focuses on goal achievement by the client(s). Accessibility means that clients are given access to the services of the CTC, as well as to all therapeutic partners of the organization.

CTC-related decisions, from the case management perspective, determine what types of services are provided and by whom. Who does forensic work? Who is subpoenable? Who is privileged? Who works best with attorneys and knows most about legal requirements, as they impact confidentiality? Some services of the CTC may be offered at satellite centers throughout a country, community, or region. Case managers may play a plethora of roles, ranging from problem-solver, advocate (as one who identifies with the weaker side to stop inequalities), broker, planner, community organizer, boundary spanner, service monitor, record keeper, evaluator, consultant (who educates others to a higher level of understanding), collaborator, coordinator, counselor, and expediter (Netting, 1992). Other roles include facilitator (keeping communication open among various groups while promoting linkages and relationships), healer (supportive leader), mediator (looking at all interests and encouraging face-to-face dialogues), arbitrator (offering mutually acceptable authoritative decisions), buffer (separator), and penalizer (giving sanctions) (Chetkov-Yanoov, 1997).

Case management, proceeding from a strengths-based orientation, recognizes that some persons who have experienced trauma are wounded and others have experienced growth, are resilient, and are able to rebound after the event has occurred. The case management (and treatment) strategies, therefore, are based "on ideas of resilience, rebound, possibility, and transformation" (Saleebey, 1996, p. 296) as well as the concept of empowerment.

Empowerment means helping clients discover, access, and utilize the resources and tools within themselves and in their various environments. Resilience means developing and utilizing the energy, skills, abilities, knowledge, and insight that a survivor possesses to solve problems and move on. Perhaps an individual develops a sense of humor or ability to be assertive through attempts to deal with the aftermath of trauma. Perhaps an individual turns to others for strength. Saleebey (1996) recognizes that resilience is "the ability to go on in spite of difficult life experiences.... (It is not) a static dimension" (p. 296).

The major characteristics of empowerment are self-efficacy or confidence (I can do it), optimism (I expect the best will happen), perceived control (I can make a difference here), purpose or aim (I am doing something meaningful), trust (I feel safe), self-esteem (through self-awareness and self renewal; I believe in myself), and causality (I have a choice). All seven characteristics can be included in the word "ownership": what one cares about, feels responsible and accountable for, and is committed to (Kurstedt, 1997). Other important aspects of empowerment are accountability (I care), stewardship (I want to serve), loyalty (I belong), and ownership (I get joy from what I do). To become self-empowered, an individual (whether leader, staff member, or client/patient) must set aside ego, confront his or her true self, expose his or her vulnerabilities, have courage and patience, have a sense of inner security, and be able to be empathic with the joy and pain of others.

The case manager also takes into account the client's cultural and personal stories, personal narrative, and folklore. This approach realizes the need for individuals to make sense of a traumatic event and find meaning in what happened to them. Generally, the client's culture is a major source of meaning, primarily through its stories and narratives.

Case management succeeds only when the CTC has a supportive administrative climate that allows for a collaborative approach between staff members and clients. CTC staff members must recognize that part of their job is to help clients access needed services that fit clients' needs, whether in the CTC or elsewhere. These staff members believe in interagency cooperation and view the client/patient as a partner in service acquisition, development, and implementation. Perhaps the client needs housing. To whom can the staff member turn? Does the staff member have a contact at the local Department of Family Services or housing authority? Is there an eligibility certification process available to become income-eligible for housing? What is available in terms of low-cost mortgages? Who provides rental assistance—churches, community organizations? These questions can be asked for other areas of need as well, for example, day care for children, respite care for adults, health care for the entire family.

WRAPAROUND SERVICES AND THE CTC

Case management may evolve into development of wraparound services. A plan to provide wraparound services is needs-driven, based on the unique strengths, values, norms, and preferences of the client(s) involved (Vandenberg & Grealish, 1997). Wraparound services are community based and developed by a community team. This team has a broad representation of agencies (including the representatives of the CTC), schools, business organizations, cultural leaders, neighborhood leaders, clergy, law enforcement personnel, and others. If the staff members of the CTC are the lead agency in a wraparound process, then those staff members identify four to ten persons who form the wraparound team. This team looks at the needs of the client family (group, organization) and produces a plan based on the family or group's needs, strengths, values, trauma, and preferences. The team then produces a crisis plan intended to prevent further crises and an outcome indicator for evaluation of service delivery. In some instances, the CTC will be the "broker agency" that coordinates the process, conducts the strengths assessment, and configures an appropriate team composed of those who know and/or work with the client and others who could contribute to that client's success and trauma resolution. The team and client(s) as part of that team then prioritize needs and develop strategies to meet those needs. Strategies that are assigned to the CTC for follow-up are accepted with a commitment for follow-through and evaluation.

A CTC provides support and protection for its clientele (Berger & Newhouse, 1991). If that CTC also functions as a community-building organization, it incorporates diversity, has a reasonable degree of shared values, promotes teamwork and effective internal communication, affirms the rights of its clientele, utilizes links beyond the organization, and shares tasks (Gardner, 1994). The focus of wraparound services also is empowerment and the wraparound plan developed for a client focuses on:

1. Collaborative partnerships between agencies with the CTC as broker for its own clients
2. Emphasis on the expansion of clients' capacities, strengths, and resources
3. A dual working focus on both the physical and social environment
4. The assumption that clients are active participants in the process of service provision
5. Channeling of energy of the CTC toward empowering disempowered client groups in particular (Weil, 1996)

THE PROCEDURES MANUAL OF A CTC

A manual for staff and others should include:

- Mission statement of the center
- Ethics statements and standards of practice
- Treatment goals and assumptions (e.g., empowerment)
- Value statements of benevolent intentions
- Flow charts

The policies and procedures manual is a written document that is regularly reviewed and revised. It is shared with all staff members of the CTC and asks for their input. It includes performance policies and written evaluation formats. It also includes salary information, hiring and dismissal information, sick leave and travel policies, time management policies, information management policies, anything about personnel issues, and an organizationally based stress reduction plan and crisis plan (Young and Stein, 1988).

TRAINING AND THE CTC

The comprehensive trauma center provides training to professionals at various levels of practice and to other persons and agencies. Deciding which of the training needs takes priority depends on the needs of CTC staff and the community, the culture of those requesting and providing training, the interests of those who are requesting training, and the specific traumas that seem to occur most frequently within the environments of the center (e.g., a natural disaster proneness, higher rates of violence, etc.). Training must be culturally competent: reflective of and responsive to the cultures served. A needs assessment can determine training needs as well, for example, is the objective acquisition of knowledge or of performance skills? Therefore, training should be designed so those trained can apply their skills and knowledge in practical settings. Skills taught in training do not automatically transfer into practice.

All staff members of the CTC need to have theoretically consistent levels of training. Mandatory trainings need to be offered in-house on a biweekly to monthly basis. Some, if not all, of this training would be eligible toward certification (through ATSS as a Certified Trauma Specialist, Certified Trauma Responder, or Associate in Trauma Support) and would give continuing education credits. Generic training might include:

- Definitions, statistics, and phenomenology of trauma
- Methods of taking a trauma history
- Differential diagnosis of acute stress, posttraumatic stress, and disorders of extreme stress
- Systematic approaches to treatment

The Maine Trauma Advisory Group's report (Jennings & Ralph, 1997) suggests that all trauma training needs to include:

1. Self-reflective components allowing trainees to examine personal biases, assumptions, ideas, beliefs bout trauma, treatment, and other pertinent topics
2. Consideration of the experiences of survivors as a guide to the work that is done; in other words, principles of treatment taught in training need to be based on the experiences of the survivors who are clientele of the CTC
3. Ways to include both professionals and survivors in the design, implementation, and assessment of the training process
4. Continual updating of content, techniques, and materials
5. A basis in a conceptual theoretical framework

Training methods need to be adaptable to a variety of cultures (Dyregrov, 1997). One necessary component of any beginning training program is an overview of trauma theory; another is the inclusion of practice sessions (Pregrad, 1997). Training sessions need to take into account a variety of cultural markers including language, physical space, religion, music, food and sociopolitical factors (Hart, 1997). Topics included in general training programs include biopsychosocial theory, stress theory, trauma theory, crisis intervention, and grief, loss, bereavement theory. The effectiveness of a training program, according to Zic (1997), can be measured on five criteria:

- Quality of implementation
- Amount and significance of new knowledge imparted/gained
- Opportunities for exchange of experience
- Personal benefits
- Professional benefits

Suncokret, the Center for Grassroots Relief Work, is a Croatian non-governmental, nonprofit organization founded in 1992 that responded to the psychosocial needs of many of the 650,000 displaced refugees in Croatia. Staff members had the opportunity to organize and participate in many training workshops, complete training assessments, and evaluate many training programs. Lessons learned by Suncokret staff members provide valuable suggestions for training offered by a CTC (Ajdukovic, 1997):

1. Experienced professionals are responsible for development and implementation of training programs, although experienced paraprofessionals might help in basic trauma training.
2. Training themes that are most important to accentuate are grief, loss, trauma, PTSD, development of communication skills, active listening, constructive feedback, problem solving, community building, empowerment, and self-help. Communication and contact are basic tools for working with the traumatized persons.
3. Short lectures followed by exercises centering on methods and skills, case consultations and casework, role plays, active support and supervision by course leaders, integration of theory with previous experience of participants are the best training techniques.
4. Feedback from training participants as to their needs must be taken into account in order to make training relevant.
5. If training participants have the opportunity to work on their own personal experiences of loss and trauma, training must make sure there is enough time to bring some type of closure to the work and must provide later support.
6. Trainees need opportunities to apply skills learned under supervision of professional experts or knowledgeable peers.
7. Training needs to be graduated, systematic, building on previous knowledge, and providing follow-up. New staff are given the same training workshops.
8. Training is a permanent process in the ideal center (Pupavec, 1997).

What do the directors of the various centers say about their training programs? Many centers offer training programs to a variety of professional groups including legal, medical, and educational professionals (Wilson). SSTAR offers a 36-hour training program to volunteers and local professionals on domestic violence and rape. Trainings range from introductory courses on trauma to advanced clinical workshops. Many centers have developed training materials or manuals (Wilson, CMI, Yule). While most of the training sessions are presented in a "live" format, Tinnin offers teleconferences as educational seminars. Others offer consultation within their settings (e.g., a hospital or university) or facilities (Homewood Hospital). Others offer consultation to outside agencies including Departments of Mental Health, Social Services (Lubin), humanitarian organizations (BNMO), victim services (TSI/CAAP), prisons (Ticehurst), law enforcement/criminal justice agencies (Cleary, Ticehurst), and public schools (Turner, Lubin, Post Trauma Resources). Some centers have developed joint programs with outside agencies. The Crisis Center in Oulu, Finland, for example, provides services to schools and workplaces, has trained and supervises 45 crisis teams throughout central Finland, and is in the process of developing a training program in posttraumatic therapy.

Objectives of consultation programs may include prevention of trauma, awareness building, or networking to build a good service base. Van der Kolk's trauma center has a 9-month certificate program to train licensed clinicians on the spectrum of trauma related issues. Centers frequently create brochures (Shalev), publish newsletters (AMCHA), have websites (Bergmann, Sanctuary, Ross, Oulu), and contribute to published articles and books (RCT). Training is the major focus of Tunnecliffe's organization; that organization conducts a multitude of courses and publishes extensive materials and workbooks. In addition, Tunnecliffe's organization offers fee-based consultation to organizations. Some organizations have Speaker's Bureaus to provide consultation to health care organizations (Ross).

MARKETING OF THE CTC

The CTC becomes known through its marketing strategies as well as through the services it provides. Word-of-mouth networking across professions is an effective means to make the CTC "known." Marketing services to potential individual, organizational, professional, and other client groups also is important as the CTC works together with other organizations in the community. As part of the community service delivery system, particularly if and when a major event occurs, the CTC makes itself known. Hospitals, hospices, schools, law enforcement, emergency services, attorneys, clergy, governmental agencies, media, the chamber of commerce, mental health centers, volunteer organizations, and others need to be familiar with its services.

COMMUNITY SERVICES OF A CTC

The CTC offers services to healthy individuals as well as to those who have been traumatized. It maintains a bookstore of materials, periodicals, videos, games, and other trauma and grief-related items and a library for both in-house use and, possibly, for out-of-building use. It may be that the CTC bookstore also contains various health-oriented items including vitamins and aromatherapy products.

Professional respondents to the State of Maine survey stated that it is important for a CTC to:

1. Make materials available to survivors in particular and community members in general that are educational and provide general information about trauma, traumatic reactions, and recovery.
2. Develop simple publications about the services offered by the CTC, whom to contact, what educational programs are offered, what resources are otherwise available in the community, and other similar topics. These materials are helpful to survivors, their families, law enforcement, clergy, physicians, emergency room staffs, other mental health professionals, victim witness advocates, volunteers, and others.

Part of the work of CTC staff members is working with multidisciplinary teams of other agencies and organizations. These "others" might include victim service providers, law enforcement officers, emergency medical responders, counselors, justice practitioners, clergy, and others (Office for Victims of Crime, 1998). These "others" need to be encouraged and assisted to establish reciprocal referral systems for times of need.

EVALUATING THE WORK OF A CTC

The goal of an evaluation program is to improve the design and performance of the CTC (Galano & Neziek, 1986). In order for an evaluation to be accurate, the program of the CTC must be clearly articulated. The program goals or service goals flow from the general mission statement, the general program goal statements, and the changing program objectives.

Evaluation of the program of the CTC may investigate the extent that services reach intended targets and whether or not service provision and delivery is consistent with the intended program design. The first step in this process is to return to the mission statement to answer the following questions, according to Galano and Neziek (1986).

Who is (are) the intended target population(s) and how is (are) the population(s) defined? Who are prioritized as target populations? What are the intended activities that constitute the program of the CTC? Who is to do what and how is that "what" to be accomplished? Answering these questions helps to set up well-defined standards and guidelines for accountability as well as methods of feedback. Furthermore, once these questions are answered, appropriate evaluation measures to be used by all center personnel can be developed. These measures may include records of service delivery, observational data, or self-report measures (through questionnaires, interviews of staff and/or clients). Evaluation of the "success" of a CTC is necessary, particularly

if obtaining funding depends on demonstration of some type of change or
outcome. Effectiveness of services can be measured, to a degree, by client
satisfaction and cost-effectiveness. Are services delivered according to the
timeline set by the CTC? To what degree do they accomplish the goals set by
center policies? Does feedback from those serviced help modify future service
delivery systems (Young & Stein, 1988)?

Perhaps one of the most efficient ways to measure the "success" of a CTC
measure change in symptom patterns, posttraumatic reactions, and coping
strategies. Assessment instruments that can be given pre- and postintervention
or at specific times across the course of intervention and service delivery can
give proof of some type of change. However, allowances have to be made for
changes in life circumstances, developmental changes, and other factors. Ideally, assessing a control group who did not use the services (e.g., did not have
treatment, did not get training, did not receive advocacy services or debriefing) would be possible, though highly unlikely in this case. Bucat et al. (1997)
note that it is possible to measure positive outcome through measurement of
anxiety and depression symptoms, PTSD symptoms, coping strategies utilized,
behaviors (medications, hospitalizations), attitudes, and interpersonal relations.

SUMMARY

The CTC operates in a shrinking world that is globally connected through
communications devices such as e-mail and fax modem services. The environment that spawns a center frequently is one of violence and disaster, tragedy
and grief, conflict and attack. Organizations such as the False Memory Syndrome Foundation try to pick away at the reality of traumatic events such as
child sexual abuse. Newly proposed techniques that are in use in a well-
rounded CTC (EMDR, TFT, and others) are under attack as well.

Any model of a CTC must be complex, not simplistic, because the model
of trauma and trauma treatment is becoming more complex, interdisciplinary,
and global. Trauma is so widespread and debilitating that nations who are not
restored to some level of functioning through intervention will suffer immen-
sely on individual, family, group, and national levels of functioning. The
culture of trauma and traumatology offers a way to look at life that describes
facts of event occurrence, explains the reactions to those events, and evaluates
the impact of the reactions and the events on the individual, family, group,
organization, and nation.

16

The Hamburg Experience

Providing Services in War-Torn Environments

Directors/representatives of 66 programs, 32 of which were outside the United States, answered the protocol questions found in Appendix II or sent information to the authors to be used in the descriptions provided in this volume. Those individuals either provided information about or discussed their centers' missions, philosophies, theory bases, and visions of an ideal center and whether the centers worked with sexual abuse survivors. refugees, asylum seekers, disaster victims, battered women, or other survivor groups. Some centers demonstrated that they were "on the way" to meeting what the directors/representatives considered to be "ideal." Others struggled to find funding, to provide minimal services under difficult (if not horrible) conditions of poverty, lack of safety, and personal risk, and "just" to survive.

THE CHALLENGE

With this context in mind, during a presentation to a variety of representatives of programs and institutions in Hamburg, Germany, on December 4, 1998, sponsored by the Institute for Social Research, several participants expressed their concerns that the model presented as "ideal" (based on recommendations of directors and authors) was a "one size fits all" model. Those participants generally worked with refugees or war-survivor populations. They appeared ready to attack any suggestion that a Western (American) model might become the "gold standard" for trauma centers. They did not see any "ideal center" model as allowing room for growth and had a difficult time listening to and grasping "gray" words or statements, for example, "these are suggestions; these are things to consider" or "what is considered to be an ideal center is very dependent upon the environments of that center."

REFLECTIONS: A DYNAMIC MODEL

The model trauma center presented in the previous chapter, as a circular model, is a flowing, dynamic model. The services offered rotate both clockwise and counterclockwise to fit the environments Those environments, designed as a blooming flower, also are growing, changing processes. The components of the model flow from the inside out in a series of foci. The choice of this nonlinear, non-left-brained model is purposeful. The various components of the model can be used individually or in a cumulative manner, as shown in Figs. 16.1 and 16.2.

CENTERS IN WAR-TORN ENVIRONMENTS

When developing trauma centers in war-torn or underdeveloped countries or in areas directly impacted by ongoing traumatic events that impact

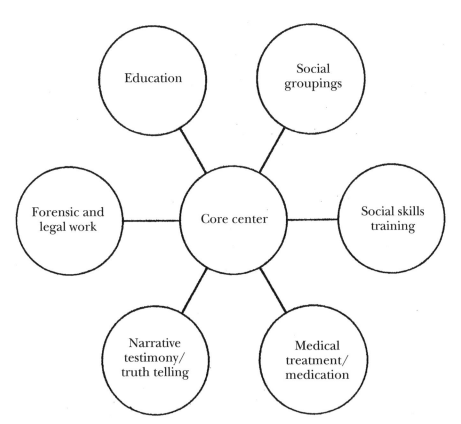

Figure 16.1. The core refugee center.

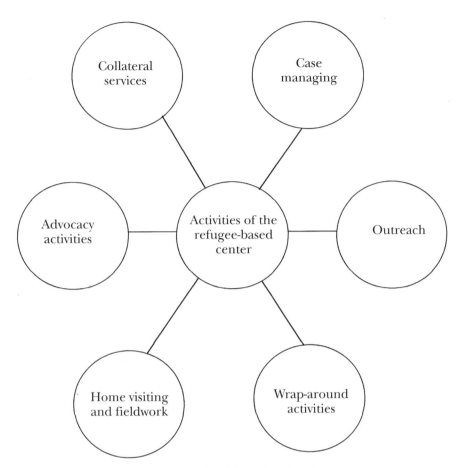

Figure 16.2. Activities of the refugee-based center.

large groups of persons (e.g., disasters), it is necessary to recognize that the ideal center may remain a farfetched, impossible-to-reach fantasy. Outsiders who come in with ideas in mind and plans in hand may find themselves frustrated, if not totally discouraged, when their plans cannot be realized. Indigenous professionals and nonprofessionals are often the real experts as to the needs of their fellow citizens and may be most knowledgeable as to the most efficacious ways to meet those needs, given the cultural, historical, political, and actual event-oriented circumstances at hand.

Needs assessments of communities and even nations must take place prior to designing any type of trauma center or services. Including indigenous peoples in the assessment and in all phases of planning leads to a more relevant, better-accepted, psychosocial approach that engenders longer-term commitment by those it aims to serve and help. The assessment will help to determine the specific characteristics of the situation as well as the most pressing needs (Bang, 1997). Local professionals have a great deal to teach any outside "experts" who may arrive "on scene" (Joshi, 1997). If internationally known professionals attempt to come in to organize and create a trauma center, it is important that those persons commit to remaining in country for an extended period of time (perhaps 6 months or more) in order to learn about the culture, develop trust from local professionals and volunteers, and conduct assessments and make plans as well as provide trainings. All too often, persons come in for a 2-week stint and then leave. If this scenario is essential, then those professionals have the responsibility to train as many indigenous persons as possible in the short time they are there, rather than try to do direct intervention. Staying in a dangerous environment for a longer period of time frequently is a risky situation that many helpers are not willing to face or experience.

How to reach out to as many persons as possible with limited resources is the reality in too many disaster or war situations. Victims need assistance at many levels and require a case management approach to intervention that is psychosocial in focus and tone. One role of a center in this situation is to train as many indigenous professionals and nonprofessionals who are qualified (e.g., teachers, nurses, religious workers) and are not direct service trauma professionals to serve the populace, in turn. Some persons are what Pregrad (1997) calls "natural helpers" who need information and skills to do what they already do best—help others. In some instances, the center, as training facility, becomes a transitional space that is safe, one that has not been damaged by personal and social traumatization (Ayalon, 1997). Going to local communities to train these persons is an essential outreach action of any center. The training cannot be totally or primarily theoretical and instead needs to be experiential and designed to integrate theory and skills. Additionally, training programs must be flexible and adapted to the particular needs of those who eventually will be served. As Mulders (1997) noted, training programs also need to contribute to "local capacity building and not create dependency on outside expertise" (p. 51). Helping organizations increase their capacity to provide services to larger numbers of traumatized persons is another aim of training.

Ajdukovic (1997) recognizes from work with survivors of the Bosnian wars that locally based trauma center programs can meet culturally specific issues more appropriately, are able to serve more individuals and groups of individuals, can provide follow-up and supervision, and become the vehicles for creating a network throughout the involved area. These centers help survivors in many areas of life simultaneously (Juul, 1997). Activities may range from provision of vocational training, help with homework, development of community initiatives, creation of support networks, and empowerment of community leaders (Ager, 1997). Activity-oriented as well as income-generating projects also are essential (Despotovic, 1997). The aim of this type of center is to create a holding environment, an environment that challenges the medical model of PTSD and recognizes that many of these survivors are victims of systematic violations of their human rights as well as war and/or disaster (Becker, 1995).

FURTHER REALITIES

In reality, a trauma center is a process, not a static object. This process aims toward an ideal that often is unreachable. Providing counseling and therapy to thousands of survivors may never be a reachable goal. Helping with provision of basic needs, training indigenous peoples in assessment and diagnosis using a nonpathogenic orientation, and working on ways to influence and modify institutions and systems may be more realistic goals. In addition, teaching coping skills for dealing with untenable situations may be a more realistic goal than is long-term therapy.

In this type of situation, the ideal trauma center is more community based and outreach oriented. Community-based projects empower local professionals and nonprofessionals alike. Ideally, according to Arcel, Folnegovic-Smale, Kozaric-Kovacie, and Marusic (1995), only the director of a center might be an internationally known individual. In this type of center, attempts to reach the greatest number of persons with minimal staff are primary. As Kos, Slodnjak, and Jovanovic (1997) wrote, "... the aim is to improve ... quality of life ... to advocate ... and to take social actions" (p. 29). Recognition of the resilience and coping capacities of many children and adults is also essential.

Many survivors of catastrophic events do not need trauma-based treatment. But they do need psychosocial intervention and help to meet their basic human needs. They do need a safe place to mourn and grieve, a predictable environment that provides some level of normalcy, and communication and contact with others like them (Pupavac, 1997). They also need triage, help with developing communication, conflict resolution, and problem-solving skills, and assistance in community building. As Pecnik (1997) noted, they need help to strengthen their coping resources and quality of life while building some degree of control through participation in planning and control of whatever resources are available. Frequently, the only type of counseling that they might accept, if any, is crisis intervention and debriefing.

WORKING IN THE FIELD

Arcel et al. (1995) has noted that individuals who work in the field in outreach satellite trauma centers, in mobile centers, or in community-based centers need to have specific roles. Some staff members (e.g., students, residents, volunteers, psychologists) may contact target groups, screen victims for PTSD, or acute stress disorder, interview victims, register basic data, refer victims to appropriate aspects of the center for treatment or to other institutions, and explain programs and activities. Mental health professionals who are on staff also make mental health assessments, design and carry out treatment plans, administer research/psychological testing, instruct and supervise field workers, participate in educational activities, and do training.

Any trauma center, no matter its location, must have clearly stated objectives, a strategy to meet those objectives, and specific activities to operationalize those strategies. As Stuvland (1997) has written that any project (center) requires "strong management, good administration, and political support (with) ... real and long term commitment." Furthermore, there is "a need to develop better tools for needs assessment, evaluation, and documentation of ... results" (p. 37).

WHAT CAN WE CONCLUDE?

A pure PTSD-based model of treatment for survivors of war, torture, and massive traumatization is not "enough." Attention to the social and economic consequences of what happened often supersedes provision of treatment, and the use of a community health approach therefore is more suitable (Wolters, 1997). Because many victims of traumatic events will not have and do not want access to what constitutes traditional treatment, creation of self-help networks supervised by trained volunteers may provide what Wolters (1997) terms "an initial safety net for the victims of extremely shocking events" (p. 57).

At the core of an initial response of a trauma center to massive traumatization is crisis intervention and situation management, not treatment. Provision of some minimal level of safety and structure in a world that may never be safe, to the greatest extent possible, is part of that process. Total team involvement and coordination is also essential to provide much attention to very concrete and practical services. Part of this intervention includes what Worthington (1997) describes as community-focused education and occupational training as part of the larger community-based psychosocial assistance program.

In a more traditional trauma program or center, psychosocial rehabilitation often is a problem-focused approach that ideally occurs after individuals have deconditioned traumatic memories and restructured schemas. This type of rehabilitation includes reestablishing secure social connections and interpersonal efficacy (van der Kolk et al., 1996) as well as teaching people how to cope using techniques that are practical, culturally-appropriate, and generalizable. Thus, psychosocial rehabilitation that occurs after the trauma is processed generally begins with a strong safety orientation and includes a strong educational component.

This type of rehabilitation is in contrast to rehabilitation that actually is more case management, particularly when traumatized individuals, groups, or communities need assistance in meeting basic needs of food, shelter, and employment. This case management may be limited to providing linkages of client(s) to service(s) to more intensive case management that is home/community based. This type of service provision is more applicable when aiding large numbers of refugees who have experienced torture, sudden dislocation, massive losses (e.g., home, country, networks, value systems). These refugees have been traumatized originally through political events and often continue to be retraumatized by the conditions they experience in exile. Making what has happened to them manageable and meaningful can be a life-long exercise.

When providing psychosocial rehabilitative services to multiply traumatized communities and societies, intervenors may recognize that fieldwork linked to the cultural and political environments in which the work occurs is the only way to reach masses of persons. This community-oriented approach brings services to the masses in culturally specific ways. It promotes accessibility through the use of mobile treatment and home-based services as well as a continuum of care ranging from medical care to (less frequently used) psychotherapy, to assistance in finding housing, education, and jobs, to provision of meals and social activities. This interdisciplinary approach to intervention looks at and attempts to impact all areas of existence: psychological damage to individuals, family disturbances, work and social impacts, spiritual impacts. The inner reality of trauma survivors may actually be treated, though less directly, when the focus of intervention is on the outer realities of survival.

CONCLUSIONS FROM SLOVENE INITIATIVES

Kos et al. (1997) recognizes, as do we, that there are many instances when the "normal" building-based trauma center does not have sufficient resources to meet the needs of victims and when the more linear, Western model of trauma treatment (client comes to the center for individual or group treatment) does not "fit." Designing community-based models of trauma intervention under these circumstances must include victims as much as is possible as partners in decision making. The victims themselves are the most familiar with ethnic, cultural, religious, educational, and coping patterns as well as customs, values, points of view, and already-existing sources of help, programs, interventions, and social resources. Kos continues, "The organization and quality of everyday life are in the aftermath period the most influential determinants of ... mental health conditions and psychosocial functioning" (p. 137). Her guidelines for the formation of psychosocial projects (as part of an outreach trauma center) also are helpful. She concludes (p. 138):

1. The design of (any) psychosocial interventions (including psychosocial-based trauma centers) depends on the concrete circumstances, needs, and characteristics of those in need as well as upon the available mental health resources.
2. The social and cultural context determines appropriate and acceptable methods of intervention.
3. Multidisciplinary teams that involve social, educational, and legal professionals are necessary to provide a holistic approach to treatment.
4. A center utilizes various helping approaches at the same time both individually and in combination.
5. Planning must be concrete and realistic as well as flexible, taking into consideration ongoing changes in circumstances and resources.
6. One of the most important components of intervention is the provision of information about the center and its program(s).
7. Any program must be evaluated and monitored consistently.
8. Fund-raising begins when intervention begins; it is a long process to get money for extra services.
9. The most efficient way to make services available to children is through the schools.
10. Volunteers are important in service delivery and can be recruited from the victim population; volunteering helps victims overcome their own traumas and sorrows (p. 141).
11. Collaboration with a large number of persons, services, organizations, and structures is an important activity in service provision.
12. When resistance to intervention exists, entering into contact through a less-threatening channel than "trauma" is more successful (p. 208).
13. The basic paradigm for giving help is an ecosocial model with community-based activities and interventions that stresses protective factors, processes, and development of coping strategies.
14. Identification of persons in the community who can act as promoters of help seeking is important, particularly when these individuals are already respected or seen as having power/authority. Integrating these persons into the team, creating a team that has a mixture of mental health professionals as well as nonmental health-oriented persons can help build acceptance and promote use of services. Avoidance of "turf" issues and competition is essential.

FINAL COMMENTS

Participating in a conference in Hamburg, Germany with representatives of many European programs was an eye-opening experience for this author. It led to a much deeper consideration of the role of rehabilitation in intervention and the conceptualization of a trauma center model that is much less "center based." The conclusions of Unkovska (1997) in her efforts to assist war-traumatized children also seem to be appropriate to note:

1. The ideal center provides services to everyone with participation by all.
2. The center uses elements from victims' traditions, culture, and religion to include habits, rituals, and other elements in psychosocial rehabilitation efforts.
3. Activities in the center are designed to fit the life experiences of victims.
4. The needs and psychological states of the victims define the center's objectives; those objectives are supportive, not directive.
5. A principal component of the work of the center, whether location based or in the field, is the building of group cohesion with stimulation of group socialization.
6. Activities of the center, both within and outside its physical boundaries, stimulate personalized expression in a process-oriented manner that is open-ended, flexible, developing, and meaningful. Ready-made solutions for treatment and intervention do *not* exist.

In conclusion, ecosocial intervention that is of a broad, social character recognizes that the social context of healing helps to determine the quality and intensity of the effects of trauma. A majority of persons exposed to traumatic events do not incur devastating effects that constitute PTSD. Protective factors from within and outside the family help to modify those effects and combine with social interventions, positive human relationships, and specific professional knowledge to lessen negative impacts (Kos et al., 1997). Adapting methods of intervention to the characteristics of the trauma and the traumatized will help to ensure more positive outcomes. As Bucat, Francěiškovic, and Moro noted (1997), healing occurs (and a trauma treatment center is effective) when interventions lead to

- Fewer symptoms of PTSD
- Positive self-concepts of those receiving help of any kind
- A more positive future outlook in survivors
- Increase in coping strategies (that are more diversified)
- Less dependency on institutional interventions
- Social participation
- Decreasing shame and guilt
- Increase in personal responsibility

It is the hope of the center directors interviewed and of the authors that any model of a treatment center will lead to these measures of effectiveness and that our work will lead to a more positive future for those a center impacts. In the words of Rev. John Calvin Little, "It can be done." The "it" of the work of a trauma center, no matter the model, is to help those who have been traumatized to refind meaning in their lives. And what will that sense of meaning entail? Perhaps, through the work of the center, individuals, groups, families, communities, and nations may develop positive relationships, give of themselves to others through service, develop more positively oriented schemas (beliefs), regain materials and rewards (home, furniture, jobs, respect, success), improve themselves, develop self-understanding, improve their physical and mental health, and find pleasure and contentment through the activities of daily life (Ebersole, 1998).

References

Ackerman, L. D. (1984). The psychology of corporation: How identity influences business. *The Journal of Business Strategy, 5*(1), 56–65.

Ager, A. (1997). Balancing skills' transmission and indigenous understandings: A conceptual framework for planning support for trauma recovery. In D. Ajduković (Ed.), *Trauma recovery training: Lessons learned* (pp. 73–82). Zagreb, Croatia: Society for Psychological Assistance.

Ajduković, D. (Ed.). (1995). *Programs of psychosocial assistance for refugee children.* Zagreb, Croatia: Society for Psychological Assistance.

Ajduković, D. (Ed.). (1997). *Trauma recovery training: Lessons learned.* Zagreb, Croatia: Society for Psychological Assistance.

Ajduković, M., & Ajduković, D. (Eds.). (1996). *Help and self-help in care of mental health care providers* (2nd ed.). Zagreb, Croatia: Society for Psychological Assistance.

Ajduković, M., Ajduković, D., & Ljubotina, D. (1997). Mental health care for helpers: A necessary ingredient of trauma recovery training and assistance in war zones. In D. Ajduković (Ed.), *Trauma recovery training: Lessons learned.* Zagreb, Croatia: Society for Psychological Assistance.

Ajduković, M., & Ajduković, D. (1993). Psychological well-being of refugee children. *Child Abuse and Neglect, 17,* 843–844.

Amani Trust. (1995). *Chivesche nurse counsellor programme: Resource manual.* Harare, Zimbabwe: Author.

Amani Trust. (1993). *Assessment of the consequences of torture and organized violence: A manual for field workers.* Harare, Zimbabwe: Author.

Amani Trust. (1998). *A trauma counseling program.* Harare, Zimbabwe: Author.

Amani Trust. (1998). *A handbook for nurse counsellors.* Harare, Zimbabwe: Author.

American Psychiatric Association. (1952). *Diagnostic and statistical manual of mental disorders* (1st ed.), Washington, DC: Author.

American Psychiatric Association. (1968). *Diagnostic and statistical manual of mental disorders* (2nd ed.). Washington, DC: Author.

American Psychiatric Association. (1980). *Diagnostic and statistical manual of mental disorders* (3rd ed.). Washington, DC: Author.

American Psychiatric Association. (1987). *Diagnostic and statistical manual of mental disorders* (3rd ed. rev.). Washington, DC: Author.

American Psychiatric Association. (1994). *Diagnostic and statistical manual of mental disorders* (4th ed.). Washington, DC: Author.

Antonovsky, A. (1979). *Health, stress, and coping.* San Francisco: Jossey-Bass.

Antonovsky, A. (1987). *Unraveling the mystery of health: How people manage stress and stay well.* San Francisco, CA: Jossey-Bass.

Arcel, L. T., Folnegovic-Smale, V., Kozaric-Kovacie, D., & Marusic, A., et al. (1995). *Psycho-social help*

to war victims: Women refugees and their families. Copenhagen, Denmark: International Rehabilitation Council for Torture Victims.

Arnold, H. J., & Feldman, D. C. (1986). *Organizational behavior.* New York: McGraw-Hill.

Ayalon, O. (1992). *Rescue! C.O.P.E. handbook: Helping children coping with stress guided group activities.*
Ellicott City, M: Chevron Press.

Ayalon, O. (1997). Creating methods offered to care-givers to prevent or deal with secondary
traumatization. In D. Ajduković (Ed.), *Trauma recovery training: Lessons learned* (pp. 161–168).
Zagreb, Croatia: Society for Psychological Assistance.

Ballard, C. G., Stanley, A. K., & Brockington, I. F. (1995). Post-traumatic stress disorder (PTSD)
after childbirth. *British Journal of Psychiatry, 166,* 525–528.

Bang, S. (1997). Psychosocial training project in Croatia. In D. Ajduković (Ed.), *Trauma recovery
training: Lessons learned* (pp. 139–150). Zagreb, Croatia: Society for Psychological Assistance.

Becker, D. (1995). The deficiency of the concept of traumatic stress disorder when dealing with
victims of human rights violations. In R. Kleber, C. Filey, & B. Gersons (Eds.), *Beyond trauma:
Cultural and societal dynamics.* New York: Plenum Press.

Becvar, D. S., & Becvar, R. J. (1988). *Family therapy: A systemic integration.* Boston: Allyn &
Bacon.

Behar, L., Zipper, I. N., & Weil, M. (Eds.). (1994). *Case management for children's mental health: A
training curriculum for child-serving agencies.* Raleigh: North Carolina Division of Mental Health.

Bennis, W. G., & Nanus, B. (1985). *Leaders: Strategies for taking charge.* New York: Harper & Row.

Berg, I. K. (1994). *Family-based services: A solution-focused approach.* New York: Norton.

Berger, P. L., & Newhouse, J. (1991). *The structure of freedom: Correlation, causes, and cautions.* Grand
Rapids, MI: W. B. Eerdmans.

Blake, R. R., & Mouton, J. S. (1985). *The managerial grid III: The key to leadership excellence.* Houston,
TX: Gulf-Publishing.

Blanchard, K., & Johnson, S. (1983). *The one-minute manager.* New York: Berkeley Books.

Bloom, B. L. (1985). *Stressful life event theory and research: Implications for primary prevention.* Rockville,
MD: National Institute of Mental Health.

Bloom, S. L. (1994). The sanctuary model: Developing general inpatient programs for the treatment of trauma. In M. B. Williams & J. F. Sommer (Eds.), *Handbook of post-traumatic therapy*
(p. 215). Westport, CT: Greenwood Press.

Bloom, S. L. (1997). *Creating sanctuary: Toward the evolution of sane societies.* New York: Routledge.

Bolman, L. G., & Deal, T. E. (1997). *Reframing organizations: Artistry, choice, and leadership.* San
Francisco, CA: Jossey-Bass.

Bowman, M. (1997). *Individual differences in posttraumatic response: Problems with the adversity-distress
connection.* Mahwah, NJ: Erlbaum.

Breslau, N., Davis, G. C., Andreski, P. A., & Peterson, E. (1991). Traumatic events and PTSD in a
urban population of young adults. *Archives of General Psychiatry, 48,* 216–111.

Briere, J. (1995). *Traumatic Symptom Inventory professional manual.* Odessa, FL: Psychological Assessment Resources.

Brown, P., & Yantis, J. (1996). Personal space intrusion and PTSD. *Journal of Psychosocial Nursing,
34*(7), 23–28.

Bryant, R., & Harvey, A. (1995). Acute stress response: A comparison of head-injured and non-
head-injured patients. *Psychological Medicine, 25,* 869–873.

Bryant, R. A., & Harvey, A. G. (1996). Initial posttraumatic stress responses following motor vehicle
accidents. *Journal of Traumatic Stress, 9*(2), 223–234.

Bucat, N., Franciskovic, T., & Moro, L. (1997). What to measure when Evaluating the outcomes of
the trauma treatment? In D. Ajduković (Ed.), *Trauma recovery training: Lessons learned* (pp.
395–403). Zagreb, Croatia: Society for Psychological Assistance.

Budman, S. H., & Steinbarger, B. N. (1997). *The executive guide to group practice in mental health:
Clinical, legal, and financial fundamentals.* New York: Guilford.

Bullock-Loughran, R. (1982). Territoriality in critical care. *Focus, 9*(5), 19–23.

Burke, W. W., & Litwin, G. H. (1989). A causal model of organizational performance. In J. W.

Pfeiffer (Ed.), *The 1989 annual: Developing human resources* (pp. 37ff). San Diego, CA: Pfeiffer & Company.

Busuttil, W., Turnbull, G. J., Neal, L. A., Rollins, J., West, A. G., Blanch, N., & Herepath, R. (1995). Incorporating psychological debriefing techniques within a brief group psychotherapy programme for the treatment of post-traumatic stress disorder. *British Journal of Psychiatry, 167,* 495–502.

Butler, R. W., Foy, D. W., Snodgrass, L., Hurwicz, M., & Goldfarb, J. (1988). Combat-related posttraumatic stress disorder in a nonpsychiatric population. *Journal of Anxiety Disorders, 2,* 111–120.

Calhoun, L. G., & Tedeschi, R. G. (1998). Posttraumatic growth: Future directions. In R. G. Tedeschi, C. L. Park, & L. G. Calhoun (Eds.), *Posttraumatic growth: Positive changes in the aftermath of crisis* (pp. 215–238). Mahwah, NJ: Erlbaum.

Callahan, R. J., & Callahan, J. (1996). *Thought field therapy (TFT) and trauma treatment and theory.* Indian Wells, CA: FFT™ Training Center.

Campbell, J. (1988). *The power of myth.* New York: Doubleday.

Card, J. J. (1987). Epidemiology of PTSD in a national cohort of Vietnam veterans. *Journal of Clinical Psychology, 43,* 6–17.

Carlson, E. B. (1997). *Trauma assessments: A clinician's guide.* New York: Guilford Press.

Catherall, D. R. (1999). Coping with secondary traumatic stress: The importance of the therapist's professional peer group. In B. H. Stamm (Ed.), *Secondary traumatic stress: Self-care Issues for clinicians, researchers, and educators* (3rd ed., pp. 80–92). Lutherville, MD: Sidran Press.

Cavallin, B., & Houston, B. K. (1980). Aggressiveness, maladjustment, body experience, and the protective function of personal space. *Journal of Clinical Psychology, 36,* 170–176.

Chemtob, C. M., Bauer, G. B., Neller, G., Hamada, R., Glisson, C., & Stevens, V. (1990). Posttraumatic stress disorder among special forces Vietnam veterans. *Military Medicine, 155,* 16–20.

Chetkov-Yanoov, B. (1997). *Social work approaches to conflict resolution: Making fighting obsolete.* New York: Haworth Press.

Cohen, P. S. (1963). Theories of myth. *Man, 4,* 337–353.

Cohen, R. E. (1995). Participating in disaster relief: What psychiatrists need to know when catastrophe strikes. www.mhsource.com: continuing education activity.

Cole, C. H., & Barney, E. E. (1987, March). *Safeguards and the therapeutic window: A group treatment strategy for adult incest survivors.* Paper presented at the 64th annual meeting of the American Orthopsychiatric Association, Washington, DC.

Colon, E. (1995). Creating an "intelligent organization" in human services. In L. Ginsberg & P. R. Keys (Eds.), *New management in human services* (2nd ed., pp. 98–114). Washington, DC: NASW Press.

Cooke, R. A., & Rousseau, D. M. (1989). *Organizational culture: Not just another name for climate. Organizational culture inventory leader's guide.* Plymouth, MI: Human Synergistics.

Cox, D., & Hoover, J. (1992). *Leadership when the heat's on.* New York: McGraw-Hill.

Creamer, M. (1996). Treatment interventions in post-traumatic stress. In D. Paton & N. Long (Eds.), *Psychological aspects of disasters: Impact, coping and intervention* (pp. 177–192). Palmerton North, New Zealand: The Dunnmore Press.

Crewdson, J. (1988). *By silence betrayed: Sexual abuse of children in America.* Boston: Little, Brown, & Company.

Daft, R. L. (1986). *Organization theory and design* (2nd ed.). St. Paul, MB: West Publishing Company.

Danieli, Y. (1988). Confronting the unimaginable: Psychotherapists' reactions to victims of the Holocaust. In J. P. Wilson, Z. Harel, & B. Kahana (Eds.), *Human adaptation to extreme stress* (pp. 219–237). New York: Plenum.

Daniele, Y. (Ed.). (1998). *International handbook of multigenerational legacies of trauma.* New York: Plenum.

Davidson, J. R. T., Hughes, D., Blazer, D. G., & George, L. K. (1991). Post-traumatic stress disorder in the community: An epidemiological study. *Psychological Medicine, 21,* 713–721.

De Andrade, Y. (1996). Psychosocial trauma: Dialogues with émigré children at schools. In G.

Perren-Klingler (Ed.), *Trauma: From individual helplessness to group resources* (pp. 205–236). Berne, Switzerland: Paul Haupt.

De Jong, P., & Miller, S. D. (1995). How to interview for client strengths. *Social Work, 40*(6), 729–736.

De la Fuente, R. (1990). The mental health consequences of the 1985 earthquake in Mexico. *International Journal of Mental Health, 19,* 21–29.

Dennert, J. W. (1998, June 5). Trauma and PTSD: Cause and effect. Response to the traumatic-stress. www.listp.apa.org.

Despotovic, M. (1997). What we have learned, and what remained to be learned. In D. Ajdukovič (Ed.), *Trauma recovery training: Lessons learned* (pp. 47–103). Zagreb, Croatia: Society for Psychological Assistance.

Dyregrov, A. (1997). Teaching trauma intervention: Lessons learned. In D. Ajdukovič (Ed.), *Trauma recovery training: Lessons learned* (pp. 49–71). Zagreb, Croatia: Society for Psychological Assistance.

Dyregrov, A., & Mitchell, J. T. (1992). Work with traumatized children—psychological effects and coping strategies. *Journal of Traumatic Stress, 5*(1), 5–17.

Ebersole, P. (1998). Types and depth of written life meanings. In P. T. P. Wong & P. S. Fry (Eds.), *The human quest for meaning: A handbook of psychological research and clinical applications* (pp. 179–191). Mahwah, NJ: Erlbaum.

Elliot, D. M., & Briere, J. (1995). Posttraumatic stress associated with delayed recall of sexual abuse: A general population study. *Journal of Traumatic Stress, 8*(4), 629–648.

Emerson, B., & Mineta, N. (1996, July 31). The disaster debacle: When disaster strikes, taxpayers get hit. Insurance is the answer. *USA Today,* p. 11A.

Eih, S., & Pynoos, R. (Eds.). (1985). *Post-traumatic stress disorder in children.* Washington, DC: American Psychiatric Press.

Erikson, K. (1976). *Everything in its path.* New York: Simon & Schuster.

Everly, G. S., & Mitchell, J. T. (1997). Critical incident stress management. In *CISM: A new era and standard of care in crisis intervention.* Ellicott City, MD: Chevron Publishing.

Fairfax–Falls Church Community Services Board. (1998). *FY 1999 community-based prevention plan: A framework for prevention services of the Fairfax–Falls Church community services board.* Falls Church, VA: Author.

FEMA. (1998). *Emergency management guide for business and industry: A step-by-step approach to emergency planning, response, and recovery for companies of all sizes.* Washington, DC: Author.

Fiedler, F. E. (1967). *A theory of leadership effectiveness.* New York: McGraw-Hill.

Figley, C. (1995). *Systemic traumatology: Family therapy with trauma survivors.* Rockville, MD: Presentation to the Maryland Psychological Association.

Fisher, R., & Ury, W. (1981). *Getting to yes.* Boston: Houghton Mifflin.

Foa, E. B., & Riggs, D. S. (1993). PTSD following assault: Theoretical considerations and empirical findings. *Current Directions and Psychological Sciences, 162,* 61–65.

Foa, E. B., Steketee, G., & Rothbaum, B. O. (1989). Behavioral/cognitive conceptualizations of posttraumatic stress disorder. *Behavior Therapy, 20,* 155–176.

Foa, E. B., & Rothbaum, B. D. (1998). *Treating the trauma of rape: Cognitive therapy for PTSD.* New York: Guilford Press.

Fontaine, J. H., & Hammond, N. L. (1994, November/December). Twenty counseling maxims. *Journal of Counseling and Development, 73,* 223–226.

Ford, J. (1998, June 11). Complicated PTSD. Response to traumatic-stress. www//list.apa.org.

Foy, D. W., Resnick, H. S., Sipprelle, R. C., & Carroll, E. M. (1987). Premilitary, military, and postmilitary factors in the development of post-traumatic reactions. In B. A. van der Kolk, A. C. McFarlane, & L. Weisaeth (Eds.), *Traumatic stress: The effects of overwhelming experience on mind, body, and society* (pp. 129–154). New York: Guilford Press.

France, K. (1996). *Crisis intervention: A handbook of immediate person-to-person help* (3rd ed.). Springfield, IL: Charles C Thomas.

Frederick, G. J. (1985). Children traumatized by catastrophic reactions. In S. Eth & R. Pynoos (Eds.), *Post-traumatic stress disorders in children.* Washington, DC: American Psychiatric Press.

French, G. D., & Harris, C. J. (1998). *Traumatic incident reduction (TIR)*. Boca Raton, FL: CRC Press.

French, J. R. P., & Raven, B. (1959). The bases of social power. In D. Cartwright (Ed.), *Studies in social power*. Ann Arbor, MI: Institute for Social Research, University of Michigan.

Fullerton, C. S., & Ursano, R. J. (Eds.). (1997). *Post-traumatic stress disorder: Acute and long-term responses to trauma and disaster*. Washington, DC: American Psychiatric Press.

Galano, J., & Neziek, J. B. (1986). *Evaluating prevention programs: A training manual*. Richmond, VA: Office of Prevention, Promotion, and Library Services, Commonwealth of Virginia.

Gallers, J., Foy, D. W., Donahue, C. P., Jr., & Goldfarb, J. (1988). Post-traumatic stress disorder in Vietnam veterans: Effects of traumatic violence exposure and military adjustment. *Journal of Traumatic Stress, 1*, 181–192.

Gardner, J. W. (1994). *Building community for leadership studies program*. Washington, DC: Independent Sector.

Gaston, L. (1995). Dynamic therapy for post-traumatic stress disorder. In J. P. Barber & P. Crits-Christoph (Eds.), *Dynamic therapies for psychiatric disorders (Axis I)* (pp. 161–192). New York, Basic Books.

Gerbode, F. A., & Moore, R. H. (1994). Beliefs and intentions in RET. *Journal of Rational and Emotive and Cognitive–Behavior Therapy, 12*(1), 27–45.

Gierowski, J. K., & Heitzman, J. (1996). *The picture and dynamics of the anxiety in victims of persecution of totalitarian system in Poland*. Krakow, Poland: Jagiellonian University.

Goenjian, A. (1993). A mental health relief program in Armenia after the 1988 earthquake: Implementation and clinical observation. *British Journal of Psychiatry, 163*, 230–239.

Goenjian, A. K., Najarian, L. M., Pynoos, R. S., Steinberg, A. M., Manoukian, G., Tavosia, T., & Fairbanks, L. A. (1994). Posttraumatic stress disorder in elderly and younger adults after the 1988 earthquake in Armenia. *American Journal of Psychiatry, 151*, 895–901.

Goenjian, A. D., Karayan, I., Pynoos, R. S., Minassian, D., Najarian, L. M., Steinberg, A. M., & Fairbanks, L. A. (1997). Outcome of psychotherapy among early adolescents after trauma. *American Journal of Psychiatry, 154*, 536–542.

Gordon, T., & Edwards, W. S. (1995). *Making the patient your partner: Communication skills for doctors and other caregivers*. Westport, CT: Auburn House.

Green, B. L. (1990). Defining trauma: Terminology and generic stressor dimensions. *Journal of Applied Social Psychology, 20*, 1632–1642.

Green, B. L. (1993). Identifying survivors at risk: Trauma and stressors across events. In J. P. Wilson & B. Raphael (Eds.), *International handbook of traumatic stress syndromes* (pp. 135–144). New York: Plenum Publishing.

Green, B. (1994). Psychosocial research in traumatic stress: An update. *Journal of traumatic Stress 7*(3), 341–362.

Green, B. L., Wilson, J. P., & Lindy, J. D. (1985). Conceptualizing PTSD: A psychosocial framework. In C. R. Figley (Ed.), *Trauma and its wake* (pp. 338–355). New York: Brunner/Mazel.

Gummer, B., & Edwards R. H. (1995). In L. Ginsbrg & P. R. Keys (Eds.), *New management in human services* (2nd ed., pp. 57–71). Washington, DC: NASW Press.

Guns, B. (1996). *The faster learning organization: Gain and sustain the competitive edge*. San Francisco, CA: Jossey-Bass.

Haas, L. J., & Malouf, J. L. (1996). *Keeping up the good work: A practitioner's guide to mental health ethics* (2nd ed.). Sarasota, FL: Professional Resource Exchange.

Hale, S., & Hyde, A. C. (Eds.). (1994). Reengineering in the public sector. *Public Productivity and Management Review, 18*, 127–131.

Hall, G. E., & Hord, S. M. (1986). *Configuration of school-based leadership teams* (R & D Report No. 3223). Austin, TX: Research and Development Center for Teacher Education.

Hallam, G. L., & Campbell, D. P. (1992, May). *Selecting team members? Start with a theory of team effectiveness*. Paper presented at the 7th annual meeting of the Society of Industrial and Organizational Psychology, Montreal, Quebec, Canada.

Hanna, R., & Ritchie, S. A. (1992). Facilities design. In A. E. Barnett & G. G Mayer (Eds.), *Ambulatory care management and practice* (pp. 488–505). Gaithersburg, MD: Aspen.

Hart, B. (1997). Transforming conflict through trauma recovery training. In D. Ajduković (Ed.), *Trauma recovery training: Lessons learned* (pp. 183–199). Zagreb, Croatia: Society for Psychological Assistance.

Harvey, M. A. (1996). An ecological view of psychological trauma and trauma recovery. *Journal of Traumatic Stress, 9*(1), 3–21.

Harvey, M. A., & Harney, P. A. (1995). Individual treatment of adult survivors. An ecological model and a stage by dimension framework. In C. Classen (Ed.), *Treating women molested in childhood* (pp. 63–103). San Francisco, CA: Jossey Bass.

Heitzman, J., & Rutkowski, K. (1996). Mental disorders in persecuted and tortured victims of the totalitarian system in Poland. *Torture, 6*(1), 19–22.

Herman, J. L. (1992a). Complex PTSD: A syndrome in survivors of prolonged and repeated trauma. *Journal of Traumatic Stress, 5,* 377–392.

Herman, J. (1992b). *Trauma and recovery.* New York: Basic Books.

Hersey, P., & Blanchard, K. H. (1982). Management of organizational behavior: Utilizing human resources (4th ed.). Englewood Cliffs, NJ: Prentice-Hall.

Hogan, R., Curphy, G. J., & Hogan, J. (1994). What we know about leadership: Effectiveness and personality. *American Psychologist, 49*(6), 493–504.

Holloway, H. C., & Ursano, R. J. (1984). The Vietnam veteran: Memory, social context, and metaphor. *Psychiatry, 47,* 103–108.

Horowitz, M. J. (1976). *Stress response syndromes.* New York: Jason Aaronson.

Horowitz, M. J., Marmar, C. R., Weiss, D., DeWitt, K., & Rosenbaum, R. (1984). Brief dynamic psychotherapy of bereavement reactions: The relationship of process to outcome. *Archives of General Psychiatry, 41,* 438–448.

Hunter, R. H. (1995). Benefits of competency-based treatment programs. *American Psychologist, 50*(7), 509–513.

Hunter, R. H., & Marsh, D. T. (1994). Mining giftedness: A challenge for psychologists. In D. T Marsh (Ed.), *New directions in the psychological treatment of serious mental illness.* Westport, CT: Praeger.

Hunty, C. (1993). *Understanding organizations.* New York: Oxford University Press.

Ingmundson, P. T. (1998, June 11). Stress and the hippocampus. Reply to www//traumatic-stress at listp.apa.org.

International Federation of Red Cross and Red Crescent Societies. (1993). *World disaster report.* Dordrecht, The Netherlands: Martinus Nyhoff.

Ivanevich, J. M., & Matteson, M. T. (1995). *Organizational behavior and management* (4th ed.). Chicago, IL: R. D. Irwin.

Jacobs, G. A. (1995). The development of a national plan for disaster mental health. *Professional Psychology: Research and Practice, 26*(6), 543–549.

James, B. (1989). *Treating traumatized children.* Boston: Lexington Books/Macmillan.

Jamieson, D. W. (1996). Aligning the organization for a team-based strategy. In G. M. Parker (Ed.), *The handbook of best practices for teams* (vol. I, pp. 299–312). Amherst, MA: HRD Press.

Janet, P. (1889). *L'automatisme psychologique.* Paris, France: Paris Balliere.

Janoff-Bulman, R. (1992). *Shattered assumptions: Toward a new psychology of trauma.* New York: Free Press.

Jennings, A., & Ralph, R. O. (1997). *In their own words: Trauma survivors and professionals they trust tell what hurt, what helps and what is needed for trauma survivors.* Augusta, ME: Department of Mental Health Mental Retardation and Substance Abuse Services, Office of Trauma Services.

Jensen, P. S., & Shaw, J. (1993). Children as victims of war: Current knowledge and future research. *Journal of American Academy of Child and Adolescent Psychiatry, 32,* 697–708.

Johnson, D. (1987). The role of the creative arts therapies in the diagnosis and treatment of psychological trauma. *International Journal of Arts in Psychotherapy, 14,* 7–14.

Johnson, D., Feldman, S., & Lubin, H. (1995). Critical interaction therapy: Couples therapy in posttraumatic stress disorder. *Journal of Traumatic Stress, 8,* 283–299.

Johnson, D. R., Lubin, H., Rosenheck, R., Fontana, A., Southwick, S., & Charney, D. (1997).

Measuring the impact of the homecoming reception on the development of post-traumatic stress disorder: The West Haven homecoming stress scale (WHHSS). *Journal of Traumatic Stress, 10*, 259–278.

Jones, J. E. (1981). The organizational universe. *1981 Annual handbook for group facilitators.* San Diego: Pfeiffer & Company.

Joseph, S., Williams, R., & Yule, W. (1997). *Understanding post-traumatic stress: A psychosocial perspective on PTSD and treatment.* Chichester, England: Wiley.

Joshi, P. T. (1997). Multi-disciplinary approach to international trauma work. In D. Ajduković (Ed.), *Trauma recovery training: Lessons learned* (pp. 169–182). Zagreb, Croatia: Society for Psychological Assistance.

Juul, J. (1997). How I happened to meet Plato and Aristotle on Ban Jelacic Square. In D. Ajduković (Ed.), *Trauma recovery training: Lessons learned* (pp. 13–26). Zagreb, Croatia: Society for Psychosocial Assistance.

Katzenbach, J. R., & Smith, D. K. (1993). *The wisdom of teams: Creating the high performance organization.* Boston: Harvard Business School Press.

Keidel, R. W. (1995). *Seeing organizational patterns: A new theory and language of organizational design.* New York: Berrett-Koehler Publishers.

Kendall-Tackett, K. A., Williams, L. M., & Finkelhor, D. (1993). Impact of sexual abuse on children: A review and synthesis of recent empirical studies. *Psychological Bulletin, 113*(1), 164–180.

Kier, K. A. (1995). *Case management in ambulatory mental health services.* Nashville, TN: Business Network.

Kinzie, J. D., Boehnlein, J. K, Leung, P. K., Moore, L. J., Riley, C., & Smith, D. (1990). The prevalence of post-traumatic stress disorder and its clinical significance among Southeast Asian refugees. *American Journal of Psychiatry, 147*, 913–917.

Kinzie, J. D., & Leung, P. (1984). Clondine in Cambodian POWs with post-traumatic stress disorder. *Journal of Nervous and Mental Disease, 177*, 546–550.

Kirkpatrick, D. G., Saunders, B. E., Amick-McMullan, A., Best, C. L., Veronen, L. J., & Resnick, H. S. (1989). Victim and crime factors associated with the development of post-traumatic stress disorder. *Behavior Therapy, 20*, 199–214.

Kleber, R. J., & Brom, D. (1992). *Coping with trauma: Therapy, prevention, and treatment.* Amsterdam, The Netherlands: Swets & Zeitlinger.

Kluznik, J. C., Speed, W., Van Valkenburg, C., & Magraw, R. (1986). Forty-year follow-up of United States prisoners of war. *American Journal of Psychiatry, 143*, 1443–1446.

Kos, A. M., Slodnjak, V., & Jovanovic, S. D. (1997). What can we learn from refugee children for child mental health protection in a non-war situation? In D. Ajduković (Ed.), *Trauma recovery training: Lessons learned* (pp. 303–318). Zagreb, Croatia: Society for Psychological Assistance.

Kos, A. M., et al. (1998). *They talk, we listen.* Lljubljana, Slovenia: The Slovene Foundation.

Koss, M. P., & Harvey, M. R. (1991). *The rape victim: Clinical and community interventions.* Newbury Park, CA: Sage.

Krystal, H. (1968). *Massive psychic trauma.* New York: International Universities Press.

Kuhn, T. B. (1962). *The structure of scientific revolutions.* Chicago, IL: University of Chicago Press.

Kulka, R. A., Schlenger, W. E., Fairbank, J. A. (1990). *Trauma and the Vietnam War generation.* New York: Brunner/Mazel.

Kurstedt, H. A. (1997, Spring). *Management systems theory, applications, and design.* ISE4016. Falls Church, VA: Virginia Polytechnic Institute and State University Northern Virginia Campus.

Laub, D., & Auerhahn, N. C. (1993). Knowing and not knowing massive psychic trauma: Forms of traumatic memory. *International Journal of Psychoanalysis, 73*, 287–302.

Lax, D. A., & Sebonius, J. K. (1986). *The manager as negotiator.* New York: Free Press.

Lazarus, R. S., & Folkman, S. (1984). *Stress, appraisal, and coping.* New York: Springer.

Leibowitz, L., Harvey, M. R., & Herman, J. L. (1993). A stage-by-dimension model of recovery from sexual trauma. *Journal of Interpersonal Violence* (September), 378–391.

Lemberger, J. (Ed.). (1996). *A global perspective in working with Holocaust survivors and the second generation.* Ramalgai, Israel: AMCHA.

Levine, P. A (1997). *Walking the tiger: Healing trauma.* Berkeley, CA: North Atlantic Books.

Likert, R. (1967). *The human organization.* New York: McGraw-Hill.

Lillenfeld, R. (1978). *The rise of systems theory: An ideological analysis.* New York: Wiley.

Lindeman, E. C. (1926). *The meaning of adult education.* New York: New Republic.

Linehan, M. (1993). *Cognitive behavior treatment of borderline personality disorder.* New York: Guilford.

Lippitt, G. L. (1982). *Organization renewal: A holistic approach to organization development* (2nd ed.). Englewood Cliffs, NJ: Prentice-Hall.

Lubin, H., & Johnson, D. R. (1997). Interactive psychoanalytic group therapy for traumatized women. *International Journal of Group Psychotherapy, 47,* 271–290.

Lubin, H., Johnson, D. R., & Southwick, S. M. (1997). Impact of childhood abuse on adult psychopathology: A case report. *Dissociation, 9,* 134–139.

MacDonald, C. (1996). Post-traumatic stress disorder: Definition and classification. In D. Paton & N. Long (Eds.), *Psychological aspects of disasters: Impact, coping and intervention* (pp. 40–53). Palmerton North, New Zealand: Dunmore Press.

Madakasira, S., & O'Brien, K. F. (1987). Acute posttraumatic stress disorder in victims of a natural disaster. *Journal of Nervous and Mental Disease, 175,* 286–290.

Mallak, L. A. (1993). *The development and application of a procedure to measure cultural strength in organizations.* Unpublished dissertation, Virginia Polytechnic Institute, Blacksburg, VA.

Markowitz., L. M. (1992). Crossing the line. *Family Therapy Networker, 16*(6), 26–31.

Marmar, C. R., & Horowitz, M. J. (1988). Diagnosis and phase-oriented treatment of post-traumatic stress disorder. In J. P. Wilson, Z. Harel, & B. Kahana (Eds.), *Human adaptation to extreme stress from the Holocaust to Vietnam* (pp. 81–104). New York: Plenum.

Marmar, C. R., Weiss, D. S., & Pynoos, R. S. (1995). Dynamic psycho-therapy of post-traumatic stress disorder. In M. J. Friedman, D. S. Charney, A. Y. Deutch (Eds.), *Neurobiological and clinical consequences of stress: From normal adaptation to post-traumatic stress disorder* (pp. 495–506). Philadelphia: Lippincott-Raven.

Marsella, A. J., Friedman, M. J., Gerrity, E. T., & Scurfield, R. M. (1996). *Ethnocultural aspects of posttraumatic stress disorder: Issues, research, and clinical applications.* Washington, DC: American Psychological Association.

Matsakis, A. (1996). *I can't get over it: A handbook for trauma survivors* (2nd ed.). Oakland, CA: New Harbinger Publications.

McCann, I. L., & Pearlman, L. A. (1990). *Psychological trauma and the adult survivor: Theory, therapy, and transformation.* New York: Brunner/Mazel.

McFarlane, A. C., & deGrolamo, G. (1996). The nature of traumatic stressors and the epidemiology of posttraumatic reactions. In B. A. van der Kolk, A. C. McFarlane, & L. Weisaeth (Eds.), *Traumatic stress: The effects of overwhelming experience on mind, body, and society* (pp. 129–154). New York: Guilford.

McWhinney, W. (1987). *Of paradigms and systems theories* (rev. ed.). Santa Barbara, CA: The Fielding Institute.

Mead, C. (1996). *Journeys of discovery: Creative learning from disaster.* London: National Institute for Social Work.

Melody, P. (1989). *Facing co-dependence.* New York: Harper & Row.

Metraux, J., & Fleury, F. (1996). Creators of their future: Group work with traumatized communities. In G. Perrin-Klingler (Ed.), *Trauma: From individual helplessness to group resources* (pp. 141–162). Berne, Switzerland: Paul Haupt.

Milgram, N., Toubinana, Y. H., Klingman, A., Raviv, A., & Goldstein, I. (1988). Situational exposure and personal loss in children's acute and chronic stress reactions to a school bus accident. *Journal of Traumatic Stress, 1,* 339–352.

Miller, K. (1995). *Organizational communication: Approaches and processes.* Belmont, CA: Wadsworth.

Mink, O. G., Esterhuysen, P. W., Mink, B. P., & Owen , K. O. (1993a). *Change at work: A comprehensive management process for transforming organizations.* San Francisco, CA: Jossey-Bass.

Mink, O. G., Owen, K. O., & Mink, B. P. (1993b). *Developing high-performance people: The art of coaching.* Reading, MA: Addison-Wesley.

Mitchell, J. (1996, May 21). Internet reply to C. Figley, "Concern over the efficacy of CISD." www/
traumatic-stress@listp.apa.org.

Mintzberg, H. (1979). *The structuring of organizations: A synthesis of the research.* Englewood Cliffs, NJ:
Prentice-Hall.

Moore, R. H. (1993a). Traumatic incident reduction: Cognitive–emotive treatment. In W. Dryden
& L. Hill (Eds.), *Innovations in rational–emotive therapy.* Newbury Park, CA: Sage.

Moore, R. H. (1993b). Innovative techniques for practitioners. In *The RET resource book for practitioners.* New York: Institute for Rational–Emotive Therapy.

Morgan, G. (1986). *Images of organization.* Beverly Hills, CA: Sage.

Mulders, M. (1997). Psychosocial health care for women war victims in former Yugoslavia: A Dutch
training and consultancy program. In D. Ajduković (Ed.), *Trauma recovery training: Lessons
learned* (pp. 351–360). Zagreb, Croatia: Society for Social Assistance.

Murphy, L., Pynoos, R. S., & James, C. B. (1997). The trauma/grief focused group psychotherapy
module of an elementary school-based violence prevention/intervention program. In J. D.
Osofsky (Ed.), *Children in a violent society* (pp. 223–255). New York: Guilford.

National Organization for Victims Assistance. (1993). *Victim assistance: Frontiers and fundamentals.*
Washington, DC: Author.

Nesbitt, P. D., & Stevens, G. (1974). Personal space and stimulus intensity at a Southern California
amusement park. *Sociometry, 37,* 105–115.

Netting, F. E. (1992). Case management: Service or symptom. *Social Work, 37*(2), 160–163.

Newman, C. J. (1976). Children of disaster: Clinical observations at Buffalo Creek. *American Journal
of Psychiatry, 133,* 306–312.

Norris, (1992). Epidemiology of trauma: Frequency and impact of different potentially traumatic
events on different demographic groups. *Journal of Consulting and Clinical Psychology, 60,*
409–418.

Nurmi, L. A. (1997, Spring). Experienced stress and value of critical incident stress debriefing
(CISD) among Finnish police officers and emergency personnel in Estonia ferry disaster.
ESTSS Bulletin, Spring, pp. 3–4.

Ochberg, F. M. (1996). The counting method for ameliorating traumatic memories. *Journal of
Traumatic Stress, 9*(4), 873–880.

Office for Victims of Crime. (September, 1996). *Third national incidence study of child abuse and
neglect.* Washington, DC: US Government Printing Office.

Office for Victims of Crime. (1998). *New directions from the field: Victims rights and services for the 21st
century.* Washington, DC: US Department of Justice.

Pace, D., Stamler, V. L., Yarris, E., & June, L. (1996). Rounding out the cube: Evolution to a global
model for counseling centers. *Journal of Counseling and Development, 74,* 321–325.

Page, H. (1885). *Injuries of the spine and spinal cord without apparent mechanical lesion.* London: J.
and A. Churchill.

Pauchant, T. C., & Mitroff, I. I. (1992). *Transforming the crisis-prone organization: Preventing individual,
organizational, and environmental tragedies.* San Francisco, CA: Jossey-Bass.

Pearlman, L. A., & Saakuitne, K. W. (1995). *Trauma and the therapist: Countertransference and vicarious
trauma in psychotherapy with incest survivors.* New York: Norton.

Pecnik, N. (1997). Training for psychosocial work with refugee and displaced women. In D.
Ajduković (Ed.), *Trauma recovery training: Lessons learned* (pp. 361–372). Zagreb, Croatia:
Society for Psychological Assistance.

Perren-Klingler, G. (Ed.). (1996). *Trauma: From individual helplessness to group resources.* Berne,
Switzerland: Paul Haupt.

Perry, B. D. (1993a). Neurodevelopment and the neurophysiology of trauma. I: Conceptual
considerations. *The Advisor, 6*(1), 14–18.

Perry, B. D. (1993b). Neurodevelopment and the neurophysiology of trauma. II: Clinical work
along the alarm-fear-terror continuum. *The Advisor, 6*(2), 14–20.

Perry, B. D., Pollard, R. A., Blakely, T. L., Baker, W. L., & Vigilante, D. (1995). Childhood trauma,
the neurobiology of adaptation and use-dependent development of the brain: How states
become traits. *Infant Mental Health Journal, 16,* 271–291.

Peterson, M. R. (1992). *At personal risk: Boundary violation in professional–client relationships.* New York: Norton.

Pfeiffer, J. (1994a). *Competitive advantages through people: Understanding the power of the work force.* Boston: Harvard Business School Press.

Pfeiffer, J. (1994b). *Theories and models in applied behavioral science: Group: TORI theory and practice.* San Diego, CA: Pfeiffer & Company.

Pichault, F. (1993). *Resources humaines et chargement strategique: Versun management politique.* Brussels, Belgium: De Boeck.

Pregrad, J. (1997). Why we decided to learn how to fish. In D. Ajduković (Ed.), *Trauma recovery training: Lessons learned* (pp. 127–137). Zagreb, Croatia: Society for Psychological Assistance.

Pupavec, V. (1997). Trauma recovery training: "Suncokret" experiences. In D. Ajduković (Ed.), *Trauma recovery training: Lessons learned* (pp. 335–343). Zagreb, Croatia: Society for Psychological Assistance.

Pynoos, R. S., & Eth, S. (1986). Witness to violence: The child interview. *Journal of American Academy of Child Psychiatry, 25,* 306–319.

Pynoos, R. S., & Nader, K. (1988). Psychological first aid and treatment approach to children exposed to community violence. Research implications. *Journal of Traumatic Stress, 1,* 445–473.

Pynoos, R. S., & Nader, K. (1990). Children's exposure to violence and traumatic death. *Psychiatric Annals, 201*(6), 334–344.

Pynoos, R. S., Steinberg, A. M., & Wraith, R. (1995). A developmental model of childhood traumatic stress. In D. Cicchetti & D. J. Cohen (Eds.), *Manual of developmental psychopathology* (pp. 72–95). New York: Wiley.

Pynoos, R. S., Steinberg, A. M., & Aronson, L. (1997). Traumatic experiences: The early organization of memory in school-age children and adolescents. In P. Appelbaum, M. Elin, & L. Uyehara (Eds.), *Trauma and memory: Clinical and legal controversies* (pp. 272–289). New York: Oxford University Press.

Quick, J.C., Quick, J. D., Nelson, D. L., & Hurrell, J. J., Jr. (1997). *Preventive stress management in organizations.* Washington, DC: American Psychological Association.

Quill, T. (1983). Partnerships in patient care: A contractual approach. *Annals of Internal Medicine, 98,* 228–234.

Rafe, S. C. (1991). *How to choose a spokesperson trainer.* Warrenton, VA: Rapport Communications.

Reilly, A. J., & Jones, J. E. (1974). Team building. In J. W. Pfeiffer & J. E. Jones (Eds.), *The 1974 annual handbook for group facilitators.* San Diego, CA: Pfeiffer & Company.

Resnick, H. S., Veronen, I. J., Saunders, B. E., Kilpatrick, D. G., & Cornelison, V. (1989). Assessment of PTSD in a subset of rape victims at 12 to 36 months post-assault. Unpublished manuscript cited in Rothbaum, B. O., Foa, E. B., Riggs, D. S., Murdock, T., & Walsh, W. (1992). A prospective examination of post-traumatic stress disorder in rape victims. *Journal of Traumatic Stress, 5,* 455–475.

Resnick, H. S., Kilpatrick, D. G., Dansky, B. S., Saunders, B. E., & Best, C. L. (1993). Prevalence of civilian trauma and posttraumatic stress disorder in a representative national sample of women. *Journal of Consulting and Clinical Psychology, 61*(6), 984–991.

Richards, B. M. (1990). *Thriving after surviving.* Murray, UT: Hartley Communications.

Richards, R. R. (1998, January). Creating a dynamic board retreat. *Association Management,* 93–97.

Ritti, R. R., & Funkhouser, G. R. (1987). *The ropes to skip and the ropes to know.* New York: Wiley.

Rosenbloom, D., & Williams, M. B. (1999). *Life after trauma: A workbook for healing.* New York: Guilford.

Ross, C. A. (1997). *Treating disorders effectively.* Richardson, TX: Ross Institute of Psychological Trauma and HiComm Productions.

Rowan, R. (1986). *The intuitive manager.* New York: Berkeley Books.

Rutkowski, K. (1996). *Situation in torture victims in Poland: Possibilities of rehabilitation.* Krakow, Poland: Jagiellonian University.

Saleebey, D. (1996). The strengths perspective in social work practice: Extensions and cautions. *Social Work, 41*(5), 296–306.

Satir, V. (1967). *Conjoint family therapy.* Palo Alto, CA: Science and Behavior Books.

Schaefer, J. A., & Moos, R. H. (1998). The context for posttraumatic growth: Life crises, individual and social resources, and coping. In R. G. Tedeschi, C. L. Park, & L. G. Calhoun (Eds.), *Posttraumatic Growth: Positive changes in the aftermath of crisis* (pp. 99–125). Mahwah, NJ: Erlbaum.

Schein, E. H. (1985). *Organizational culture and leadership.* San Francisco, CA: Jossey-Bass.

Schneider, W. (1994). *The reengineering alternative: A plan for making your current culture work.* Burr Ridge, IL: Irwin.

Schwartz, E. (1998, January). Mission: Possible. *The Costco connection,* pp. 26–27.

Senge, P. M. (1990). *The fifth discipline: The art and practice of the learning organization.* New York: Doubleday/Currency.

Shalev, A. (1992). Posttraumatic stress disorder among injured survivors of a terrorist attack: Predictive value of early intrusion and avoidance symptoms. *Journal of Nervous and Mental Disease, 180,* 505–509.

Shalev, A., (1996). Stress versus traumatic stress from acute homeostatic reactions to chronic psychopathology. In B. A. van der Kolk, S. McFarlane, & L. Weisaeth (Eds.), *Traumatic stress: The effects of overwhelming experience on mind, body, and society* (pp. 77–101). New York: Guilford Press.

Shalev, A., & Mintz, H. (1989). Combat stress reactions. In N. D. Ries & E. Dolu (Eds.), *Manual of disaster medicine* (pp. 169–182). Berlin, Germany: Springer-Verlag.

Shapiro, F. (1995). *Eye movement desensitization reprocessing: Basic principles, protocols, and procedures.* New York: Guilford.

Sink, D. S., & Tuttle, T. C. (1989). *Planning and measurement in your organization of the future.* Norcross, GA: Industrial Engineering and Management Press.

Smith, P. (1985). *Disaster: A manual for public mental health professionals. Mental health involvement in the aftermath of a disaster or tragedy.* San Diego, CA: San Diego County Mental Health.

Solkoff, N., Gray, P., & Keill, S. (1986). Which Vietnam veterans develop post-traumatic stress. *Journal of Cognitive Psychology, 42,* 687–698.

Sperry, L. (1996). *Corporate therapy and consulting.* New York: Brunner/Mazel.

Steele, F. I. (1973). *Physical settings and organizational development.* Reading, MA: Addison-Wesley.

Stuvland, R. (1997), Trauma projects and the future. In D. Ajduković (Ed.), *Trauma recovery training: Lessons learned* (pp. 361–372). Zagreb, Croatia: Society for Psychological Assistance.

Sugarman, B. (1989). The well-managed human services organization: Criteria for a management audit. *Administration in Social Work, 12*(4), 17–27.

Swiss, J. E. (1992). Adapting total quality management (TQM) to government. *Public Administration Review, 52,* 356–360.

Teki, H. (1992). *Promoting mental health for those living in contaminated areas.* San Diego, CA: Nears Press.

Teter, H. (1996). Mass violence and community treatment. In G. Perren-Klingler (Ed.), *trauma: From individual helplessness to group resources* (pp. 71–86). Berne, Switzerland: Paul Haupt.

Trice, H. M., & Beyer, J. M. (1992). *Cultures of work organizations.* New York: Prentice-Hall.

Tunnecliffe, M. (1996a). *Crisis intervention support manual.* Palmyra, Australia: Bayside Books.

Tunnecliffe, M. (1996b). *Emergency phone response course manual.* Palmyra, Australia: Bayside Books.

Tunnecliffe, M. (1997, February). Are traumatic events the norm for humans? *Emergency Support: A Newsletter on Critical Incident Stress Response, 3*(1), 2.

Tunnecliffe, M. (1997a). *The crisis support first aid kit: What everyone should know about helping others in times of emotional stress.* Palmyra, Australia: Bayside Books.

Tunnecliffe, M. (1997b). *Peer support training manual.* Palmyra, Australia: Bayside Books.

United States Department of Justice. (1996). *Third national incidence study of child abuse and neglect.* Washington, DC: Author.

Unkovska, L. K. (1997). One model of helping war-traumatized children: Many ways to understand them. In D. Ajduković (Ed.), *Trauma recovery training: Lessons learned* (pp. 319–334). Zagreb, Croatia: Society for Psychological Assistance.

Ursano, R. J. (1981). The Vietnam-era prisoner of war: Perceptively personality and the development of psychiatric illness. *American Journal of Psychiatry, 138,* 315–318.

Ursano, R. J. (1987). Comments on "post-traumatic stress disorder: The stressor criterion." *Journal of Nervous and Mental Disease, 178,* 273–275.

Vandenberg J. E., & Grealish, E. M. (1997). *The wraparound process: Orientation manual.* Pittsburgh, PA: The Community Partnerships Group.

Van der Hal, E., Tauber, Y., & Gottesfeld, J. (1996). Open groups for children of Holocaust survivors. *International Journal of Group Psychotherapy, 46*(2), 193–208.

Van der Hart, O., & Horst, R. (1989). The dissociative theory of Pierre Janet. *Journal of Traumatic Stress, 2,* 397–414.

van der Kolk, B. (1989). The compulsion to repeat the trauma. *Psychiatric Clinics of North America, 12*(2), 389–411.

van der Kolk, B. A., & McFarlane, A. (1996). The black hole of trauma. In B. van der Kolk, A. C. McFarlane, & L. Weisaeth (Eds.), *Traumatic stress: The effects of overwhelming experience on mind, body, and society* (pp. 3–23). New York: Guilford.

van der Kolk, B. A., McFarlane, A., & van der Hart, O. (1996). A general approach to treatment of posttraumatic stress disorder. In B. A. van der Kolk, A. C. McFarlane, & L. Weisaeth (Eds.), *Traumatic stress: The effects of overwhelming experience on mind, body, and society* (pp. 417–440). New York: Guilford.

Vroom, V. H. (1964). *Work and motivation.* New York: Wiley.

Vroom, V. H., & Jago, A. G. (1988). *The new leadership: Managing participation in organizational culture.* Englewood Cliffs, NJ: Prentice-Hall.

Vroom, V. H., & Yetton, P. W. (1973). *Leadership and decision making.* Pittsburgh, PA: University of Pittsburgh Press.

Walsh, W. F., & Donovan, E. J. (1990). *The supervision of police personnel: A performance-based approach.* Dubuque, IA: Kendall/Hunt.

Wanger, D. B., & Spencer, J. L. (1996). The role of surveys in transforming culture: Data, knowledge, and action. In A. I. Kraut (Ed.), *Organizational surveys: Tools for assessment and change* (pp. 67–87). San Francisco, CA: Jossey-Bass.

Warner, B. S., & Weist, M. D. (1996). Urban youth as witnesses to violence: Beginning assessment and treatment efforts. *Journal of Youth and Adolescence, 25,* 361–377.

Weil, J. O. (1996). Community building: Building community practice. *Social Work, 41*(5), 481–499.

Weisbord, M. R. (1976). Organizational diagnosis: Six places to look for trouble with or without a theory. *Group and Organization Studies, 1,* 430–447.

Weiss, S., & Durat, N. (1994). Treatment of elderly Holocaust survivors: How do therapists cope? *Clinical Gerontologist: The Journal of Aging and Mental Health, 14*(3), 81–98.

Williams, M. B. (1990). *Post-traumatic stress disorder and child sexual abuse: The enduring effects.* Doctoral dissertation, Fielding Institute, Santa Barbara, CA.

Williams, M. B. (1992). A systems view of psychological trauma. *Journal of Contemporary Psychotherapy, 22*(2), 89–105.

Williams, M. B. (1994). Creating safety in survivors of severe sexual abuse. In M. B. Williams & J. F. Sommer, Jr. (Eds.), *Handbook of post-traumatic therapy* (pp. 162–178). Westport, CT: Greenwood.

Williams, M. B., & Sommer, J. F., Jr., (Eds.). (1994). *Handbook of posttraumatic therapy.* Westport, CT: Greenwood.

Wilson, J. P., & Keane, T. (Eds.). (1997). *Assessing psychological trauma and PTSD: A handbook for clinical, medical, and legal practitioners.* New York: Guilford.

Wolfe, B. (1989). *New research: Audiotape of panel discussion.* Rockville, MD: Phobic Society of America.

Wolfe, V. V., Gentile, C., & Wolfe, D. A. (1989). The impact of sexual abuse on children: A PTSD formulation. *Behavior Therapy, 20,* 215–228.

Wolters, W. (1997) Extremely shocking events: Counseling the parents. In D. Ajduković (Ed.), *Trauma recovery training: Lessons learned* (pp. 427–435). Zagreb, Croatia: Society for Psychological Assistance.

Woody, R. H. (1988). *Protecting your mental health practice: How to manage legal and financial risk*. San Francisco: Jossey-Bass.

Worthington, P. (1997). The experience of men: A presentation of the issues.

Wright, D. C., & Woo, W. L. (1997). *Outcome of inpatient treatment of chronic PTSD: One year follow-up*. Guelph, Ontario, Canada: Homewood Health Center.

Yehuda, R., & McFarlane, A. C. (1995). Conflict between current knowledge about posttraumatic stress disorder and its original conceptual basis. *American Journal of Psychiatry, 152*, 1705–1713.

Young, M. A. (1993). *Victim assistance: Frontiers and fundamentals*. Dubuque, IA: Kendall/Hunt Publishing Company.

Young, M. A. (1998, February). Keynote presentation at the annual meeting of the Association of Traumatic Stress Specialists, Oklahoma City, OK.

Young, M. A., & Stein, J. H. (1988). *Model victim assistance program brief*. Washington, DC: National Organization for Victim Assistance.

Zealberg, J. J., Santos, A., & Puckett, J. A. (1996). *Comprehensive emergency mental health care*. New York: Norton.

Zic, B. (1997). The influence of psychosocial programs during the war on social work practice in Croatia. In D. Ajduković (Ed.), *Trauma recovery training: Lessons learned* (pp. 231–240). Zagreb, Croatia: Society for Psychological Assistance.

Zinner, M. B., & Williams, M. B. (Eds). (1999). *When a community weeps: Case studies in group survivorship*. Philadelphia, PA: Taylor & Francis/Brunner Mazel.

APPENDIXES

I
Terms and Abbreviations

AA	Alcoholics Anonymous
AAMFT	American Association of Marriage and Family Therapists
ACD	Alliance for Creative Development (Quakertown, PA, USA)
ADD	Attention Deficit Disorder
ADHD	Attention Deficit Hyperactivity Disorder
ASD	Acute Stress Disorder
ATSS	Association of Traumatic Stress Specialists
CAPS	Clinician Administered PTSD Scale
CARE	Crisis Amelioration Response Effort of ITRA
CASA	Court Appointed Special Advocates
CEO	Chief Executive Officer
CIRTS	Critical Incident Response Teams
CISD	Criticial Incident Stress Debriefing
CNS	Central Nervous System
COPIN	Caring of Persons in Need (Buffalo, NY, USA)
CPS	Child Protective Services
CSDI	Constructivist Self Development Theory
CSVR	Centre for the Study of Violence and Reconciliation (Johannesburg, South Africa)
CTC	Comprehensive Trauma Center
DDIS	Dissociative Disorders Interview Schedule
DDNOS	Dissociative Disorders Not Otherwise Specified
DES	Dissociative Experiences Scale
DESNOS	Disorders of Extreme Stress, Not Otherwise Specified
DID	Dissociative Identity Disorder
DMV	Department of Motor Vehicles
DRS	Dissociative Regression Scale
FCTS	Forensic Center for Traumatic Stress (Cleveland, OH, USA)

FTS	Family Trauma Services, Inc. (Alexandria, VA, USA)
HRD	Human Resource Development
IAA	Injury Adjustment Assessment
ISTSS	International Society for Traumatic Stress Studies
IPTS	Institut Psychotrauma Switzerland (Visp, Switzerland)
ITR	IInternational Trauma Recovery Institute (Mesa, AZ, USA)
LCSW	Licensed Clinical Social Worker
LPC	Licensed Professional Counselor
MD	Medical Doctor
NECTR	Northeast Center for Trauma Recovery (Greenwich, CT, USA)
PTR	Post Trauma Resources (Columbia, South Carolina USA)
PTSD	Posttraumatic Stress Disorder
PTSR	Posttraumatic Stress Reaction
RCT	Rehabilitation Center for Torture Victims (Copenhagen, Denmark)
REBT	Rational Emotive Behavioral Therapy
SA	Survivors Anonymous
SCID	Structured Clinical Interview
SCL	Symptom Checklist
SE	Somatic Experiencing
SIA	Survivors of Incest Anonymous
SPA	Society for Psychological Assistance (Zagreb, Croatia)
SSTAR	Stanley Street Treatment and Resources, Inc (Fall River, MA, USA)
TAS	Toronto Alexithymia Scale
TCISM	Trauma Critical Stage Intervention Model
TED	Traumatic Event Debriefing
TM	Transcendental Meditation
TR	Traumatic Reaction
TREATI	Trauma Research, Education and Training Institute, Inc. (South Windsor, CT, USA)
TRI	Trauma Recovery Institute (Morgantown, WVA, USA)
TSI	Traumatic Stress Institute (South Windsor, CT, USA)
TSR	Traumatic Stress Reaction
WIRC	Wound and Injury Recovery Center (Salt Lake City, UT, USA)

II
Trauma Centers
and Their Addresses

PRIVATELY DEVELOPED CENTERS

Traumatic Stress Institute/CAAP/TREATI
Center for Adult and Adolescent Psychotherapy
22 Morgan Farms Drive
South Windsor, CT 06074
860-644-2541 Fax: 860-644-6891
Laurie Anne Pearlman, PhD, Research Director
Kaye Saakvitne, PhD
www.tsicaap.com

The International Trauma Recovery Institute, LLC
233 No. Val Vista Drive, Suite 680
Mesa, AZ 85213
602-832-4789 Fax: 602-832-4789
E-mail: ItriJBell@aol.com
Janet Bell, PhD, Director
janetbell@asu.edu

Porter and Porter, Inc. A Center for Stress and Trauma
6121 South Cowan Road
Muncie, IN 47302
1-800-996-2906 Fax: 317-823-2906
Pamela Porter, PhD, Director

Post Trauma Resources
1811 Bull Street
Columbia, SC 29201
803-765-0700 Fax: 803-765-1607
L. H. Bergmann, President
www.posttrauma.com

Northeast Center for Trauma Recovery (NECTR)
38 Lake Avenue
Greenwich, CT 06830
203-661-9393 Fax: 203-661-9342
Charles H. Rousell, MD

The Center for the Treatment of Traumatic Life Situations, Inc.
94 Ward Avenue
Staten Island, NY 10304
718-720-9173
Deborah L. Cosentino, CSW

Trauma Recovery Institute
314 Scott Avenue
Morgantown, WV 26505
304-291-2912
Louis Tinnin, MD
trauma@access.mountain.net
http://web.maintain.net/~/trauma/

Dr. Robert H. Moore & Associates
575 S. Duncan Avenue
Clearwater, FL 33756
727-443-1120

The Trauma Center
227 Babcock Street
Brookline, MA 02146
617-731-3200 x 421 Fax: 617-277-5322
Bessel van der Kolk, MD, Clinical Director
Kevin Becker, PhD, Program Director
bvanderk@traumacenter.org

The COPIN Foundation
5622 Buffalo Avenue
Niagara Falls, NY 14304
716-283-5622 Fax: 716-283-5912
Sharon L. McGrath, RNC

Post-traumatic Stress Center
19 Edwards Street
New Haven, CT 06511
203-624-2146
Dr. Haddar Lubin, MD
David Read Johnson, PhD
Lubin—Johnson.PTScenter@compuserve.com

Stanley Street Treatment and Resources, Inc. (SSTAR)
397 Stanley Street
Fall River, MA 02720
508-679-5222
Dr. Rhonda Sabo, Contact person and clinician

CENTERS WITH AFFILIATIONS AND CENTERS IN PROGRESS

Center for Stress and Trauma
Four Commerce Park Square
23200 Chagrin Blvd Suite 325
Cleveland, OH 44122
216-292-6007 Fax: 216-292-7352
John P. Wilson, PhD, Director

Forensic Center for Traumatic Stress
2368 Tudor Drive, Suite 200
Cleveland Heights, OH 44106
Toll Free 888-440-3287 216-932-0965
Dr. Thomas A. Moran, Chief Operating Officer

National Institute for the Prevention of Traumatic Stress Disorder
Wound and Injury Recovery Center/America (WIRC/America)
3760 S. Highland Drive, Suite #500
Salt Lake City, UT 84106
801-273-3943
Barry Richards, LCSW

Victims of Violence Program at the Cambridge Hospital
1493 Cambridge St.
Cambridge, MA 02139
617-492-3539 Fax: 617-491-8151
Mary Harvey, PhD
harveymr@aol.com

Trauma Recovery Institution and Resource Center (TRIARC)
1642 Fell Street
San Francisco, CA 94117
415-923-1630
Kate Garay, Director
Kgaraytri@aol.com

The Center for the Study of Genocide, Violence, and Trauma
315 Whitney Avenue, 3rd Floor
New Haven, CT 06511
203-624-1897
203-397-5077 Fax: 203-397-1699

and

Yale University School of Medicine
Department of Psychiatry
30 Ranch Road
Woodbridge, CT 06525-1912
860-347-0367
Dori Laub, MD

PRIVATE AND NOT-FOR-PROFIT CENTERS AROUND THE WORLD

TraumaTys
87 Blvd St. Joseph West
Montreal Quebec H2T2P5 Canada
514-272-3326 Fax: 514-272-8973
Louise Gaston, PhD
www/traumatys.com

ERGOS—Privates Institüt zur Transformation und Integration der
        Folgen von Schock und Trauma GmbH
Schellingstrasse 78
80799 Munich, Germany
89 27 81 82 24 Fax: 89 27 81 82 22
Tania Kuchler, Director

Institüt für Traumapädagogik und Therapie
Carmerstrasse 10
10623 Berlin, Germany
49 30 46 421 85
Oliver Schubbe, Diplom-Psychologie
http://traumatherapie.ole

Trauma Centers in Russia (Mari-El Republic)
PO Box 1038
North Sebago, ME 04029
207-787-2172
Dr. David Niles

Kriisikonsultointi-Ja Koulutuskeskus (The Crisis Consultation and
    Education Center)
Koulukatu 20
90100 Oulu, Finland
358 8 340 848 Fax: 358 8 344 866
E-mail: crisis.cons@va.netppl.fil
Paivi Saarinen, Contact

Emergency Support Network, Tunnecliffe & Associates, Pty.
PO Box 106
Palmyra, Western Australia 6157
09 430 4377 Fax: 90 430 5017
Michael Tunnecliffe
miket@ivantree.com.an

Psychosocial Trauma Program PTSD Istanbul
Istanbul Medical School Department of Psychiatry
Topkapi
Istanbul, Turkey
212 534 00 00 x 2374 Fax: 212 631 24 00
Dr. Sahika Yüksel
sahikayuksel@turk.net

NONRESIDENTIAL AFFILIATED CENTERS
THROUGHOUT THE WORLD

The Center for Traumatic Stress at Hadassah University Hospital
PO Box 12000
il 91120 Jerusalem, Israel
02 6777111 Fax: 01 643 4434
Arieh Shalev, MD
ashlev@bisji.ac.il

Post Traumatic Stress Disorder Unit
University of New South Wales
School of Psychology
University of New South Wales
NSW2052 Sydney, Australia
61-2-3853640 Fax: 61-2-3853641
Richard A. Bryant, PhD
r.bryant@unsw.edu.au

Wits Trauma Clinic
The Center for the Study of Violence and Reconciliation
PO Box 30778
Braamfontein 2017 S. Africa
University of the Witwatersrand
Private Bag 3 WIT52050
Johannesburg, South Africa
11 403 5102 Fax: 11 339 6785
Mary Robertson, Director
www.wits.ac.za/csvr

Center for Victims of Political Persecution
Jagiellonian University
Department of Social Pathology
ui Kopernika 21
31-501 Krakow, Poland
48-12-21-31-29 Fax: 48-12-21-56-95
Dr. K. Rutkowski

The Sinai Centre
Jewish Mental Health Service
RIAGG
Laan 1914 nr 23
Postbus 66
3800 AB Amersfoort, Netherlands
33 464 0640 Fax: 33 461 9616
Dr. H. I. Elzas
www.riaggamersfoort.nl

BNMO Centre, Stress and Social Rehabilitation Center
Heijting en Weerts
Westhaven 45
NL-2801 PL Gouda, Netherlands
31 182 521 086 Fax: 31 182 581 211
E-Mail: heijweer@antenna.ni
Jos Weerts, MD
www.bnmo.nl

Camden and Islington Community Trust
VCL Medical School
Traumatic Stress Clinic
73 Charlotte Street
London, W1P 1LB, England
44-171-530-3666 Fax: 44-171-530-3677
Stuart Turner, MD
E-mail: sturner@canditse.demon.co.uk

Stresscare
Caroline Keane
20 Parkwood Road
Tavistock, Devon
PL1901-11-1 England
Phone/Fax: 44 1822 610546

Uppsala Academic Hospital Trauma Program
Tom Lundin, MD
Uppsala University Hospital
Outpatient Clinic Psychiatry
Sparrisgatan 2
Uppsala, Sweden 575446
46 18 178822 Fax: 46 18 257508

CENTERS SPECIALIZING IN TRAUMA AND THE WORKPLACE

Crisis Management International, Inc.
Eight Piedmont Center Suite 420
Atlanta, GA 30305
1-800-274-7470
Bruce Blythe, President and CEO

Occupational Services of Australia
PO Box 408
Eisternwick, Australia 3185
61 3 9525 9751 Fax: 61 3 9525 8707
e-Mail: Lesposen@vic.bigpond.net.au
Les Posen, PhD

SIAM: Gesellschaft für Sicherheitstechnik und Arbeitsmedizin mbH
Society for Occupational Security and Medicine, LTD
Gotenstrasse 23
D68259 Mannheim, Germany
621 71 1312 Fax: 621 71 1380
Dr. A. Reinecke

HOSPITAL-BASED TRAUMA CENTERS

The Benjamin Rush Center
614 S. Salina Street
Syracuse, NY 13202
315-428-0925
Dr. Karen Wolford, Clinical Supervisor
wolford@oswego.edu

The Center: Post-Traumatic Stress Disorders Program
Psychiatric Institute of Washington
4228 Wisconsin Avenue NW
Washington, DC 20016
202-965-8456 Fax: 202-965-8452
Dr. Joan Turkus, Dr. Christine Courtois,
Dr. MaryAnn Dutton, Directors
the center@pico.com

Sheppard Pratt Trauma Disorders Services
6501 N. Charles Street
Baltimore, MD 21204-6819
410-938-5075 Fax: 410-938-5072
Dr. Richard Lowenstein, Director

The Sanctuary @ Friends Hospital
Alliance for Creative Development
1110 N. West End Blvd
Quakertown, PA 19851
215-538-2686 Fax: 215-538-7622
Sandra Bloom, MD
Lyndra Bills, MD
wlow@sanctuarysage.com

The Meadows
1655 Tegner Street
Wickenburg, AZ 85390
1-800-395-8833
Ellen Anderson, Community Relations
703-708-7158
www.themeadows.org

The Collin A. Ross Institute for Psychological Trauma
Tiniberlawn Mental Health System
1701 Gateway Blvd Ste 349
Richardson, TX 75080-3546
214-918-9588 Fax: 214-918-0969
Forest View Mental Health Services
1055 Medical Park Drive SE
Grand Rapids, MI 49546-3671
800-949-8439
rossinst@rossinst.com

Homewood Health Centre Program for Traumatic Stress Recovery
Adult Survivors of Childhood Trauma Unit
150 Delphi Street
Guelph, Ontario N1E 6K9 Canada
519-824-1010
Dr. David Wright
www@homewoodhealth.com

Ticehurst House Hospital Treatment Center
Ticehurst
North Wadhurst
East Sussex TN5 7FHJ England
1580 200391 Fax: 1580 201006
Dr. Gordon Turnbull, Clinical Director

CENTERS FOR HOLOCAUST SURVIVORS AND THEIR FAMILIES

Group Project for Holocaust Survivors and Their Children
345 E. 80th Street, Apt 31 J
New York, NY 10021-0644
212-737-8524 Fax: 212-628-2086
Yael Danieli, PhD
yaeld@aol.com

Café 84: Day Program for Jewish Survivors
Sjobacken 44
Hässeiby S-16565, Sweden
Phone/Fax: 46-838-1888
Hedi Fried, MA, Founder and Director

AMCHA Center
23 Hillel J. M. 9481 Israel
02-250-634
or Ramatgai, Israel
SIMA Weiss-Haeshal 7
972-3-6725112
Dr. Daniel Brom
www//amcha.org

CENTERS DESIGNED TO WORK WITH REFUGEES

Slovenska Filantrapija
Center for Psychosocial Help to Refugees
Levstikova 22
1000 Ljubljana, Slovenia
386 421 2600 Fax: 386 421 2605
slovenska.fondacija@quest.arnes.si

The AMANI Trust
PO Box 5465
Suite 3, 1 Releigh St KOPJE
Harara, Zimbabwe
263 4 792222 Fax: 263 4 737509
Priscilla J. Mbape, Program Director
www.oneworld.org/amani
amani@echoicon.co.zw

The Bellevue NYU Program for Survivors of Torture
%Division of Primary Care Medicine
NYU Medical Center
550 First Avenue
New York, NY 10016
212-263-8269 Fax: 212-267-8234
Dr. Allen Keller
ash45@aol.com

Direct Consultancies: Healing Community Trauma and Mass Violence
Counseling, Consultation, Training
461 Frederick Street
San Francisco, CA 94117
415-564-2695 Fax: 415-681-0848
Holbrook Teter, Director

Institute für Psychotrauma Schweiz (Suisse, Switzerland)
Napoleonstrasse 16b
3930 Visp, Switzerland
PO Box 189
41 31 333 0477 Fax: 41 28 463423
Dr. Gisela Perren-Klingler
1 pt perren@swissonline.eh

The Society for Psychological Assistance
University of Zagreb School of Social Work
Nazorova 1
10000 Zagreb, Croatia
Fax: 385 1 4821 206
Dean Ajduković
www.dpp.hr
spa@dpp.hr

Center for the Prevention and Resolution of Violence
Qa Tutsawinavu Hope Foundation
PO Box 65720
Tuscon, AZ 85728
520-628-7525 or 575-1308 Fax: 520-797-8656
Amy Shubitz, MA

Government of the Republic of Croatia
Office for Victims of War
Ulica Republike Austrije 14
HR-10000 Zagreb, Croatia
385 1 177580 Fax: 385 1 177 701
Zavonimir Knezovic

The International Rehabilitation and Research Center for Torture
    Victims (RCT)
Borgergade 13 PO Box 2107
Copenhagen, Denmark 1014
003 376 0600 Fax: 003 376 0500
Inge Genelke, MD, Secretary General
Mr. Gens Anderson, Managing Director
rct@rct.dk

The Center for International Trauma Studies at New York University
114 East 32nd Street, Suite 505
New York, NY 10013
212-889-8117 Fax: 212-226-8403
Jack Saul, PhD
traumastudies@nyu.edu

TRAUMA CENTERS FOR CHILDREN

CIVITAS Child Trauma Program
Department of Psychiatry and Behavioral Sciences
Baylor College of Medicine
One Baylor Plaza
Houston, TX 77030
713-770-3751 Fax: 713-770-3747
Dr. Bruce D. Perry
bperry@bcm.tcm.edu

KidsPeace National Centers for Kids in Crisis
1650 Broadway
Bethlehem, PA 18015-3998
1-800-8KID123
E-mail: www.kidspeace.org

Family Trauma Services, Inc.
21 1 1 Eisenhower Avenue #204
Alexandria, VA 22314
703-549-4000
Laurie Rosser, MSW, Program Director

Children's Crisis Treatment Center
Intensive Trauma Assistance Program
1823 Callowhill Street
Philadelphia, PA 19130-4197
215-496-0707 Fax: 215-496-0742
Eileen M. Clery, PsyD, Director
marchwin@msn.com

The Child Trauma Stress Clinic
Department of Psychology
University of London Institute of Psychiatry
De Crespigny Park
London SES 8AF England
011 44 171 7083497
William Yule, PhD
w.yule@iop.hpmf.ac.uk

The UCLA Trauma Psychiatry Services
Department of Psychiatry UCLA Neuropsychiatric Institute
300 UCLA Medical Plaza #2235
Los Angeles, CA 90095
310-206-8973 Fax: 310-206-4310
Dr. Robert Pynoos
rpynoos@npik.medsch.ucla.edu

GOVERNMENT-FUNDED TRAUMA CENTERS

Program for the Defense of Personal Liberty
Bogotá, Colombia
10155 Collins Avenue #1104
Bal Harbour, FL 33154
305-868-0256 Fax: 305-868-6150
Referral through Dr. Frida Spiwak

Swedish Rescue Services Agency
Räddnings Verket/Statens Räddningserk
Karolinen
65 1 80 Karlstad, Sweden
Lars Osterdahl
4654 10 4000

The Northern Virginia Veterans Outreach Center
8796 E. Sacramento Drive
Alexandria, VA 22309
Robert Tecklenberg, Team Leader

The National Center for War-Related PTSD
ARMC Locked Bag I
West Heidelberg, Victoria, 3081 Australia
613-9496-4329 Fax: 613-9496-2830
Mark Creamer, PhD

III
The Research Protocol

THE STRUCTURE OF THE ORGANIZATION

Name
Location and setting: First World, Third World? Urban, rural, suburban?
Population(s) served as primary victims, secondary (family) victims and tertiary (caregivers) victims?
Who needs this organization? Who are the needy?
If resources are limited, how are services prioritized and triaged?
How do you identify who needs you most?
Whom do you over- and underserve?
At what points do those you serve have input into services provided?

Present Staffing

Gender, profession
What specific disciplines do you need (social work, medicine, psychology, management)?
What are your generic needs for staff?
In what ways do you utilize lay caregivers and volunteers?
Who provides psychosocial support for your organization?
Do trauma survivors or survivor–professionals have a role?
Do you provide any type of medical care directly or indirectly through referral?
What are your minimum staffing standards?
Who provides supervision?
Who maintains levels of quality control over staff? Who evaluates staff and the service staff provides?
How are staff needs met to prevent burnout and compassion fatigue/ secondary trauma?
What is the level of cooperation among staff members?

How secure are jobs (in terms of tenure as well as actual physical security)?
How loyal is the organization to employees?

Qualifications and Training of Staff

What qualifications and training are specific to trauma?
Are staff licensed and/or certified? By whom? What are the qualifications?

Safety of the Setting

Is it a safe setting in a safe country?
Do you serve evacuees, refugees, survivors of unsafe settings at a distance from
   the trauma?
Is your setting unsafe, at-risk, putting helpers at risk?

About the Organization

What led to the creation of the organization?
What needs were seen that led to its creation?
What is the mission statement?
What is the philosophy?
What is the history of the organization?
What descriptive materials do you have or have you created in the past? Send
   them.
What is the organizational structure? Send a chart.
With what other agencies do you network, cooperate?
How do you market your services and publicize your existence? Send materials.
What size, type of population do you serve? What are the demographics?
How is your organization funded?

   • By the state or government? A branch of the government?
   • With government support or opposition?
   • As a commercial venture?
   • As a private practice?
   • As a for-profit organization? A nongovernmental organization? A
     charity-sponsored organization?

What statistics have you gathered about the populations you serve and the work
   you do?

THEORY BASE

What is the model of trauma upon which your organization is based? For
   example, cognitive–behavioral, contextualistic, psychodynamic, eclectic,

etc.? Do you do counseling (individual and/or group), psychotherapy, advocacy, system intervention/political action, provision of medication?

What theoretical principles do you follow?

If you do debriefing, what theory(ies) do you use?

Have you collected statistics demonstrating its effectiveness or non-effectiveness?

How does your debriefing method(s) work?

How do you evaluating how the work of debriefing is being done?

What are the treatment goals of the organization as they relate to your theoretical stance?

What has your organization contributed to the theory of PTSD/PTSD treatment? What publications? Theoretical models? Research instruments? Studies?

Where have your personnel received their theoretical training about PTSD? From whom?

PRACTICE-RELATED ISSUES

How and from whom do you get your referrals?

Do you advertise?

What is the timing of your intervention(s) with victims/survivors? How do you identify which stage of trauma survivorship is evident?

- Acute intervention during an event/incident?
- Early postevent?
- Late postevent?
- Distant and very late intervention (e.g., AMACS, World War II survivors)?
- Do those treated need to admit the existence of the trauma?

What is your view of repressed memory?

Must claims be seen as valid to be treated?

How do you respond in times of acute need? Do you have enough resources or have your resources been overwhelmed?

How do you assess and respond to intermittent need? Chronic need?

Do you provide services to persons with ongoing need over long periods of time while adding new clients?

Is there an end point in length of time service is provided?

How do you deal with the "reluctant needy"?

What types of assessment do you do?

What is your time line for assessment?

What instruments do you use?

What instruments have you developed?

What procedures do you use/follow and what are your criteria for a PTSD-positive diagnosis?

What other diagnoses do you see occurring most frequently comorbidly?

Who does the assessment?

How do you diagnose the nature and extent of trauma?

What is your record-keeping format?

What are your policies on confidentiality?

Do you keep records for insurance purposes?

How do you keep records for forensic purposes?

What research have you done on assessment?

What purposes do your assessments have? To plan for treatment, for commitment, as forensic evaluations, for determination of disability claims?

Treatment Options

What treatment options do you offer?

How do you triage clients/patients for type of treatment?

What type(s) of short-term treatment do you do and with what method(s)?

What type(s) of long-term treatment do you do and with what method(s)?

Do you do crisis intervention?

Do you do debriefing? If so, with either or both of these interventions, when, using what model, and what techniques or methods?

Do you do defusing?

Do you offer training to clients?

Training, Consultation

Do you offer training to professionals, laypersons?

What are the principles you follow for training?

How do you select persons to do the training?

Who sets training standards?

What are your specialty areas for the training you offer?

Do you offer continuing education units or other creditation formats?

Have you developed training materials? If so, would you share them?

Have you developed curricula?

Do you offer consultation? To whom? Under what circumstances?

What prevention activities do you do? With whom (schools, media, lawyers, doctors, EAPs, others)?

What type of inoculation or public education do you do? If you do any of these activities, please describe the services you give in detail.

Do you do forensic work? In what types of cases?

Who among you are expert witnesses? In what area?

Do you do negotiation/mediation? Conflict resolution for active conflict? In what areas and with whom? Do you do hostage negotiations?

To what degree are you involved in community action, advocacy, and social change?

Please provide one or more illustrative cases that demonstrate the uniqueness, as well as the normal range, of the services you provide and offer to traumatized persons/groups/organizations/communities.

LOOKING AT THE PAST, PRESENT, AND FUTURE

What do you believe the "state of the trauma world" to be at the present time?

Is trauma more evident? More intense? More frequent?

What traumatic event(s) have you dealt with as an organization (e.g., natural disasters, plane crashes, mass shootings, etc.)?

What are the biggest challenges to your organization as an entity at the present time?

What are the biggest challenges to the field of posttraumatic therapy?

Index